Dedicated to Christine Goans,
For the kindest friendship, love, and support, even when things have not been straight forward.

To Tina Jones, in recognition of your bravery as a grandmother and creativity with slow cookers!

And for Sandra Shuff, creator of the most glorious lavender oil, because every dusty book I opened brought your face to mind. Maybe it was memories of Utah that made me giggle or perhaps it's just the cannabis. Either way, loads and loads of smiles.

All Rights Reserved. No part of this publication may be reproduced in any form or by any means, including scanning, photocopying, or otherwise without prior written permission of the copyright holder.

Copyright © 2017 Elizabeth Ashley - The Secret Healer

Introduction

"This is a game changer," breathed the journalist, staring incredulously at the chemical analysis in his hands. I can only imagine the explosion of electricity powering through Fred Gardner's body, that moment in 2009, as his mind struggled to calculate the endless possibilities a cannabis medicine, that didn't make you high, could offer humankind.

For in his hand was the GC report for a verified CBD dominant chemotype of medical marijuana, Soma-A-Plus. Cannabidiol (CBD) weakens or neutralises the effects of "The High Causer" THC when it interacts with the CB_1 receptor in the brain. This genetic innovation by cannabis farmers heralded the sunrise of a new era of wellness for our species.

Ten years prior, the British government had funded a joint venture between GW Pharmaceuticals and a Dutch seed company founded by expatriate cannabis experts Robert Clark and David Watson, Hortafarm. Their mission, to seek out CBD rich cannabis strains and to isolate the molecule from them. Whispers of their success rippled across the Atlantic and were picked up by Steve D'Angelo at Harborside Health in Oakland. Using Steep Hill Laboratories, together they made the first official verifications of chemical dominance of CBD in strains using gas chromatography.

Thanks to prohibition in the 1930s, Western medicine has become completely estranged from cannabis, a plant that has provided people with food, medicine, and comfort since the dawn of time. These innovations put her smack bang into the healing spotlight, where she should always have been.

"Well..." smiles Cannabis, as she straightens out the ruffles in her skirt...

"Looks like I'm back, at least for a while."

A very long while, Sister, if my guess is right.

Because genuinely, at this point, I can't see how at least 70% of the population can achieve wellness without her.

It's *that* important.

And then probably even more important than that too!

And that's strange, because before Dr. Robert Pappas first introduced me to Hemp CO_2 at last year's NAHA conference, I hadn't even known we had an essential oil, let alone a whole booming industry capable of transforming someone's entire existence. After a year of study, I am ready to show you what I have learned.

I promise you...

The medicine of this plant is going to blow your mind...but that's okay, you're in a safe space...

Because one of the most important aspects of cannabis is how it *protects* the brain from damage and then helps it to repair.

And if you doubt that, you might want to look up a 1998 patent taken out by the US government, derived from a pre-clinical study and funded by the National Institute of Health, outlining the neuroprotective and anti-oxidant properties of *Cannabis sativa* and its potential uses for Alzheimer's disease, Parkinson's disease, HIV, and dementia.

And that's only the start. The list goes on forever. You can tell that by the length of this book! I have had to shorten it because my publishing house only has the capability to manufacture books up to 499 pages. Trust me, this book could have grown to thrice its size, at least.

And my Goddess, it has been hard work!

But if you smelt a certain sickly, sweet stench as you walked past my shed door, and wonder what secrets may be healed inside, then let me first show you that the aroma is not what it may have seemed. No lighted spliff, no leaves upon a campfire, only an evaporator full of hemp oil, or a massage oil oozing CBD. For these are the hempen tools of this therapist, and superlative ones they are too.

My studies find this to be a plant beyond compare. The strangest coincidence has evolved it to mend a biological system few of us even knew existed, let alone understood was broken. And yet, in more people than not, the endocannabinoid system (our primary endocrine system) is just that: fractured, dysfunctional, kaput! It is curious and inviting to try to understand more.

Understand.

Now *there* is a word. How much do we understand about *Cannabis sativa?*

The answer to that is two-fold. We know inordinate amounts, and yet we know nothing. And I promise you that is frustrating. We want answers... Well, certainly *I* do... but they remain elusive.

I could give you concrete explanations of how and why cannabis works, but if I did that I'd be better employed earning spectacular commission selling oils for a famous MLM. Because the answers just *aren't* there. Not yet. They are fragmented, like the most frustrating jigsaw you have ever done. There are clues to something revolutionary, hints that make your eyes pop and take your breath away with excitement for what we may yet find.

But for the most part, anecdotal evidence trumps science.

Much as we hate it, we need to accept that.

The strategy to overturn anti-drug propaganda has been to collate indisputable evidence of the plant's physiological effects through data collection, test tube analysis, and animal experiments. The protective wall scientists have created is unassailable. Cannabis is supremely safeguarded from the nay-sayers by a fortress of evidence. It is undeniable that cannabis heals in the most extraordinary ways. In ways, unsurpassed by any other plant or even in many cases, any pharmaceutical drug either. But so far clinical trials have been few.

Inside the fortress walls, dwell many types of people. Men in white coats, yes. Scholars? Yes, they are there too. In some parts, there are even politicians holding court. But here, in this space, those in pain rest peacefully and tiny children play. Tiny children, whose parents had all but given up hope of ever seeing their joyful games.

Take Kalel Santiago, for example. This remarkable little boy from Puerto Rico is rather a special child. By the time he had reached the age of three, he had already fought and overcome a rare childhood cancer: neuroblastoma. He had spent more than two years of his little life suffering surgeries, chemotherapy, and radiation treatments. Surely, this little family had endured enough heartache? Especially since the tiny angel suffered in total silence, never uttering a single word. When cancer treatment concluded, the family took on the next battle, searching for a reason behind his silence and his other unusual behaviours. Their worst suspicions were confirmed when he was diagnosed with severe, non-verbal autism.

I couldn't help but marvel at the serendipity of this boy being born into his particular family. They researched autism tirelessly, and sought potential treatments for him. It was at a fundraiser for surf therapy, when he was 9, still silent, that they encountered a specialist in high CBD hemp oil. Just two days after using a mouth spray they had been given, Kalel uttered his first sounds at school enunciating the vowels: A, E, I, O, U. His teacher, astonished, recorded the marvel and sent it home. Very quickly he started to join the sounds using consonants and then declared: "amo mi mama," *I love my mom.*

His parents, Gladys and Abiel, can only pinpoint the difference in his care as being CBD.

It's one story out of millions, all reporting radical changes in autism.

So clearly high CBD hemp oil treats autism.

But *why*?

Well, the difficulty is that no-one really understands *what autism is,* or why numbers of children being diagnosed with it are rocketing. The Centre for

Disease Control suspects that one in 68 children in the US may now be born somewhere on the spectrum. It has been found that a certain receptor (CB_2), seems to be upregulated in children with autism, but is *that* why these people exist?

Their endocannabinoid system seems to signal in a rather disrupted fashion, but whether that's what gives them such symptoms as hypersensitivity to noise and a fragile digestive system, we still could not say (although CBD would be indicated for both these symptoms).

Is that why cannabis helps?

Maybe…

Probably…

We don't know.

That's just one observation found about autism, and believe me, there are hundreds. Some are fascinating, like the rodent discovery of two genetic mutations that prevent the brain from deleting synapses, thereby skewing memory cues. Is this how cannabis is helping? Potentially, because it *is* an endocannabinoid dysfunction. Is it an insight into what *causes* autism? The media would tell you, absolutely! It is a massive breakthrough. Some doctors, however, hold their hands up, begging us to exercise caution in that assessment, because in their opinion it doesn't even prove definitively it causes autism in *rats,* let alone in humans.

Can you see the problem?

Answers about cannabis always lead to more questions.

You have been warned!

I have endeavoured to elucidate the science as well as I am able, but tales from the dark side of complementary medicine are far more compelling than any test tube in this book is, I can tell you. That's why it's important its story be told, and why I have persisted with the book even though it has almost defeated me more than a hundred times.

It is the stories of the parents who have refused to give up that have spurred me on. Like little Kalel's parents…

Like Paige and Michael Figi, the parents of Charlotte Figi, the namesake of the high CBD hemp strain, Charlotte's Web. She had developed Dravet's Syndrome as a tiny dot, and had had her first epileptic seizure when she was having her nappy changed at just three months old.

Dravet's is a very rare genetic disease, predisposing children to incredibly frequent and prolonged seizures and then reducing development in speech and thought, as well as heightening their disposition to infection. There is between a 15-20% mortality rate for children with this disease.

One day, presumably at the end of her tether, seeing no improvement from the doctor's treatment, Charlotte's mother went to see some medical marijuana growers. The Stanley Brothers (Joel, Jesse, Jon, Jordan, Jared and Josh...) had become well known in the State of Colorado, where cannabis is legal. Joel had created a cannabis oil after his cousin fought a losing battle to cancer using the doctor's pharmaceuticals. Their successes with cancers and other diseases made the brothers' *Realm of Caring Dispensary* infamous. Compassionately, they listened to Paige's heart-breaking tale of Charlotte's illness and vied to create a strain of cannabis with very little THC - thus avoiding psychoactive effects - to treat the little girl. The product went on to be called Charlotte's Web.

Now, because of her oil, Charlotte is now practically seizure-free. Apart from the amazing change in the seizure activity there have been fundamental changes in the child's general demeanour and mental health too; her brain is beginning to work in a very different way. After six months, she began to laugh again. She has regained her ability to talk and no longer cries incessantly. Her parents fervently believe it is CBD that is responsible for returning their beloved daughter to them.

Throughout the book you will see me draw from a book written by a marijuana activist, Regina Nelson. I have also watched many videos of conference lectures she has given. She is beautiful, brave, and fearless. I am sure she will not mind my sharing the story of her own daughter, who at the age of 26 was diagnosed with stomach cancer, and was told she was going to have to have three quarters of her stomach cut away. Her mum begged her to move to Colorado where she would be allowed to use cannabis oil, which she eventually did, as well as drinking cannabis juice. One day, she was rushed to the emergency room, vomiting up blood and matter. Things looked very grim. When she was scanned, however, a miracle revealed itself. Her tumour was hanging by a thread. What she was actually throwing up, was the tumour itself, as it left the body cancer free.

Now, marijuana is different to our high CBD hemp. It has different chemistry, rich in the psychoactive component THC (although there are high CBD marijuana strains too, which I will address at the end of the next chapter). Read enough internet pages, you may conclude that it is scientifically proven that only smoking pot can get rid of cancer. Further, the message implies the labs all say cannabis *cures* cancer. It's a very, very tangled web. It is more complicated and more beautiful than that.

Part of the importance of writing the book for me was to try to understand the truth behind cancer claims since I had ignored my brother's pleas to give my dad cannabis when bowel cancer was eating him alive. Now better educated, I want to say to John that I should have listened. I am sorry that I didn't. You didn't have the whole story, and even though you were only partly right, I think that would have been enough. It will take me a long time to forgive myself. Both my dads (father and step father) suffered dreadfully at the end of their precious times in this world. Had I researched this book earlier, I might perhaps have been able to alleviate some of their pain. I would certainly have used the oils outlined in this book.

Not all cannabis medicine is executed through the CB_1 and CB_2 receptors of the endocannabinoid system. It has many mechanisms. However, I have chosen to elucidate this system as thoroughly as I can, since it has an irrefutable function as a bridge between the emotions and the physical body. *Clinical Endocannabinoid Deficiency Syndrome* might yet be proven to be a cause behind stress-exacerbating diseases such as fibromyalgia, Chronic Fatigue Syndrome, and migraine (to name a few). First proposed by Dr. Ethan Russo in 2004, evidence supporting his theory stacks ever higher and giving credence to the millions of people who use cannabis to ease their hypersensitivity to pain.

Just as the test tube results are frustrating, the history may also make you want to scream. For the archaeological evidence of ritual is compelling, yet it is so very nebulous and elusive. Samples of immaculately preserved green herb have been found in tombs dating back several thousand years. Partnered with antiquities made from the most glorious golden metalwork, we still can't completely grasp what the weed was placed in the grave for. Were smokers in conversation with their deity, or simply trying to escape a reality too painful to perceive? Was the cannabis a tool to project the user out of linear time, into the shamanic no-time dimension, known to the ancient Greeks as chiros, or were they simply checking out for a while? It's the stuff of the most romantic science fiction...and yet...these are fragments of a jigsaw... nothing more.

But the stories are enchanting, they are wild and erotic. The heroes of the story are brave and fearless warriors, rulers of great kingdoms and travellers to other realms. As the smoke clears and we see our own peers approach, I'd ask you all to doff your caps and give a little courtesy. Many have risked prison, prejudice, and pain to bring you this medicine, and I promise you wholeheartedly, you will be glad that they did.

Table of Contents

Contents
Introduction 2

Table of Contents 9

Chapter 1 What is Cannabis Oil? 3

   Cannabis Strains 5

      Cannabis sativa 5

      Cannabis indica 5

      Cannabis ruderalis 6

   Differences in properties...7

      Cannabis sativa 7

      Cannabis indica 7

      Cannabis ruderalis 7

   The Cannabis Medicines: Understanding the Differences 8

      CBD-Rich Hemp Oil 8

      Hemp Essential Oil 8

      Cannabis Carrier Oil 9

      Hemp Seed Carrier Oil 9

      High CBD Medical Marijuana versus High CBD Hemp 9

      Does it show in drug's testing? 9

Chapter 2 - History 11

   China 11

   Chinese Medicine 14

   The Steppe 20

   Siberian Medicine 27

   Egyptian Medicine & Antiquity...28

- Unani Medicine 33
- Contraindications in Ayurveda 38
- Cannabis in the Bible 40
- Rastafarianism 44
- British Herbal 45

Chapter 3 The Endocannabinoid System 55
- Functions of the eCS 55
- Receptors 56
  - CB_1 57
  - CB_2 59
  - Endocannabinoids 61
  - Anandamide 62
  - 2-AG 62
  - The Other Players 63
- Degradative Enzymes 63
  - FAAH 64
  - DAGL & MAGL 64
  - ECLs 64
- Transport Proteins 64

Chapter 4 Hemp's Healing Components 66
- Phytocannabinoids 67
  - THC - Delta 9-tetrahydrocannabinol 67
  - CBD - Cannabidiol 69
  - CBN – Cannabinol 72
  - CBC - Cannabichromene 72
  - CBG - Cannabigerol 72

  THCV - Tetrahydrocannabivarin 73

  CBDv - Cannabidivarin 73

  Terpenes 74

  B-Caryophyllene 74

Chapter 5 Properties and Interactions of CBD 76

 Orphan Receptors 76

  GCPR55 76

  GPCR 18 79

  GPR119 80

 Signalling Protocols 80

  Presynaptic Signalling 80

  Postsynaptic Signalling 80

  Orthosteric and Allosteric Sites 81

  Tonic and Phasic Signalling 82

  Imbalance 82

 Gene Transcription 83

  MAP/ERK Pathway 84

  PPAR System 84

  COX Pathways 87

  TRPV 87

Chapter 6 The Nervous System 90

 The Electrical Nervous System 90

  Dendrites 90

  Axons 90

  Myelin 90

  Neurones 91

- Synapses 91
- Brain 91

Glia 92
- Neuroepithelial Cells 97
- Ependymal Cells 97
- Oligodendrocytes 97
- Tanycytes 97
- Microglia 98
- Astrocytes 98
- Depolarisation 100
- Calcium Ion Channels 101

The Chemical Nervous System 104
- Serotonin 105
- Dopamine 106
- GABA 108
- Glutamate 112
- Glutathione 119
- Adenosine 127
- Glycine 127
- Acetylcholine 128

Chapter 7 Lessons from Homeopathy 129
- Cannabis in Homeopathy 129
  - Miasm 129
  - Psora 130
  - Syphilitic 131
  - Sychotic 131

- Sychotic Miasm 132
  - Physical properties 133
  - Psychological 137
  - Sychotic Challenges 139
- Mental 139
  - Mind Body Perception 140
  - Cosmic Ordering 141
  - The Rise of Sychosis 142
  - Connective tissue 144

Chapter 8 Clinical Evidence 145

- Bioavailability 147
- Psychological 148
  - Stress 148
  - Depression 149
  - Anxiety 149
  - PTSD 150
  - Sleep Disorders 161
  - Addiction 163
  - Schizophrenia and Psychosis 165
  - Bipolar 169
  - OCD 169
- Neurological 170
  - Epilepsy 170
  - Neurodegeneration 174
  - Autism 175
  - ADD/ADHD 176

- Multiple Sclerosis (MS) 176
- Parkinson's Disease 178
- Alzheimer's Disease 181
- Huntington's Disease 182
- Prion/Mad Cow Disease 187
- ALS 187

Mind Body Interface 188
- Inflammation 188
- Atopy 193
- CEDS - Chronic Endocannabinoid Deficiency Syndrome 194
- Chronic Pain 195
- Arthritis & Rheumatism 195
- Cancer and Tumours 196

Appetite and Metabolism 202
- Anorexia 202
- Atherosclerosis, Diabetes, and Metabolic Syndrome 203
- Diabetes 205
- Stroke and TBI 206
- Heart Disease 207
- Liver Disease 208
- Hepatitis 210
- Kidney Disease 211
- Nausea 211

Respiratory Distress 213
- Asthma 213

The Tissues 213

  Glaucoma 213

  Osteoporosis/Bone Health 214

  Skin – Acne & Psoriasis 216

  Spinal Cord Injury 216

 Immunity 217

  Antibiotic Resistance 217

Chapter 9 Care of the Endocannabinoid System 219

Chapter 10 Spiritual Dimensions of the Essential Oil 229

 The Archetype of Cannabis 240

  Writing 243

  Time 243

  Recording 244

  Measurement 244

  Death 246

 Uranus and Neptune 249

  Anatomical correlations 254

  Physiological correlations - Uranus 255

  Additional anatomical correlations - Uranus 255

  Understanding Uranus Medicine in the Birth Chart 257

Chapter 11 Cannabis in Aromatherapy 261

 Hemp Seed Oil (Carrier Oil) 261

 Topical Use 263

 CBD Oil 264

 Hemp Essential Oil 265

  Physical Medicine 265

  Inflammation 265

- Symptoms of neurological inflammation 266
- Pain 266
- Emotional and Spiritual Medicine 266

Chapter 12 Resources 268

- Where to buy High CBD Hemp CO2 268
- Create a Carrier 268
- Recipes 269
  - Acne 270
  - ADD & ADHD 271
  - Addiction 271
  - Alzheimer's Disease 273
  - Appetite Stimulant 274
  - Arthritis 274
  - Asthma 275
  - Atherosclerosis 275
  - Autism 276
  - Chronic Cystitis 278
  - COPD 279
  - Diabetes 280
  - Depression 280
  - Cancer care 281
  - Dermatitis 282
  - Diverticulitis, Crohn's, IBS, and Coeliac Disease 282
  - Dystonia 283
  - Epilepsy 283
  - Hashimoto's Disease 284

- Hepatitis ... 284
- Herpes ... 285
- High Blood Pressure ... 285
- Insomnia ... 285
- Lyme's Disease ... 286
- Headaches and Migraine ... 286
- PTSD ... 287
- Sarcoidosis ... 287
- Pain ... 288
- Fibromyalgia ... 288
- Joint pain ... 288
- Muscle Pain ... 289
- Nerve Pain ... 289
- Muscle Cramps ... 289
- Leg Weakness ... 290
- Spasticity ... 290
- Meditation blends ... 291

Conclusion ... 293

CANNABIS TRAINING ... 297
- FREE bonus training ... 297
- Professional Training ... 297
  - Your Cannabis Life ... 297
  - Your Cannabis Practice ... 297
  - Cannabis Future ... 297
- Cannabis Medicine Support ... 297
  - The Secret Healer's Introduction to Aromatherapy ... 298

- Other Books by The Secret Healer...299
  - Book 1:- The Complete Guide to Clinical Aromatherapy & Essential Oils for the Physical Body (Free to download)...299
  - Book 2:- Essential Oils for Mind Body Spirit...299
  - Book 3:- The Essential Oil Liver Cleanse...299
  - Book 4:- The Professional Stress Solution...299
  - Book 5:- The Aromatherapy Eczema Treatment...299
  - Book 6:- The Aromatherapy Bronchitis Treatment...299
  - Book 7:- 50 Easy Recipes for Dry Skin...299
  - Book 8:- 75 Easy Christmas Aromatherapy Recipes...299
- The Secret Healer Oils Profiles...299
  - 1: Monarda – A Native American Medicine...299
  - 2: Vetiver – An Ayurvedic Medicine...299
  - 3: Holy Basil – An Ayurvedic Medicine...299
  - 4: Rose – Goddess Medicine...299
  - 5: Sweet Basil – The Oil of Empowerment...299
  - 6: Clary Sage- Natural Estrogen?...299
  - 7: Spikenard- A Woman Washes Jesus's Feet. Was It our Oil of Aromatherapy? ...299
  - 8: Helichrysum – For The Wound That Will Not Heal...299
- Business Training for Professional Aromatherapists...299
  - Sales Strategies for Gentle Souls...299
  - About the Author...300
- References...304

Chapter 1 What is Cannabis Oil?

Cannabis belongs to the genus ***Cannabaceae,*** the **hemp** family. Plants are dioecious, meaning a plant is either male or female. Pollen drifts on warm summer breezes, or is carried on the feet of intoxicated insects from the male plant to the female for fertilisation. In rare cases, plants might also be monoecious, containing both male and female characteristics. Nature has evolved these plants in the most remarkable way to pollinate between themselves.

The differently sexed plants look dissimilar. The male grows tall with extraordinarily fibrous tissues. The smaller female creates blossoms laden with trichomes, which create the sticky resin containing the psychoactive component known as THC. Eventually, these buds surround seed pods and ancient peoples have grown hemp seed for sustenance for millennia.

For obvious reasons, the female plant, known as marijuana, gets all the good press, but male plants are also extremely useful. Their long fibrous stems make fantastic textile. If you watch Grand Designs, you may have seen that hemp is enjoying a renaissance in the construction industry, being utilised as an organic binder to toughen concrete.

Its use as a textile is nothing new - it makes wonderful clothes and paper. History attributes the first piece of hemp paper to a Chinese official Cai Lun. Legend tells of his creation using mulberry and mixing them with other bast fibres, scraps of fishnets, old rags, and waste bits of hemp. The earliest hemp paper example is a map dating from 179-41 BC found at Fangmatan in the Gansu Province.

Interestingly, some of the most famous documents in history were written on hemp. In the 15th century The Gutenberg Bible, and the 17th century, King James Bible, were both printed onto hemp. The philosopher Thomas Paine's works: The Rights of Man, Common Sense, and The Age of Reason, some of the first writings of America's independence, were printed onto hemp.

In 1776, the Declaration of Independence was drafted onto Hemp paper, then fourteen years later The U.S. Constitution was printed onto it too. Great authors Mark Twain and Victor Hugo both printed onto hemp, as was my most beloved book, Lewis Carroll's Alice's Adventures in Wonderland.

So that's the male plant, but what about the female? What does she look like? Well, we might say she has hips, bless her. She is curvier and of course a little more risqué than the boys! The female plant is shorter and stockier than the male and this renders it useless for fibre, but of course, she has properties of her own. She produces hemp seed and is often grown for the strange body and mind effects induced when trichomes are burned.

Trichomes are the small resin glands whose name comes from the Greek word meaning *growth of hair*. Comprised of a stalk and a head, these are microscopic, mushroom-like protrusions, emanating from the surface of buds, fan leaves, and in far lesser numbers, the stalk.

The psychoactive constituent, THC, synthesizes in the heads of these trichomes and brings about marijuana's infamous psychedelic trip, as well as some important aspects of its medicine. This derivative word, marijuana, originated as a 1930s propaganda term to incite the fear of cannabis. Deliberately linked to the immigration of Mexican refugees of the Civil War in 1910, scaremongering films and posters hawked the perceived dangers of smoking the herb with madness and violence brought by "those people." Prior to the Mexican influx, cannabis was hardly known as a recreational drug in America. More often, it was found as an active component in medicines. More than 30% of 1930's American over-the-counter medications contained cannabis. Many empty cannabis medicine bottles are still found today, commanding high price tags by collectors. The marijuana bad press all but wiped the herb out of the dispensary.

Cannabis is an exceptionally ancient plant. Isolating exactly *how* old is very difficult to do. Where normally there might be fossilised remains of plants, very few remains of *cannabis sativa* have ever been found. Fossils belonging to related species show that cannabis sativa probably originated in Germany between 82.5 and 66 million years ago, during the Late Cretaceous period. The plants of the *Cannabaceae* genus share very little in common except for an evolutionary origin. There are only 11 classes in the genera. For example, cannabis is a herbaceous plant, whereas a sister genera *Celtis* contains only trees. Hops are a very close cousin of cannabis as indeed are nettles, all hailing from the plant order of Urticales.

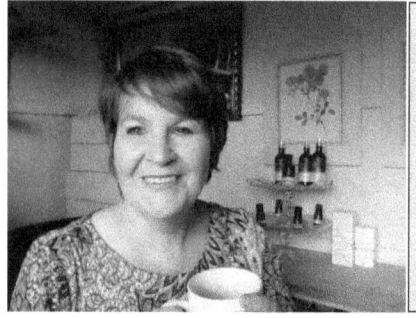

Wondering about the person speaking to you? I would be! So, I made a little video to introduce myself. It would be great to make your acquaintance.

Click here, so I can say hi!

https://buildyourownreality.lpages.co/lets-meet-up/

Cannabis Strains

There are three main strains of cannabis:

- *Cannabis sativa*
- *Cannabis indica*
- *Cannabis ruderalis*

There is disagreement as to whether these are three individual species or whether *indica* and *ruderalis* might be subspecies of sativa. I think we can leave them to argue that out because it really does not affect our medicine, and for the purposes of keeping differences in properties straight in our mind it is easier to consider them separate.

From these three "master species" (my term!) derives literally hundreds of subspecies strains, all bred for their different effects. The difficulty is that just like anything you get to know about cannabis/hemp/marijuana, strains can have many names, so this means not every strain is unique (that is, it might have three or four different names). At this point, don't let that concern you or you will be dragged down the White Rabbit's Hole. Just know that there are lots of subspecies…and let that sit with you for a while.

We'll start by looking at the "master species" because it is quite interesting to see how they have evolved.

Cannabis sativa

The most popular family of cannabis is the *sativa*. Originating from equatorial countries, these cannabis plants evolved to take advantage of the low fluctuations of sunlight; once they flower, cleverly they continue to grow. *Sativa* tend to hang looser, looking airier (leggy almost) than other cannabis families. Their evolutionary trickery results in a longer flowering time and a proportionally higher yield of flowers and seeds. All cannabis leaves have a seven-fingered leaf, a common trait for plants originating from harsh climates, optimising their biology to take best advantage of the light. *Sativa* leaves resemble long spindly fingers, and these fingers are the ones commonly associated with the usual representation of the plant.

Cannabis indica

Indica plants are shorter and stockier than their sativa counterparts. Originating from subtropical areas around Pakistan and Afghanistan, it is the latter country you will often find reflected in strain names (Afghan Kush, for example). Where *sativa* plants grow best around 30 degrees north and south of the equator, *indica* plants grow further out, at latitudes of between 30 to 50 degrees north and south of the equator, meaning they have needed to evolve to react to sudden light fluctuations. As soon as they reach their ideal height, every iota of the plant's energy then goes into producing flowers. Hence the strain's shorter stature.

To utilise sunshine to the best of its ability, *indica* produces wider leaves to increase surface area. They flower far faster than sativa too. It's an economic crop, taking up little space and producing precious flowers quickly, offering an attractive crop for growers looking to make a quick buck.

Cannabis ruderalis

Growing in frigidly cold areas of the world, usually above 50 degrees north of the equator in China and Russia, *ruderalis* flowers automatically, meaning the crop largely looks after itself. Evolutionarily, it's an extremely intelligent strain. These regions have very short growing periods, with only three months of growing weather. Neither *indica* nor *sativa* would survive in these icy climates, but *ruderalis* has cleverly adapted by creating this automatic growing cycle.

Days are short in the freezing north, and summer lasts barely a few weeks. *Ruderalis* is small, compact, and efficient, producing small leaves and tiny side branches. It gets to work very quickly, germinating speedily, and then immediately sets about a frantic growth cycle, allowing plants to flower and seed in just ten short weeks.

Each strain has their own properties too, because each subspecies has developed its own unique chemistry in response to the climate challenges it was exposed to. THC's function in the plant, for example, is as a UV filter for the plants as well as an insect deterrent.

Different challenges, different resulting chemistry.

Differences in properties

Cannabis sativa

Generally speaking, *sativa* plants naturally tend to have very high concentrations of THC and far lower levels of CBD. Traditionally, the marketplace values high THC strains, particularly for smoking. For the most part *sativa* properties will look thus:

- energising and uplifting
- motivating
- inspiring creativity
- generates a cerebral head buzz
- combats nausea
- chases away depression
- generates a sense of well-being
- stimulates appetite

Cannabis indica

Indica strains have a reputation for having a much higher CBD content than *sativas*. Later, you will learn that one of the main functions of CBD is to modulate the effect that THC has on the body and mind. *Indica* properties are very different to the *sativa*. Rather than being a cerebral buzz this is a body buzz. It also:

- Relaxes muscles
- Reduces inflammation
- Acts as an analgesic
- Has sedative properties
- Increases appetite
- Relieves stress and anxiety
- Increases dopamine

Cannabis ruderalis

Ruderalis has been largely ignored throughout history as it is less psychoactive than other species. More recently though, it has become a popular means of genetically bolstering subspecies for other properties.

C. ruderalis contains about the same number of cannabinoids as C. indica and C. sativa do, but the amount of THC is considerably lower. About 70% of the alkaloids you find in sativa can be identified as THC, but in ruderalis plants this tops out at about 40% or less. Hybridising with ruderalis also means faster growing crops need far less attention during cultivation. It's a grower's dream!

The Cannabis Medicines: Understanding the Differences

CBD-Rich Hemp Oil

This is a CO_2 extract from cannabis. For any readers new to aromatherapy, this means carbon dioxide has been used to separate the chemicals from plant matter. CO_2 has a state, existing between liquid and gas, known as hypercritical or supercritical. When the pressure of CO_2 is released, the gas escapes and the producer is left with a beautifully pure extract. It is, as the name suggests, high in CBD – cannabidiol - and completely free from psycho-activity.

This CO_2 extract is recommended for oral consumption, but it can also be added to massage oils, creams, and lotions. You can buy it diluted into carrier oils like hemp seed oil or coconut oil. It is a dark orangey colour and usually comes in a needleless syringe for you to decant the desired amount. This is a very small dose, the size of a grain of rice.

When you read the section on the endocannabinoid system you will understand that this product is vital to your therapy, and you or your patient probably needs to be taking daily doses of this CBD-rich hemp oil for a short period.

I have included recipes where CO_2 maybe blended into treatments too. It has a deep note, very earthy and heavy, and lends a very grounding effect to the blend.

Hemp Essential Oil

Cannabinoids are fat soluble molecules. They are hydrophobic and thus will not pass through distillation. **They do not appear in the essential oil**.

It is, however, bursting with terpenes and flavonoids, each with their own spectacular sorcery. In my opinion, this is a very simple and easy product to use. Again, no psycho-activity, but this has a very high ethereal vibration. It is gloriously happy, vibrant, and energetic. It is mischievous and likeable.

For clarity, most of the book focuses on High CBD hemp oil (the CO_2). Don't expect to see much about the essential oil until the end.

It's only fair to tell you…

In my opinion, both the CO_2 and essential oil smell… Well, frankly, *vile,* but they have the uncanniest blending capacity. Seeming to disappear, they fortify the prowess of their friends. The essential oil, in particular, creates spectacular fragrance profiles, and just like the spiritual lessons we learn later about the oil, she is completely without ego, always seeking to amplify those around her. I think you will really enjoy the blending when we get to it later.

Cannabis Carrier Oil

You can't buy this, it requires homemade preparation. I heartily recommend you experiment and create this most delightful witch's brew. Remember that the cannabinoids are fat soluble? This means you can leech them into coconut oil just as you would for, say, calendula. I'll give you a recipe for this later, but know that we can easily and excitingly create a cannabis carrier for topical use that will still give us access to the precious CBD.

If you do happen to buy a fairly large bottle of hemp oil, it is likely to be...

Hemp Seed Carrier Oil

Taken from the seeds. Different thing entirely. Buyer beware. Quite often this will be labelled *Hemp Carrier Oil*. There is, however, a giveaway.

"Method of Extraction" – Cold pressed? Then it must be from seeds.

High CBD Medical Marijuana versus High CBD Hemp

There is a subtle distinction.

Apart from the million and one medicinal reasons for using cannabis, like vetiver, it is a phyto-remediating plant: it cleans soil. Experiments show that both hemp and cannabis draw cadmium, nickel, and lead from the earth, cleansing it for future generations. The heavy metals travel up the plant and are stored within the leaves. Now naturally, medical marijuana has a far higher yield of CBD than hemp, thus, fewer leaves need to be used to make the extract. If you can get your hands on high CBD medical marijuana, this is going to be better.

Does it show in drug's testing?

Ah well there's a question and I'm sitting firmly on the fence, because I always promise you I'll tell you the truth as I see it.

The official line is **no, it doesn't show up in drug's tests.**

Levels of THC are so low in the small qualities you take, that they would not be picked up. That's what I would have told you when I started writing this book, and there is only one thing that makes me doubt this. When we get to the aromatherapy section you'll see some reports of errant sprinkles of THC finding their way into hemp *seed* oil. It defied explanation. They weren't supposed to be there...but nevertheless the oil tested positive for THC.

Now, in America, if you ask your physician for a prescription for medical marijuana, (providing you in one of the states where it is exempt, of course) then you would have evidence to put you in the clear, even if the test did come back positive. But that probably won't wash here, in the UK if you are in the armed forces etc. So, even though the official line is no...and I don't doubt that's right, I'm going to tell you the line I have taken. My daughter should be taking it...she's like a walking advert for all the reasons why it would be good for you. But her job depends on a clean drug's test so I've asked her not to take it. Perhaps I am being overcautious but it seems like too big a risk when your livelihood is on the line.

Want a closer look at the different medicines?

I'll show you them on this video:

https://buildyourownreality.lpages.co/recognise-your-hemp/

Chapter 2 - History

The moment where we meet cannabis will never be at the beginning, for its roots were planted way before those first written words of history. And yet in some ways, attempting to glimpse those early tendrils of smoke feels like the only way to truly witness the medicine of the plant. As months pass, its scent becomes more than just a fragrance, a scent drifting across the room, as the aroma draws back curtains of mystery.

The story of cannabis lies in these pages, but nothing more. My writing bears no testament to how it can make you feel. How grief is washed away in its bath, or how boundaries between this world and the next are stripped away. But even using the essential oil, you'll begin to recognise the tingle, the inexorable allure as her fingers dance across the periphery of your consciousness and associations flit across your mind. It's so fleeting, so quick, you'll wonder if Tinkerbell caught her toe as she swerved through your mind. No sooner have you registered a connection – or could it be a memory…?

It's gone.

And yet it is there - this knowing – an inner smile and the soul seems to sigh… *I remember.*

It's incredibly odd.

But there is no escaping it.

China

Let's journey far into the past to a small village on the banks of the Yellow River in China.

Sitting outside small round mud houses with thatched millet roofs, people feast on root vegetables from bowls of glossy polished stone. Over the fire, fish gently roast on stick spits. The warm humid weather is broken by the softest of breezes filling the air, with the rustling of crops in the fields.

The men, wearing loin cloths, have their hair tied into tight tidy top knots. Exhausted from their hunting and farming, they are hardly aware of the merry chatter of the females. Later their women, dressed in little more than a piece of cloth, will wander down to the settlement to feed the sheep and pigs. But for now, their job is to tend to the needs of their men and children. One passes her man a heavy amphora filled with drink. It's a beautiful and decorative piece. The rich-coloured clay has been carefully hand-crafted, adorned with a simple yet attractive pattern. On closer inspection, it is clear to see that the decoration has been made by careful diagonal indentations of rope.

By and by, this pot will break and become the very earliest archaeological evidence of hemp agriculture. Found in Taiwan, it dates back 10,000 years to the Neolithic period. It seems likely that man cultivated hemp as a foundation for his existence long, long before *civilisation* even took place. Ancient China, often referred to as "the land of hemp and mulberry," held hemp as one of its earliest agricultural crops.

Ancient Chinese history is sumptuously overlaid with the story and culture of hemp. Written circa 16th century BC, The Xia Xiao Zheng contains a collection of seasonal rituals and describes hemp as one of the main Ancient Chinese crops. The Book of Songs, *the* oldest extant collection of *Chinese* poetry, lists six crops in circulation: "he, su, dao, shu, ma, and mai." 'Ma' is hemp. Archaeological finds of fibres and seeds from around the Yellow and Yangtze rivers verify this data.

The *Shih Ching,* or Book of Odes, was written during the Western Zhou dynasty (1100 to 256 BC). An ancient manual for people, living south of present day Beijing in the 11th to the 6th century BC, it advises using cannabis to improve the soil when cultivating the land for hemp fibres and seeds. Here we find one of mankind's oldest records of potash fertilisation.

It reads:

"Hoe up all the weeds in the field during the summer solstice (June 21), let them dry in the sun, and then burn them into ash. All these ashes will permeate into the soil after a heavy rain and the soil will be fertilized."

The Essential Arts for the People, *Qi Min Yao Shu,* is one of China's most treasured scientific legacies. Dating back 1,400 years, it summarises Ancient Chinese best practice for cultivating hemp. It describes seed collection, optimum sowing time, and crop rotation suggesting adzuki beans should always follow hemp. Every possible aspect influencing hemp quality is considered.

The meticulous detail portrays an early yet comprehensive understanding of the difference and relationship between the cannabis plant sexes. Remarkably, this predates any written evidence of similar knowledge in Europe by at least a millennium and a half.

It reads:

"If we pull out the male hemp before it scatters pollen, the female plant cannot make seed.

Otherwise, the female plant's seed production will be influenced by the male hemp plants scattering pollen, and during this period of time the fibre of the male hemp plant is the best."

Confucius describes the vital crop as *"the cloth of the peasant masses"* in *The Book of Rites*. He teaches how mourners of the dead are expected to wear the cloth symbolically. In many parts of China this tradition still survives today, as people are mindful to stay in the good graces of ancestors. Ancient manuscripts repeatedly decree that the nation must continue to grow hemp as a guarantee of cloth supply for its people.

The *Shu King* is a collection of documents dating from 2350BC. One of the five Chinese classics, for 2000 years it has formed the basis of Chinese Literature. It tells the story of the mythical Yu the Great (2200-2101 BC) and his challenges controlling the waters of China. Plagued by floods, China was failing as its crops were ruined by water damage time and time again. Originally, Yu's father, Gun, had been tasked with the unenviable job of controlling the floods. A thankless task, naturally it was doomed for failure. For five years he built fantastic dams to stem the flow, but to no avail: the water just careered through them. Yu's succession to the throne must have seemed little more than poisoned chalice. But as he ascended to power, Yu had an epiphany.

Suddenly, he saw clearly that damming the flow would be pointless, and instead set about constructing an intricate network of canals to irrigate the crops. It was a long and arduous project, and for 13 years Yu worked tirelessly with his men, eating and even sleeping with them.

Try to imagine, if you will, the enormous cost an undertaking such as this would bring. Gargantuan amounts of money were filtered into the economy to pay for it, via a taxation system of "tributes" in which hemp played a vital part. Each geographical area was to provide tributes as a means of funding their local engineering.

The tribute consisted of salt, matting, and marine produce of various kinds. The Tae Valley produced silk, hemp, lead, pineapples, and choice stones. The Lae (mountain) foreigners worked the fields and their tribute vessels were stored with Mulberry and silks.

One might be forgiven for thinking that only the poorest enjoyed the benefits of hemp but the Retrospective Decree, Section 3 of the Shu King, illustrates the stark contrast of it also being used by the very wealthiest. It reads:

The King, in a hempen headgear and chequered robe of state, ascended the reception staircase, while the learned nobles and the Princes of the States, with hempen headgear and dark robes, entered and took up their stations. The Great

Protector, the Great Historian, and the Great Master, all vested with hempen caps and scarlet robes of state.

The hemp hats, signs of mourning of their old king, Ching Wang, and the vibrant scarlet of the new king, Khang Wang's hempen robe of celebration. It's stirringly beautiful imagery.

Chinese Medicine

But I know you didn't come here to learn about cloth, or probably even seeds. So, let's see how the Ancient Chinese used cannabis in their medicine (and in fact, some still do). Incense, of course, formed the basis of medicine, but also of worship of the deity and even seduction of a lover.

Traditional Chinese medicine regards food and medicine itself as being inextricably linked. Naturally, better tasting medicines became beloved foods, and those not-so-great remained necessary evils, stored away for desperate measures in times of dire illness. Nevertheless, essentially, they are the same thing. It's impossible to separate the two, just as it has been with plants we have looked at in other books – most notably spikenard and rose; early ritual and medicine were one and the same. We can only really assume the mind-altering aspect of the drug by looking at the way the person consumed it, or indeed if they were using it in ritual celebration.

Incense, or more specifically smoke, holds a very special space in Ancient Chinese religion, drifting up to the wide blue expanse of sky and carrying prayers and offerings up to the gods. The indigenous being, The Supreme Deity Shang Di, was the highest of all gods. Too distant from mere mortals, it was the job of the Emperor to make offerings and commune with Shang Di. Each year he would make a special journey to the Temple of Heaven to make offerings of jade, silk, wine, and incense, and the most perfect sacrificial calf.

The finest of musicians journeyed with him, with glorious sets of bells and instruments, who then played exquisite music to welcome Shang Di and thank him for his presence. Majestic songs of praise and adoration were sung unto the creator, exalting him and promising him of their love. The music drifted up to Him on deeply aromatic smoke.

The song:

I hope this smoke from the fire will transport your offering to your place in Heaven.

All are praising your great name. The Heavens, The Earth, the plants, and the animals

The mountains, and the rivers

All are present and singing songs of praise to you.

The Emperor, usually commanding the country and issuing edicts, then assumed his place in the rightful order of the universe, offering himself prostrate in subservience to the only being superior to him. He entered into prayer of his plans for the coming year. Representing all creatures under the sky, he took their hopes and wishes to Shang Di. Asking for forgiveness for the nations transgressions he entered lengthy discourse with his god.

Standing patiently and reverently, he watched the calf burn and the smoke curling up into the Heavens. Knowing that Shang Di would soon smell the offerings of his people, he waited for the Supreme Deity to enjoy his gifts. An enormous 50 pounds of incense was thrown up onto the fire.

Then, taking the promises of protection from the Highest One back to the people, he was assured of success and care of China. It was to be guaranteed if every aspect of the ritual had been performed in the most meticulous detail.

So, what was in the incense?

In truth, we don't know. Documents from the Han Dynasty explain that foreign incenses like frankincense, agarwood, and spikenard were all imported to make ever more glamorous incense, whilst local ingredients were saved as offerings for the poor. This might imply that cannabis was not used, but I sense that's probably unlikely. The Emperor's discourse with Shang Di was unusual, special, which infers some sort of altered reality. To me, that suggests an entheogen, some kind of psychoactive substance that generates the divine, within. Certainly later, by the time polytheistic Taoism had taken its place, cannabis had become one of the most established ways to speak with the gods.

The Chinese clearly understood, very early, cannabis's power to affect one's mind. Several hundred pieces of jade and stone "oath documents" dating to the Eastern Chou Dynasty (770-221 BC) attest to this. Found in the Shansi Province, they are inscribed in red and attach the character *"ma"* to a symbol meaning "negative." They seemed to connect it with something bad.

The Ready to Use Pharmacopeia, the *zhenglei bencao,* draws on very ancient sources to describe its plants. Of cannabis, the author tells a story we will see many times.

"Those who wish to see demons should take it with other certain drugs for up to 100 days."

In *The Origin and Use of Cannabis in Eastern Asia,* botanist Li explains shamanism was widespread throughout China; cannabis enabling journeys to other dimensions. Unsurprisingly, medicine held all manner of connotations of sorcery in people's minds. Medicine men were practicing magicians, wielding wands made from hemp stalks carved with serpents. They must have been terrifying people to meet.

In *Cannabis and The Ancient World,* Chris Bennet explains this shamanic relationship with cannabis lasted several centuries, and over time filtered through into Taoism. A fifth century Taoist priest spoke of how they ate seeded buds in ritual: *"Magician technicians (shu chia) say if one consumes them with ginseng it will give preternatural knowledge of events of the future."* Further, in the Manual of Five Viscera, *Wu Tsang Ching* urges: *"If you wish to command demonic apparitions to present themselves, you must constantly eat the inflorescences of the hemp plant."*

So, eating the inflorescences, the flowers, allows a person to have knowledge superseding what is normal or natural...

Freaky!

Fourth century texts, the *Yuanshi shangzhen zhongxian ji* – Records of The Perfected Mortals - show cannabis being used as an incense in censors. They advise:

"For those practicing Tao, it is not necessary to go to the mountains. Some with purifying incense and sprinkling and sweeping, are able to call down the Perfected Immortals."

The Taoist Encyclopaedia, Supreme Secret Essentials *Wushang Biyou,* describes Taoists experimenting with different types of hallucinogenic smoke. Historian Joseph Needham illustrates how these rituals formed the beginning of Taoist creed.

"The chain of events which led to the establishment of Mao Shan...as the first permanent centre of Taoist practice, began in +349 or slightly earlier with visitations by immortals to a young man named Yan His. In a series of visions, there appeared to Yang a veritable pantheon of celestial functionaries, including the lady Wei and the Mao (brothers). In the course of these interviews, aided almost always by cannabis, Yang took down in writing a number of sacred texts which the immortals assured him were current in their own supernal realm, as well as oral elucidations and answers to Yang's queries about various aspects of the unseen world.

Considerable evidence points to cannabis also being used extensively by a sect called The Way of Infinite Harmony. These worshipped the Daoist goddess Magu, also known as The Hemp Maiden. The symbolic protector of females, Magu is often painted as a beautiful young lady with long birdlike fingernails, and often associated with caves. She wears a shimmering gown, not of this Earth, and not woven in any way we can conceive.

There's little surprising about the use of cannabis to bring about an alternate reality, and yet to our twenty first century Westerner brains, it may jar. We... no, let's say I... *I* experienced difficulties absorbing this aspect of the medicine of the plant, considering it to be a "side effect." And an undesirable one at that.

Yet, natural medicines don't have side effects, do they Elizabeth?

Only main effects.

It is as important an aspect of the healing as any other we encounter.

This, being out of it - being off your head, if you will - has its own very real uses. It removes a person from pain, emotionally, spiritually...and as we see now, physically.

Grant me, please, the honour of introducing you to Hua T'o, a doctor of the greatest note.

According to the official history of the Eastern Han Dynasty (25-221CE) "History of the Later Han", Hua T'o successfully completed an extremely complicated intestinal resection anaesthetising his patient with "Ma Fei San", a concoction of "cannabis boiling powder" and wine.

Notes from the biography of Hua T'o lead us by the hand into his gruesome second century operating theatre.

But if the malady resided in the parts on which the needle [acupuncture], cautery, or medicinal liquids were incapable of acting, for example, in the bones, in the stomach or in the intestine, he administered a preparation of hemp [ma-yo] and, in the course of several minutes, an insensibility developed as if one had been plunged into drunkenness or deprived of life. Then, according to the case, he performed the opening, the incision or the amputation and relieved the cause of the malady; then he apposed the tissues by sutures and applied linaments. After a certain number of days, the patient finds he has recovered without having experienced the slightest pain during the operation.

Would you like me to type up a referral?

Goodness, it must have been a hefty amount of weed to numb the body that much, but there is also a theory the wine may also have helped to extract and concentrate the active cannabis compounds. Sadly, he demanded his notes be destroyed before his death and so the recipe has been lost in the annals of time. We can only guess at the quantities and methods used.

The ingredient named in early texts, *Ma yo* literally translates to *hemp* oil, but, confusingly, the modern translation could also be *sesame* oil. Nineteenth century scholar M. S Julien disagrees on both accounts, suggesting the mixture was most likely to be cannabis **resin** mixed with the wine.

A disciple of Hua T'o, Wu Pu, makes clear distinctions between and *ma ze* non-toxic hemp seeds and *ma fen,* the toxic resin in subsequent writings.

In ***The Origin and Use of Cannabis in Eastern Asia,*** Li suggests linguistic evidence points to the stupefying effect of cannabis being very much "old news."

The word *Ma* can translate to hemp or cannabis but it might just as correctly be interpreted as "numbness, senseless or tingling." *Mamu* can also mean numb and the Chinese word for anaesthetics and narcotics is *mazui*. Clearly, they share a common stem. Thus, when you read the term **_Ta ma,_** the translation should be psychoactive cannabis.

Li also translated *Cheng Lei Pen Ts'ao,* or the Cheng Lei Herbal, originally written by Tang Shen Wei in 1108 CE.

He finds that Ma Fen has a spicy taste and is used for:

- Waste diseases and injury
- Clearing the blood
- Reducing temperature
- Relieving fluxes
- Reversing rheumatism
- Discharging pus

But the first euphoric medical applications appeared long, long before this in the *Materia Medica Sutra* or *Pen Ts'ao*, supposedly written by the Emperor Shen Nung.

Shen Nung is reputed to have lived somewhere between 3494-2857 BCE, and is certainly someone worth meeting. He is credited with inventing agriculture, no less, and with teaching medicine to the Chinese.

Shen Nung had watched with quiet fascination as sick people endlessly visited priests, even though their rituals seemed incapable of curing. A keen farmer, he decided to look more closely at the plants used to see if he could understand the situation better to improve it.

Now this, ladies and gentlemen, was a most opportune moment in Chinese history because legend has it that Shen Nung was the bearer of a belly of no ordinary constitution.

It was translucent! (Can you imagine?!).

He could investigate every process taking place during his dining. Apparently, every day he would ingest a different *seventy* plants, investigating their poisonous attributes and their antidote qualities.

The original text of *Pen Ts'ao* no longer exists (and indeed, it might never have done) but an unknown first century author compiled another herbal and explained that he had drawn references from this strange and marvellous work.

This "First" edition, *Pen Ts'ao Ching,* was published at the end of the Han Dynasty (ca 1800 BPA). Containing 365 medicines, including the oldest written proof of cannabis usage, this provides evidence that medicinal knowledge of the plant spans two thousand years. It reads:

"*Ma fen (Cannabis seed) . . . if taken in excess will produce hallucinations (literally 'seeing devils'). If taken over a long term, it makes one communicate with spirits and lightens one's body.*"

The text explains the drug became so popular because it contains elements of both yin and yang; soft, yielding, and passive feminine and the hot, active male principle. Since both male and female plants have yin and yang elements to them, Shen Nung then determined only *female* plants should be cultivated for medicine.

Eventually, *Pen Ts'ao* was to become the standard Chinese medicine authority. The Chinese people deified Shen Nung and heralded him "Father of Chinese Medicine." I feel reassured he probably knew what he was talking about.

According to him, cannabis should be prescribed to patients suffering from **a deficiency of yin.**

It's so bizarre how I go in circles writing these books. The very first one I wrote, *The Professional Stress Solution,* talks of how cannabis makes someone very yin and outlines the problems of yin disease. You might want to cross reference here. I found it useful going back. To cut a very long story short, this would be aggressive people and those that cannot forget (since poor memory is very yin) amongst other aspects.

Nung lists indications of Ma Fen (the resin made from the female plant) as:

- Menstrual fatigue
- Gout
- Rheumatism
- Malaria
- Beri-beri (Vitamin B_1 deficiency)
- Constipation and absent mindedness

(Taylor 1963, Li 1975)

The *Pen Ts'ao Ching* also includes cannabis in the "**Drugs of First Class**", a list headed up by Ginseng.

"Of the first class of drugs, there are 120 sorts, which are considered to perform the function of Kün or sovereigns. They support human life and thereby resemble Heaven. They are not poisonous. Whatever quantity you take and howsoever you use them, they are harmless. If you wish to have a body light, to improve the breath, to live an old age without growing old, make use of these drugs of the first class. These include ginseng, jujubes, oranges, Job's tears, Discorea (glutinous yams). Benincasa cerifera (ash ground) Amaranthus blitumm, Cannabis sativa, Kadsura."

Nowadays, we have a slightly different perception, understanding that prolonged or excessive use of cannabis will eventually do harm by pushing the endocannabinoid system out of kilter.

Gradually, throughout the fourteenth and fifteenth centuries, trade and relations broke down between China, Korea, and Japan. Each civilisation looked inward to their own cultural pathway. Nevertheless, Japan and Korea continued to send students to China to learn agriculture, science, and medicine, so cannabis then reached its influences outwards.

In Japan, *tai ma* is viewed as one of the *Sanso*. The Three Plants: cannabis, along with *red safflower* and *indigo*, symbolise long life. Traditional Japanese uses are like Chinese and draw heavily on their pharmacopeia. They are thought to provide the following benefits:

- Laxative
- Relives asthma
- Soothes poisonous bites
- Worms pets
- Treating skin ailments
- General tonic and promoting vigour

The Steppe

On the website, Ancient-Origins, Bryan Hill describes a 1997 discovery of a hemp rope in Czechoslovakia. Dating it at 26,900 BC, he placed it as the oldest known cannabis object in existence. Disappointingly, original dig papers have thus far evaded me but there is no doubt in this remote and unforgiving landscape that cannabis has dwelt for the longest of times.

In *"Researches"* (450 BC) the Ancient Greek historian Herodotus depicts a strange and unusual scene witnessed on his explorations around the Black Sea, the area he refers to as Scythia. If we looked at a map today, this is areas stretching from the Ukraine right up to the borders of India. An enormous space.

His strange and enigmatic narration is one of our most compelling glimpses into funeral rites.

"After the burial, those engaged in it have to purify themselves, which they do in the following way. First, they will soap and wash their heads; and in order to cleanse their bodies, they act as follows: they make booths by fixing on the ground three sticks inclined towards one another, and stretching around them wooden felts, which they arranged so as to fit as close as possible. Inside there are bronze dishes placed upon the ground into which they put a number of red-hot stones and some hemp seed."

The Scythians were a terrifying nomadic tribe from the modern-day area that would have been Northern Iran. It stands a good chance that the spread of the popularity of cannabis throughout the globe may be down to its important status in Scythian life. So much so that in the ancient world, hemp earned the title "Scythian Fire."

Who were these terrifying peoples, the Scythians?

Reader, get ready to be fascinated. I feel robbed we never learned about them at school.

They seemed to rule from 9th Century BC to 4th Century AD (yes, you did read that right. It's a phenomenal length of time, isn't it!), though no-one really knows where they came from. A shamanic tribe, they left behind them an inordinate amount of art and treasures to learn from. The area they ruled was called Scythia, although historians disagree whether this was in fact the area of one large tribe or perhaps a collective name used to describe many unrelated peoples of this geographical area.

It is thought that in the 8th Century BC they raided Zhou, China, and then expanded westwards, dislodging the Cimmerians, the existing rulers of the Pontic Steppe. With the Cimmerians out of the way, the Scythians looked triumphantly out of their wagon windows to survey their realm.

And what a realm it was!

It spread from the Black Sea up to the Caspian Sea, across to Moldova, then to Western Ukraine to the Volga district of Russia. So, if you trace that on a map, it runs from 30 degrees to 55 degrees east longitude!

Vast!

A nomadic people, they raised herds of cattle, horses, and sheep. Living in tent-covered wagons, they were some of the first warriors to master the art of mounted warfare. They were extraordinary metalworkers, fighting with bows and arrows whilst seated on horseback. Seemingly, Cimmerian foot soldiers stood little chance against such skilled warriors and trained horses.

The Scythians created a vast trade network between Greece, Persia, India, and China. By the seventh century BC they crossed the Caucasus, (the border of Europe and Asia, to heathens like you and I), and were frequently recorded as raiding the Middle East. In short, these were scary, *scary*, **scary** people.

Herodotus continues...

"Hemp grows in Scythia, it's very like flax; only that it is much coarser and is a taller plant. Some grows wild in the country, some is produced by cultivation. The Thracians cloth themselves with garments made of the hemp; so well resembling Flax, that a man must have great experience in those materials to distinguish one from the other: and he who had never seen this hemp would think their cloths were wrought out of Flax.

The Scythians, as I say, take some of this hemp seed, and creeping under the felt coverings throw them upon the red-hot stones; immediately it smokes and gives out such a vapour no Grecian vapour bath can exceed. The sing, delighted, shout for joy, and this vapour serves instead of a water bath; for they never by any chance wash themselves with water."

This seems to have been a description of a ritual to help the deceased's family accompany them into the next life. If that were true, how lovely to be unburdened of the worry that they may have gone to a better place; a beautiful ritual to overcome sorrow and to prevent depression *collectively*. It's likely this was the reason that hemp was given the name "Scythian fire." In a 1998 paper *"Düftender rauch für die seele"* Fred Wollner suggested cannabis may have been one of the oldest plants ever used for fumigation.

Numerous significant excavations have proven Herodotus's explanation to be entirely accurate. A discovery from 2015 sent the media into a complete frenzy when it was announced that archaeologists had found bongs in Russia dating back 2400 years. The discovery was kept under wraps for two years to ensure the site was protected from looting, and no wonder!

Stavropol-based archaeologist Andrei Belinski had begun to excavate the kurgan (a mound placed over a burial chamber), called Sengileevskoe-2, as a precaution to make way for a new network of powerlines. The team didn't really expect to find a great deal because it was clear that someone had looted the kurgan at some point in the past, probably in the 19th Century. After digging for a few weeks though, they came across a very thick layer of clay. Beneath that they found a large rectangular chamber which had been lined with wide flat stones. Inside the chamber was treasure beyond compare.

Apart from the bong there were also three gold cups, a large ring for the finger, two rings for the neck, and a gold bracelet. When the gold had been cleaned it weighed around 7 pounds, or 3.2 kilograms.

As residue was cleaned from the gold vessels, startling ornate decorations emerged, revealing what seems to be Scythian understandings of their underworld. One vessel depicts griffons ripping a horse and stag apart. The other, an elderly bearded man slaughtering virile young warriors.

Experts believe this vessel may be recounting the story of the "bastard wars" also described by Herodotus. He had related that the Scythians had been warring with the Persians for 28 years. When finally returning home, they found their tents full of strangers. Slowly the horrible truth dawned that their lonely wives had cavorted with their slaves. These strangers they met were the bastard children of the interludes. The children, now grown, sought to engage the returning heroes in battle. It was a massacre with unrivalled loss of life.

Herodotus relates that one warrior returned to his fellows saying: *"What are we doing Scythians? We are fighting our slaves, diminishing our own number when we fall, and the number of those that belong to us when we fall by our hands. Take my advice - lay spear and bow aside and let each man fetch his horse whip and go boldly up to them. So long as they see us with arms in our hands, they imagine themselves are equals in birth and slavery; but let's then behold us with no other weapon but the whip, and they will feel that they are slaves, and flee before us."*

Belinski feels the pictures depict a more metaphorical belief that power struggles exist when a ruler or king dies. *"When a king died, there was chaos. The spirit world was upset by the death of the King, and order had to be born anew."*

It's thought that similar ritual use probably occurred amongst the Assyrians and various ancient tribes such as the Thracians, a pale skinned and red haired nomadic race. Herodotus provides us with another story, this time from Assyria, found in his *"Books of History"*:

"Of the river Araxes... When many people have come together, they light a fire, sit around it in a circle and they throw these fruits into the fire. When the smell of the burning fruits enters their noses, they become inebriated like the Greeks from their wine. They throw more and more fruits into the fire, so that they become more and more inebriated and finally jump up and begin to dance and to sing. This is what is said about the way they live."

In 1929 Professor S. I. Rudenko, a Russian anthropologist, unearthed the remains of a Scythian burial site hidden in the Altai Mountains on the border of Siberia and Outer Mongolia. The trench that he found measured about 160 feet squared and about 20 feet deep. Along the perimeter were the skeletons of a number of horses. Also inside was the body of an embalmed man. There he found a bronze cauldron with burnt remains at the base, later confirmed to be cannabis seeds.

Rudenko's team also found shirts made from hemp and metal censors apparently for inhaling marijuana, although he could attach no ritual significance to them. Potentially, then, they had been using them for recreational use. Some of the cauldrons were very small. Others weighed as much as 75 pounds! Most had solid bases shaped into a cone, presumably so that hot fire could be heaped around the base. Fixed to the rim, opposite each other, the upper section of the largest bowl had animal-shaped handles. Other finds indicated that potentially women participated alongside the men.

This is a short description of an extraordinary archaeological dig that is now a UNESCO world heritage site. If you want to have a closer look at the excavation and some of the most extraordinary metalwork made by the Scythians have a look at this link: https://goo.gl/Df4NSd.

In 1993, a spectacular discovery was made of the so-called "Siberian Ice Princess", or the "Ukok Princess", also uncovering ancient cannabis. The young woman, aged about 25 years old, was found in Pazyryk in the Altai Mountains of Siberia. The tomb is believed to date back to the 5th Century. Completely preserved by permafrost, miraculously "The Princess" was covered in the most spectacular bodywork of tattoos. They are considered the most detailed and most colourful ever found from the ancient world. Works of the finest artistry, they depict griffons and panthers as well as other fantastical beasts. Unbelievably her clothes were also preserved, showing her to be immaculately dressed in a silk skirt and gloriously ornate, long sleeve boots.

The tattoos served as one of the ways to date her. It has been suggested that the animals indicate a sacred language of the Pazyryk, that depicted the person's innermost thoughts. It is also thought the longer a person lived the more tattoos were added. There have been discoveries of Pazyryk warriors being tattooed over their entire body, but they were older people. Since the woman only had tattoos over her arms, it led to the understanding that maturity would lead to more artwork. In the same manner, it suggests the picturing might also allude to her status in society.

These glorious animals are also seen in other modes of art but historians believe that these bodily tattoos were used as a means to pass more easily from this life to the next and as a means of identification – like a passport, if you will - in both lives. In the after-life, the pictures would make it easier to identify and join loved ones who had passed over.

She was buried, as was customary for Scythian burials, with her horses. For a commoner one horse would usually have sufficed, but this lady was special, warranting six, each with their saddles and bridles attached as a means of a suitable escort to the underworld. This, it is thought, alludes to status. Unusually though, she had been buried alone. Usually, men and women would have been buried together, with families all in a row. But this lady seemed to be unusual, warranting an isolated burial. Researchers think this might indicate celibacy, which is known to have been usual for shamans and cult servants.

Was the cannabis for ritual use? Yes, perhaps, but it also seems very likely that she was in an inordinate amount of pain. An MRI, conducted in Novosibirsk, revealed that the 'princess' had suffered from osteomyelitis, an infection of the bone or bone marrow, from childhood or adolescence. Then, near the end of her life, she sustained injuries when falling from her horse. Lastly, she had breast cancer, which ravaged her into a dreadful state of emaciation. Her decline seems to have been slow, the tumour in her left breast and metastases in her lymph, glands taking five years to eventually overcome her. The cannabis she was taking seemingly allowed her to commune with spirits and to act as a conduit between the community with the spirit world.

The intricacies of the investigation will astound you. Scientists can see that she arrived in Ukok in October, in the fourth stage of cancer. Struggling with pain and heavily drugged with painkillers, she had weakened terribly. In this vulnerable state, it seems likely she fell from a horse and was seriously injured. The MRI shows that she fell on her right temple, right shoulder, and right hip, although she was clearly alive for a while after the fall because oedema formed around her injuries.

Anthropologists believe that the migration to the winter camp might have been the only thing powerful enough to motivate this very sick and frail lady to get onto a horse. It's very notable that her people didn't leave her to die, or even kill her, given that she would have made their dangerous journey even more arduous. Instead, they felt impelled to take her with them to camp, showing just how important she must have been. It seems likely she never left her bed when she reached the winter camp. Pathologists believe the people stored her body before the funeral, probably for about two to three months. Tests on the horses' stomachs alongside show their last meal was eaten in June, most likely when she was buried, even though scientists feel she probably died in January or even March. She was buried in the spring, as the ground softened. As it re-hardened an air pocket had formed, encasing the Ice Princess in permafrost and preserving her for two and half millennia.

This poor woman was probably so ravaged with pain that sniffing cannabis was her only way to get through the day. In her altered state of mind, it seemed she could speak to other beings and became important and cherished by the tribe. It would certainly explain why they took so much care for her and buried her in a way not that dissimilar to royalty.

Although she was called Princess, shaman is more likely. The term Ice Princess was given to her by the media: researchers call her *Devochka,* meaning "Girl".

The people of the Altai Mountains still attribute great powers to her. They believe earthquakes have happened because her body was removed. They remember that the helicopter, taking her away, almost crashed. She has been returned to the area where she came from, and now resides in a specially designed glass coffin.

Weed has been found in the Yanghai Tombs (also spelled Yang-Hai) in northwest China.

Nestled at the base of the Fire, or Flaming, Mountains (*Huoyan Shan*), Yanghai lies right in the foothills of the Heavenly Mountains (Tian Shan) on the edge of the gloriously fertile Turpan Oasis. People have been drawn to this beautiful area for thousands of years, and this is the burial grounds of an ancient nomadic people called **Gushi**, (sometimes seen as Jushi.) Many of the finds seem to share similarities with the Scythians, leading experts to suspect that perhaps the Gushi were somehow connected to Scythia.

Historical evidence tells us these people *"lived in tents, followed the grasses and waters, and had considerable knowledge of agriculture."* They were farmers, owning cattle, horses, camels, sheep, and goats. They were accomplished horsemen and archers and spoke an extinct language called *Tocharian,* thought to have been similar to Celtic.

The Yanghai Tombs had a long history ranging between 3000 and 2600 years old. Since the region is so arid, the mummies of the dead and other organic materials were immaculately preserved and were found in the most amazing condition when the 250 tombs were excavated at the turn of this century. There have been many striking insights into the people who lived here because of this fabulous preservation. Not least to us, the man found in "Room 90".

Surprisingly, for a tomb found in China, a 2,500-year-old man found buried here was Caucasian with blue eyes. It is thought the Gushi had originated from Russia. Sadly, his body, reduced to a skeleton, was not as well-preserved as others that have been found. Most of the objects that had been buried with him seemed to be connected with horsemanship, although there was also a musical instrument, bows and arrows, and some wooden cups. An open leather basket lay near the man's head and was filled with immaculately preserved fruits, leaves, and shoots. Next to it lay a wooden bowl of cannabis, still green after all these thousands of years.

"The deceased was laid out on the bottom of this tomb on a little bier," explained Dr. Ethan Russo, in his study published in the Journal of Experimental Botany. The bier was a movable frame on which a coffin or a corpse had been placed before burial or cremation and presumably carried the deceased to their grave. Russo continues:

"This individual seemed to be very high status because of the variety and quality of the grave goods, including the equestrian equipment, the archery equipment and the large amount of cannabis." (Large amount is specifically 789 grams. That's nearly 2 pounds. Ladies and gentlemen, this is a *seriously* large stash, suggesting this had been collected over a time and not simply taken from one plant).

Closer examination showed they were female flowers, discounting any possibility that the hemp might have been intended for rope and leading researchers to suspect he was probably a shaman. Archaeologists didn't recover any kind of pipe so it is probable that he would have eaten it or perhaps thrown it onto the fire and taken a jolly good gulp of the fumes. What was it for? Pain relief maybe, divination perhaps. It's interesting to contemplate that the flowers had been laid *by his head*, so scholars wonder if this is significant and that perhaps he intended to continue his work here in the afterlife.

When the hemp underwent radiocarbon dating, it was deemed to be 2,495 years old. Although it had retained its green hue, the volatiles must have evaporated because it no longer exuded its characteristically sweet weedy smell.

Siberian Medicine

The female inflorescences of *Cannabis ruderalis* are frequently found as being used as fumigants in sweat lodge ceremonies, as well as being dried and then smoked or inhaled. Christian Ratsch describes a local recipe for psychoactive shamanic incense in his *Encyclopedia of Psychoactive Plants: Ethnopharmacology and its Applications*. A concoction of equal parts hemp flowers, juniper branch tips, thyme, and wild rosemary, he relates that wormwood, mugwort, or other species of Artemisia might also be included.

The cookery fanatics among you might relish experimenting with baking with *C. ruderalis*. A sedative and aphrodisiac, cannabis is blended with psychoactive ingredients then sweetened with saffron, nutmeg, cardamom, and honey in traditional Russian delicacies.

In the Altai region, "bagaschun" is considered to be the universal panacea. Recipes for this Mongolian folk medicine consists of hemp and juniper being blended into bat guano.

Delightful!

The hemp/guano mix is a beloved tonic in Russian folk medicine too. Sadly, I have been unable to ascertain how one should administer such a spectacular thing. Your homework is to create me 16 easy recipes of hemp and guano and to post it onto the internet. Obviously, I'll have to insist on seeing case history pictures of it being used!

C. ruderalis is the chosen prescription for depression in Russia and Mongolia.

Egyptian Medicine & Antiquity

Although cannabis is rarely seen in ancient Egypt, as a medicine it does have a hieroglyph, Shemshemet. Dr. Lise Manniche recommends we pronounce this "Shm- Shm Tu" or "sm sm". It literally means *medical marijuana plant*. Some scholars have previously suggested that the term might sometimes be easily confused with sesame, but although cannabis is an unusual medicine it is always recommended for *external* use, whereas sesame is usually ingested.

The Ebers papyrus is the oldest complete herbal in history. Although it is not the earliest reference to cannabis, it lets us glimpse ancient Egyptian medicine at around 1600 BC. It gives a fascinating insight into cannabis being used for gynaecology. In formula 821 (96:7-8) we see a recipe for mother and child:

"SuSm-t ground in honey and introduced into her vagina."

Mechoulam, arguably the world's most important cannabis researcher, suggests this might have been to prevent haemorrhage after childbirth.

Then, in Formula 618, honey, ochre, hemp, and other ingredients are blended together for a remedy for a poorly finger or toenail.

Ramesseum III is again a medical papyrus, probably dating back even further to 1700 BC and the reign of Ramses II. It belongs to a collection of texts spanning a wide range of subjects and dates. They form the archive of the tomb in which they were found and have been described as the "most precious single find of papyri" from pharaonic Egypt and now are housed in the British Museum in London.

Because they are so fragile and fragmented it has been difficult to conduct studies of them in detail thus far. Luckily, the section describing cannabis is in relatively good repair. It prescribes:

"A treatment for the eyes: [blended with] celery, hemp is ground and left in the dew overnight. Both eyes of the patient are to be washed in the morning."

A twist though, because I suspected that the physician may have realised the potential of the herb against glaucoma (and probably he has) but another section of this papyrus also seems to describe the eruption of the Santorini volcano in 1600 AD. Could this wash be to cleanse the eyes of volcanic dust? I dunno.

Interesting, isn't it?

The Chester Beatty VI Papyrus is dated to c. 1200 BC and is thought to be the world's oldest treatise on anorectal disease (affecting the anus and rectum). It is one of several papyri, acquired by philanthropist Chester Beatty in the 1920s. This one comes from Thebes, and was also donated to the British Museum. I like this one because it feels like you see Egyptian studies unfolding before your eyes. Some words are still not yet understood (underlined and in bold), maintaining the nebulous and mysterious meaning of the recipes.

See what *you* make of it.

What do you think the patient might have been suffering from?

*"Another remedy for the part of the body named sâq, the bladder to drive away the **chenefet** substances and whatever other anal affliction of a man or women [....]*

*If the problem manifests itself in a fashion due to divine action, both abscesses of the bladder, some **setet** of the joint, then he will lose water between his buttocks, then he will have a fever on account of this that he has sustained, his urine will flow, the evacuations will be painful, his anus is heavy, the flow from the abdomen is without end, you must say to the patient "It is a heaviness of the anus, a problem that I can treat." This remedy you must prepare for him until he is cured: goose fat 5 ro; honey 50 ro; human milk 15 ro. This will be placed four days following.*

*Another remedy, which is prepared after this; water of wheat **mimi**; 1 cannabis juice; 1 juice of a **quebou** plant; 1 goose fat; 1 lotus leaves; 1 acacia leaves. This will be prepared in a homogenous mass and placed in the anus four days following."*

I'm not sure what the affliction is, but it sure ain't good!

Be careful whom you describe this recipe to. I feel sure if I showed it to The Strong Silent One, he would find his voice next time I ask "Does my bum look big in this?" He'll answer, "Yes, but maybe that's because your anus is heavy."

And I won't even have a quebou plant to rectify that either!

So, the question everyone seems to want to know is did the ancient Egyptians use cannabis psycho-actively?

Oh, my goodness what a can of worms...

Probably!

There are many mentions of The Smoke Eaters at Thebes (which was the main Holy centre of Egypt) and their use of cannabis in mortuary rites, although I cannot find much out about them at all. Diodorus Siculus, a Greek historian from Sicily, describes how the women of Thebes used cannabis to dispel sorrow and bad humour, although whether the two are the same I cannot decide.

But Pandora's Box first opens in Paris in 1976.

At Le Bourget airport, a line of military wait with all the pomp and circumstance of a state visit because a very important king is about to grace their runway.

This is not such a rare occurrence, only this particular visitor had been dead for over 3000 years. The mummy of Ramses II had been flown to Paris's Ethnological Museum to undergo treatment for funguses and bacteria that had been gradually degrading his body whilst on display in the Cairo museum.

While the mummy was in Paris, various specimens were given to several local eminent Egyptologists to work on to bring in their own varying disciplines of investigations in a bid to learn more about the great king, but also ancient Egypt in general.

Dr. Michele Lescot, a well-respected scholar from Paris's own Museum of Natural History, was given a piece of the burial linen to study. When she reported findings of a pollen granule of tobacco her work was met with derision and scorn and accusations of shoddy workmanship abounded. It was insisted that one of her colleagues must have been smoking a pipe and contaminated the linen because tobacco would not be seen in Egypt until Columbus had brought it back to Europe from the Americas.

I have to say I have worried a bit about Dr. Lescot and how she must have felt after such sorry remarks and what it did to her career, because the belief that she had screwed up remained in circulation until another great woman, Dr. Svetlana Balabanova, took up the fight six years later.

Now people, let me tell ya, Dr. B. is nobody's fool. She is a forensic toxicologist with police training and even pioneered some of the drug tests used in sports competitions today. If there is good sh*t to be found in human tissue, Dr. B is the gal to find it.

She did.

Taking up Lescot's trail, she asked to see intestinal tissues from inside of the cadaver of Ramses the Great. There she found pollens of cannabis, coca (cocaine), and tobacco. These ran through and around the body cells "like rings on a tree."

Then, in 1992, she had the opportunity to take the studies further when a "super team" was gathered to look at new findings in archeo-cadavers. Seven mummies were despatched to her and the findings were the same. Each one had evidence of cocaine and nicotine and all but one showed evidence of cannabis consumption. Since that time, she has investigated over 3000 ancient bodies and virtually every royal mummy shows evidence of so called "Divine plants", that is shamanic plants that help you commune with the gods.

So, you would have thought it was conclusive, but guys if you thought people on aromatherapy forums are nasty to one another (there, I said it!) we ain't got nothing on Egyptology! The haters really started to hate, coming out of every possible orifice of sarcophagus woodwork. Some authorities said that perhaps these had been absorbed as people smoked around the mummies as they had viewed the exhibits and that the only way to see if it had really been ingested was to examine different depths of it in the scalp. That perhaps she had been duped by later "fake" mummies that had been painted with black tar...

It goes on and on.

Balabanova and her team have stood their ground. One by one, they have overcome each argument in turn. At the moment, the results of the tests still stand, but one can see why they are very hard to absorb.

Just how did tobacco or cocaine get from the Americas to ancient Egypt? Is everything we know about the ancient trade routes wrong?

We know that hemp was in the country because it is recommended in the Pyramid texts as a material to make rope. Further, hemp was stuffed into crevices in rock faces. When water was added the hemp expanded to break open the rock and make bricks to build with. A sample of hemp fabric was also found in the tomb of Akhenaten. Whether it actually *grew* there is uncertain, until it is documented that the Roman emperor Aurelius taxed it, but that doesn't arise until the third century AD. There is also no doubt they used psychoactive ingredients like mandrake and blue lotus so yes, I think taking the odd puff or two also seems very likely.

Antiquity

Another papyrus we have at our disposal is newer, around 2nd century AD, the Vienna Papyrus which discloses writing of Galen and Pliny. This idea of recorded information from further and further into the past is very important (and of course, what I am doing now!). It is a valuable record of the use of hemp, but the danger of this is always going to be Chinese Whispers. Each telling of hemp's tale has its own slant and dimension added to deepen intrigue, but also in today's world to circumnavigate copyright! This is very interesting here. Have all accounts been construed and correctly related?

Pliny wrote in 77 AD that *"Esparto – made of a species of course grass - was used at sea, but on land they prefer ropes made of hemp."*

Galen and Ephippus both describe how seeds can be cooked and eaten as a delicacy, and here Galen hints at psycho-activity:

"There are some who fry and consume [the seed] together with other desserts. I call "desserts" these foods that are eaten after dinner in order to stimulate an appetite for drinking. The seed creates a feeling of warmth and if consumed in large amounts affects the head by sending to it a warm and toxic vapour."

Given that most of the writings we find from Galen are reworks of things other people have written, it is not outside the realms of possibility that he too misunderstood what someone else has written. I say this because hemp seed is not psychoactive and it doesn't actually give you the munchies. It is, however, very drying, and it definitely gave me a headache when I worked with it! It can also make you inordinately thirsty, so perhaps he is not describing some kind of hashish delicacy at all. Maybe it is just the seeds.

Both he and Dioscorides are keen to point out that not only is it fantastic for earache but it will also reduce potency. In *De Alimentorum facutatibus,* Galen compares hemp to Vitex Agnus Castus, the Chaste Tree, the sacred tree of Hera, saying it is similar in appearance, which I thought was interesting but nothing more.

He also advises *"The seeds dispel wind from the lower abdomen and dry the user to such an extent that when eaten in excess sexuality is extinguished."*

He continues:

"Some squeeze the juice from green seeds to use as a remedy for blockages in the ear."

Over the centuries, especially in British medicine, you will see Galen's words regurgitated repeatedly in different texts:

"Earaches and desiccant of men's seed."

Pseudo Apuleius, in his fourth century herbal *Herberium Apulei Platonici,* breaks the mould a little bit and advocates using the herb mixed with grease for

swellings of the chest and mixing cannabis with nettle seeds and vinegar for **cold sores** (ow, ow, ow... Surely that stings?)

Unani Medicine

Collated from an eloquent monograph in 1965 by Shri. C. Dwarakanath for the United Nations Office and Drugs and Crime, the following terms form part of their efforts to assess the safety of using cannabis in the traditional medicine disciplines, Ayurveda and Unani- Tibbi. Officers' understanding of the herb was greatly enhanced by Sanskrit's erudite descriptions of its actions.

Bahuvadini - Causes excessive garrulousness

Bhang - Arrests the functions of the brain in excessive doses

Chapala - Causes vacillation of the mind

Dafe-a-tashanj - Anti-convulsive

Harshini - Stimulates a pleasurable sensation and causes elation of mind

Madini - Induces narcosis

Mohini - Causes mental confusion

Moras-hi-zan - Causes delirium

Mujafifmani - Devitalising

Mumsik - Retentive

Munawam - Hypnotic

Muqavi mehda - Stomachic

Mushtai - Appetiser

Muskan alm – Pain-killing

Mussakar - Intoxicant

Nuqavi bah - Aphrodisiac

Quabiz - Induces constipation

Ranjika - Causes excitement

Samvida manjari - Inflorescence causes garrulousness

Tandrakrit - Causes drowsiness

Trailokya vijaya - Causes a state of mind in which the subject feels that he is capable of conquering "the three worlds"

Vijaya - Causes a feeling of being unconquerable

Virapatra - Means "potent leaf" India & Ayurveda

Ayurvedic medicine seeks to balance three functional elements, the doshas, what the human body is composed of, and is commonly represented as Vata or Vayu (ether or air), Pitta (fire and water), and Kapha (phlegm or water and earth).

In Dr. K. M. Nadkarni's *Indian Materia Medica* Volume 1, we benefit from the term "Vipaka" being described more succinctly than the usual "wind, bile, phlegm" annotations that western scholars might usually provide.

"...the word Vayu does not imply 'Wind' in Ayurvedic literature, but comprehends all the phenomena which come under the functions of the Central and Sympathetic Nervous Systems; that the word Pitta does not essentially mean 'Bile' but signifies the functions of Thermogenesis or heat production and metabolism, comprehending in its scope the process of digestion, coloration of blood and formation of various secretions and excretions and that the word Kapha does not mean 'Phlegm' but is used primarily to imply the functions of Thermo-taxis or heat regulation and secondarily formation of the various preservative fluids, e.g., Mucus, Synovia, etc."

Good health depends on a perfect balance between these three doshas.

Cannabis has a very long history in Ayurveda. Its Sanskrit name is Bhanga and it is classified as a **stimulant for all three doshas**. The ancient medicinal texts use it for purification, but at the same time **class it as a toxic substance.** A reference is made to bhanga in *Ashtadhyayi of Panini* (a very ancient paper about Sanskrit grammar) showing that cannabis was known in India as early as the fourth and third centuries BC.

Historically, the Brahmins used the herb to bring about both relaxation and an altered state of consciousness, and to enable them to sink deeper into their meditations. These holy men used the herb in myriad ways to induce different effects. On some occasions, they might inhale smoke from the marijuana hash. On others, they might ingest a delicious milk concoction blended with the spices and leaves from the plant. Also famously known as bhang, this drink is still often consumed in India during the Holi festival. Partaking of "the bhang" supposedly leads the drinker up a stairway to enlightenment, effortlessly peeling back the layers of consciousness and revealing their true nature.

I managed to find a recipe for bhang on the Ayurveda College website:

- 2 cups water
- 4 cups warm milk
- 1/2 to 1 teaspoon rosewater
- 1 oz bud (of marijuana flowers)
- 3/4 to 1 cup sugar
- 2 tablespoons blanched almonds

- 1/8 teaspoon garam masala
- 1/4 teaspoon ginger powder

I had to experiment a little and made it with some hemp flowers, and even though it should normally be made with marijuana for its psychoactive effects I can still see how one could easily become hooked. It is utterly scrumptious and feels incredibly indulgent and exotic. Did it still reveal my true nature? I reached for a second cup, thus radiating my pitta greediness. I'm not sure my good girl's version did much else, no.

Historically, it's likely that the very earliest written reference to cannabis in India can be found in the Atharvaveda (remember the gorgeous book of hymns we spoke about in the Holy Basil book that told scholars so much about life 4000 years ago?). This first mention would date to about 1500 BC.

It lyrically pleads: *"We tell of the five kingdoms of herbs headed by Soma; may it, and kusa grass, and bhanga and barley, and the herb saha, release us from anxiety."*

We also find the prowess of bhang acknowledged in ancient medicinal texts: **Chakara Samhita** (translates to *the internist*) and the **Sushrata Samhita** (*the surgeon*).

The Sushrata Samhita advises using cannabis for phlegm, catarrh, and diarrhoea.

What's interesting though, is that unlike the usage in China, when the subject of anaesthesia arises for surgery, both books relate that alcohol is their preferred method of dulling the senses, rather than cannabis. Was the plant still being used as a religious instrument, we wonder? Perhaps the psychoactive properties had not yet been discovered by the time they had been written (dates of authorship are unknown but we are probably talking around 2nd century and 6th century BC, respectively).

It seems likely that the first unambiguous regard to cannabis being a drug appeared in the 11th century from *Cikitsasarasangraha* by the Bengal author Vangasena. He portrays the herb as a *"drug-like opium whose mode of action is to pervade the whole body before being absorbed and digested."*

*T*he *Dhanwantari nighantu,* written in the eighth century AD, explains bhang entered Indian medicine because of its **intoxicating stimulation to digestion,** because it was **hot and diuretic**, and because of its **expectorant and aphrodisiac properties.**

In the 13th century the materia medica of Ayurvedic plants, *Rajanighantu,* detailed several new characteristics of the cannabis plant unlisted in earlier works.

Cannabis is described as:

- *balyatva* (strength-giving)
- *katutva* (acridity)
- *medhakaritva* (inspiring of mental power)
- *samgrdhitva* (astringency) & *kashayatva* (astringency) (I can't seem to distinguish between the two)
- *sreshthadipanatva* (the property of a most excellent excitant)
- *tiktatva* (pungency)
- *ushnatva* (heat)
- *vakpradatva* (speech giving)
- *vatakaphapahatva* (removing wind and phlegm)

Translations of the work tell us that its effects on man are described as:

- Excitant
- Heating
- Astringent
- Destroys phlegm
- Expels flatulence
- Induces costiveness (I had to look that one up. It either means not generous, or means constipation. I suggest here it probably means the latter, but one can never be sure!)
- Sharpens the memory
- Excites appetite

Another compendium of therapeutics dating to the thirteenth century AD *Sharangadhara Samhita* also lists several prescriptions titrated with *bhang*.

Generally, early Ayurvedic practitioners used cannabis and preparations of bhang for **diarrhoea, dysentery,** and **insomnia**.

In addition, it was administered for **skin diseases** where patients might take cannabis internally as well as using it externally.

Often bhanga was added to **herbal vaginal pessaries** prescribed for ladies suffering from "**contracting vaginas.**" It took me a while to decipher that this is vaginismus, a condition where ladies tense up, causing painful penetration during intercourse.

The twelfth century text *Ananda Kanda* lists several different texts for erectile dysfunction. These include:

- *Curna*
- *Vatika*

- *Leha*
- *Paka*
- *Dugdhapaka,*
- *Kvatha*
- *Modaka*

Madan Modaka and Kameshwar Modaka are both sweets made from bhanga, prescribed to alleviate the strain of sexual debility. As with many Ayurvedic preparations, these foods are created with many purposes in mind. A recipe for Madan Modaka contains many herbs, but notably hemp leaves with flowers and seeds fried in clarified butter, equal in weight to all other ingredients. This was also used for coughs, chronic bowel complaints, and impotence.

Many instances are found in folk medicine where juice has been extracted from the cannabis leaves or a paste made from them. In Ayurveda, this juice was **applied to the head to remove dandruff** but also to get rid of every infant school child's mother's nightmare, **nits!**

Powdered leaves **are dusted over open fresh wounds to help them to scab over.**

Poultices were made from the plant and applied to **areas of local inflammation**, to **soothe neuralgia** and to ease the pain of **haemorrhoids.**

The Rasa shastras are the ancient Ayurvedic alchemy texts containing medicinal preparations created from metals, minerals, and toxic plants. The end effect is always the same as it is in any alchemy, that of transformation. Here cannabis is identified, changing the condition of those who have lost their appetite, have failing digestion, intestinal spasms, poor blood circulation, and heart disease.

In his book *Rasa Shastra: The Hidden Art of Medical Alchemy* Andrew Mason pairs cannabis with soapstone for treatments. Where he describes the dynamics of cannabis as being hot, he attributes the dynamics of soapstone as being cold. He states that cannabis should be purified using rosewater, aloe vera juice, or salt water and used for internal/external bleeding, skin diseases, vaginal discharges, diarrhoea, dysentery, menorrhagia, leucorrhoea, gonorrhoea, heart pains, cough, and pyorrhoea.

(Honestly, the words they missed out of our school spelling tests – that list was impossible to type! Still, can you imagine being examined on that delightful list of abnormally heavy bleeding, thick whitish-yellow vaginal discharge and a venereal disease involving inflammatory discharge from the urethra or vagina, and lastly a virulent inflammation of the gums and tooth sockets? On second thought, that may not be the sort of exposure any teacher wants to subjugate

themselves to in front of a class of 13-year-olds. In this case, perhaps some things are best left to the spell checker!).

The *Rajavallabha*, written in the 15th century by Sutradhar Mandan for the famed ruler and military leader Rana Kumhha of Mewar, gives a vivid description of cannabis: *"Indra's food (i.e. ganja) is acid, produces infatuation, and destroys leprosy. It creates vital energy, the mental powers and internal heat, corrects irregularities of the phlegmatic humour, and is an elixir vitae."*

The Vegetable Materia Medica of Western India by William Dymock (1884) explains: "The Rahbulubha alludes to the use of hemp in gonorrhoea." Sadly, I could not find the original text to tell you anything about it, but please, underline gonorrhoea and leprosy, because when we get to the homeopathic section and the section on glia…boys and girls, you are gonna freak out!

Contraindications in Ayurveda

Ananda kanda (where we found the erectile dysfunction recipes) dedicates an entire chapter to toxicity. No-one really knows who wrote it or when, but it's thought to date from about the 12th century, mainly based on the fact that there seem to be no references that bhang had any toxic effects before 1000 AD.

The name of the book means "Root of Bliss" and describes how using cannabis with eight other herbs guarantees you a life of 300 years. Sadly, of course, we don't know if the author reached his aspired years. Just for larks I paged the oracle to see who the longest living person on record was. Sadly, his name is not Raja. Her name was Jeanne Calment of France (1875–1997), who lived to the ripe old age of 122 years, 164 days. Apparently, she famously met Vincent van Gogh when she was 12 or 13, who was reputed to be a big hemp and absinthe man. Perhaps he taught her a thing or two about cannabis!

Ananda kanda outlines the differences in purification and overuse. Cannabis is listed in Ayurvedic literature as one of the *upavisha*. These are like a class-two drug that, unlike herbs such as monkshood, will not kill instantly, but over time become toxic to the body.

These very powerful drugs exert great levels of healing and thus should only be used for illnesses that will not respond to other methods.

It describes nine successive stages of marijuana toxicity. Whilst we do not expect to see these with hemp oil, I think as a practitioner it is useful to know them to recognise escalation to marijuana.

Signs the text recommends you look out for are redness in the eyes, complete forgetfulness, and then finally in the ninth stage: *"shouting, fainting, rolling on the ground, difficulty in speaking, disclosure of secret feelings, misery, extreme prostration."*

The texts are clear.

When cannabis is used inappropriately, it will aggravate all three of the doshas: vata, pitta and kapha (it reduces pitta and heightens kapha and extreme use heightens vata too).

- It should ***always*** be used in combination with other plants and for only a very short amount of time. The same warning themes run right through Ayurveda. The general view on cannabis is that it is toxic to the liver, the blood, and the reproductive system.
- Extended applications cause constipation and dryness of the skin, connective tissues, and organs.
- It depletes immunity, reduces strength and energy, and robs the person of all motivation and happiness; it also weakens sexual desire and renders their body unable to heal.
- Long-term use will eventually cause impotency and infertility.
- It has a *tamasic* dulling effect, and *rajasic,* meaning it dulls the mind.

It's impossible to know how many of these main effects we can level at THC. Whether they will affect long-term users of CBD oil or even hemp essential oil is unclear, but I think as a practitioner there is a duty of care to assume that we may possibly be, and should always be, on the lookout for these happening to the patient over time.

All texts insist that long-term use of cannabis diminishes will and ambition and leads to dullness, confusion, lethargy, and depression. They fervently believe that cannabis clogs the mind as well as the subtle channels. Everything about __misuse__ of the drug is deemed to be in complete contradiction to the meditative and spiritual practices which aim for a peaceful and purely tranquil sattvic mind that we researched so thoroughly in the Holy Basil book.

A powerful medicine then, especially when used in combination with other magical plants... To you and I, it should be used as a synergist to improve other healing, but it should be a short sharp shock to the system.

Nothing more. Nothing less.

If there *has* been an overuse, the best recommendation seems to be bed rest and sleep it off. It's also recommended that cooling foods such as milk, ghee, and sugar are used both internally and externally. So we might see these in Ayurvedic food recipes, but they also appear in "beauty" creams, lotions, and other preparations.

Ayurveda very helpfully offers us a list of healing herbs to reduce the effects of cannabis overuse. These are:

- Camphor
- Cloves
- Sandalwood

It also recommends a mouthful of the sourest lemon juice, as well as tamarind, to counteract narcotic effects of marijuana.

Calamus neutralises the toxins of marijuana and removes the accumulation of drugs from the body in general. What I find really beautiful is that it will work on the nervous system and the mind to diffuse the emotional problems which possibly lead to the abuse in the first place. Gloriously poetic healing. Plant medicine, how I love thee.

However, where plants like vetiver, holy basil, and even spikenard are truly beloved in Ayurveda, I felt there was probably significance in an old Hindu curse. Apparently, hemp grows prolifically around disused buildings in India. *"May hemp grow around your house"*, means I want so many bad things to happen to you that you need to abandon your home and leave it to nature.

Not nice, is it?

It doesn't feel like people look on hemp kindly!

That gives me pause.

Cannabis in the Bible

I couldn't remember having been shocked by the presence of cannabis in the Bible when I studied Old Testament archaeology for my A Levels. When I can remember the ins and outs of the Epic of Gilgamesh and the fall of Jerusalem, it seemed a little bit strange that cannabis might have passed the 17-year old me by.

Well, the reason is, it's not there. That's why. But the question is... Was it ever?

Sula Benet (1903-1982) was a Polish anthropologist and expert in Polish and Judaic history in culture. In 1936, she proposed a compelling argument in her paper *Early Diffusion and Folk Uses of Hemp* that the term *Kaneh Bosm* had been wrongly translated to *calamus* in the 5th century when it had been placed into the Greek version of the Bible, The Septuagint. She says that *Kaneh Bosm* is more likely to be hemp. Every translation since then, including Martin Luther's in the reformation, had retained the incorrect word. If her theory is correct, cannabis had previously been very much alive and well in the Old Testament but has since been eradicated.

I must say, this section contradicts a great deal of what is written in my Spikenard book, because I, too, have taken *Kaneh Bosm* to be *calamus* there, but the more I think about her argument, the more I wonder if she might be right.

There are several places where the term arises. Originally, the term *Cannabis* was thought to come from Scythian usage, but Benet describes how it is more likely to come from Hebrew or other Semitic languages. She takes her translations right back to the Aramaic version of the Torah called the *Targum oncelos,* which dates to the first century AD.

The word **Kan,** she says, has a double meaning. It can mean either *Reed* or *Hemp*. **Bosm** means aromatic. Sometimes we will see the word **Kaneh** used alone, in places where the plant seems to relate to rope, fabric, or texture, and we see Bosm added at times where an incense seems to be implied.

The first time we "meet" cannabis, it is merely an inference. It appears in a familiar Old Testament passage most of you will recognise, with the prophet Moses, just as he is beginning to become Shamanic. We read: *"Moses discovered the angel of the Lord in flames of fire from within a bush."*

Smiling?

Yes, it made me smile too. It is almost too obvious, isn't it?

Does that imply he was high? That seems a scandalous suggestion.

I think I need to move to safer ground.

The next mention is actually of Kaneh bosm and as I said, we encountered it in the recipe for Holy Incense that we worked so hard to understand in the Spikenard book. So, we had said calamus is in the recipe, but the amounts suggested for Kaneh Bosm are enormous. Like cannabis, Calamus is also psychoactive, but nowhere near as "benign" as cannabis. It constitutes 75% asarone, which is a precursor to trimethoxyamphetamine. In doses of the scale used in the Holy Anointing recipe, it would be hideously toxic. That's pretty interesting, but there is more.

In Genesis 41:22 we see Kaneh Bosm appearing in a dream that Pharaoh asks Joseph to interpret for him. First, he sees seven healthy cows and then seven skinny ones eat them, but they still look ravaged. Pharaoh is troubled and then the next night he has a similar dream, but this time it's a cereal (it's two parts... It's a serial... Corn...geddit? No? Oh, never mind...).

He describes:

"In my dream, I saw seven heads of grain, full and good, growing on a single stalk. 23 After them, seven other heads sprouted—withered and thin and scorched by the east wind. 24 The thin heads of grain swallowed up the seven

good heads. I told this to the magicians, but none of them could explain it to me."

Could *"A stalk with seven heads of grain coming from it"* be a description of hemp? I think it could, and it would be a very *in*accurate description of calamus, which is not a grain but more like a reed.

The word Kaneh arises in several places throughout the Bible as either a foodstuff, a rope, or a textile. Calamus is none of these things.

It is very hard to find direct references in the Bible, but Benet argues, perhaps conveniently, that this is because of translational changes throughout history. One example that she gives is just as the ancient Chinese had a requirement that the dead be buried in clothes made of hemp, so did the Hebrews, but later translations changed the word into "linen."

In a Greek translation of the story of Solomon, dating from somewhere between 1st and 5th century AD, we read:

"I commanded her to spin the hemp for the ropes used in the building of the House of God. She was brought to stand night and day spinning the hemp." Strong ropes they must indeed have been to build the gargantuan House of God. A reed just could not have held the weight.

You see, it *is* easy to see how the confusion may have arisen, because when you read Hebrew it is ultra-perplexing because they only write in consonants. It is up to the reader to decide how these words are pronounced. In *God's Gift,* Rev. Burgess Shale radically appraises the Old Testament by isolating the terms "*qaneh*" or "*qnh*". In particular, he translates a passage in Ezekiel, and he argues *qnh* should not be "reed" as is traditionally read, but instead "Hemp measuring rope." Armed with this new translation tool, he was able to find an amazing 62 references to quaneh.

If this is in fact true, then Benet *is* correct, that qnh must be an object both textile and an ingredient in anointing oils.

So, let's say Benet is right, and cannabis is indeed part of the Holy Incense, then we must follow the smoke signals and find references aplenty. Using this new evidence, it is hard to ignore that every time Moses communes with God, either he has lathered himself with the anointing oil or he seems to hear God in some smoke.

Could it be true? Was Moses acting as shaman under the influence of a marijuana high? It seems highly *un*likely that the Hebrews know nothing of cannabis when their neighbours openly enjoyed it so reverently and the shamanistic link of seeing a deity in smoke would certainly not be unusual either. Later, in the 6th century BC, another monotheist Zoroaster would speak to his deity Ahura Mazda in shamanic ecstasy produced by cannabis. Likewise, the ancient Greek Oracle of Delphi appeared to followers behind a veil of intoxicating smoke.

Let's add to this and cast our minds back to the erotic and languorous Song of Songs we studied in the Spikenard book. Perhaps we might meet cannabis again.

"Come with me from Lebanon, my bride, come with me from Lebanon.

Descend from the crest of Amarna, from the top of Senir, the summit of Hermon.

How delightful is your love, my sister, my bride!

How much more pleasing is your love than wine, and the fragrance of your ointment than any spice!

The fragrance of your garments is like that of Lebanon, your plants are an orchard of pomegranates with choice fruits with henna and nard, nard and saffron, kaneh and cinnamon, and every kind of incense tree."

Song of Songs 4:8-14

Now, I am testing your memory a bit here, but you may remember how, in the Spikenard book, we spoke of Song of Songs possibly being a hymn to the Phoenician goddess Astarte, or as she was also referred to, the Queen of Heaven. In their book, *The Temple and the Lodge*, Michael Baigent and Richard Leigh describe how Astarte was always worshipped at the top of hills and mountains. This seems very reminiscent of how the Scythians journeyed to caves in the hillside to worship their own goddess, Hestia-Tabiti.

Baigent and Leigh point us to a quote from 1 Kings 3:3:

"Solomon loved Yahweh; he followed the precepts of David his father, except that he offered sacrifice and incense <u>on the high places</u>."

Then in 1 Kings 11 v 45 an even stronger clue that Solomon's heart may be tied to Astarte arises. It reads: *"But King Solomon loved many strange women, together with the daughter of Pharaoh, women of the Moabites, Ammonites, Edomites, Zidonians, and Hittites."*

Then...

"As Solomon grew old, his wives turned his heart after other gods, and his heart was not fully devoted to the Lord, his God, as the heart of David his father had been." (1 Kings 4:11)

Had Solomon become a follower of Astarte, the goddess of the Sidonions? If so, then we know that smoke would most certainly have derived from a lighted cannabis plant.

This behaviour of offering sacrifices to other gods could not be without consequence, and in Isaiah 43:24 we feel the wrath of God towards his people. He has serious concerns about their usage of Kaneh Bosm and here we take from the traditional translation. He accuses them *"You have not bought any fragrant calamus for me, or lavished on me the fat of your sacrifices. But you have burdened me with your sins and wearied me with your offenses."*

In Jeremiah 6:20, he demands: *"What do I care about incense from Sheba or sweet calamus from a distant land? Your burnt offerings are not acceptable; your sacrifices do not please me."*

So far, I was fairly convinced until this point. It's this reference to "sweetness [calamus]" I have an issue with. I am not sure about it at all. We are all familiar with the sweet smell of marijuana drifting out of doorways, but taste... No, it's not sweet! Ayurveda says pungent, I say the devil's armpit! It's unspeakably vile, in my opinion. Far be it from me to question the word of the Lord, but...

I don't know. Let's investigate further.

So, if all this *were* true, then should we not find plenty of archaeological evidence for cannabis in the Holy Land dating from the Exodus?

Well, I would expect we should, but there's not a jot.

The earliest evidence we find in Israel dates to the fourth century AD, thousands of years later, to a very sad tomb near Jerusalem. The body of a young girl with a full-term foetus in utero was interred there. The baby was clearly too large to be born. It seems as if cannabis may have been used in a similar way to the ancient Egyptian methods for birthing. The fumes had not been enough. The girl and baby had both died and been buried together with the incense.

Rastafarianism

Of course, if it were true that cannabis was in the Bible, then it would be of no surprise to one particular sect of Christianity, who have always kept cannabis as their sacrament, the Rastafaria. They use several names for cannabis: herb, weed, kaya, sinsemilla (Spanish for "without seeds"), or ganja (from the Sanskrit word *ganjika* that is used in ancient Nepal and India). All of those we are familiar with and these open up a whole new realm of possible nuances in the scriptures.

Genesis 1:11: *"And God said, Let the earth bring forth grass, the herb yielding seed, and the fruit tree yielding fruit after his kind, whose seed is in itself, upon the earth: and it was so."*

Genesis 1:29: *"And God said, Behold, I have given you every herb-bearing seed, which is upon the face of all the earth, and every tree, in the which is the fruit of a tree yielding seed; to you it shall be for meat."*

Genesis 3:18: *"... thou shalt eat the herb of the field."*

Psalms 104:14: *"He causeth the grass to grow for the cattle, and vegetation for the service of man."*

Proverbs 15:17: *"Better is a dinner of herbs where love is, than a stalled ox and hatred therewith."* [44]

Revelation 22:2: *"the river of life proceeded to flow from the throne of God, and on either side of the bank there was the tree of life, and the leaf from that tree is for the healing of the nations."*

Certainly, it feels to me that Revelations might be speaking about cannabis here.

Rastas smoke ganja as a spiritual act, usually whilst studying the Bible or discussing philosophical truths. The sacrament cleanses the body and mind, they say. It heals the soul, exalts their consciousness, brings peacefulness and pleasure, and brings them closer to gaining insight from Jah. Sacramental use of cannabis in celebration of the Rastafari faith became legal in Jamaica on April 15, 2015. I find it amusing that it does not surprise Rastas that ganja is illegal for other purposes, recognising it as capable of opening people's minds to the truth. I feel like I am becoming ever more like them, ang-ree at the materialistic and closed minds of the authorities they call Babylon. Of course, they holler, Babylon would not want everyone to have that power.

British Herbal

British hemp cultivation seems to date to around 800 AD, and the earliest evidence is of pollen found in a well in York. In early documents, we see it with the name Hænep. For the most part, it seems like it was grown mainly in coastal areas for ease of transport for ropes, fishing nets, sails, and cordage to neighbouring ports. Usage grew readily until about the 12th century, when agriculture diversified and farmers became more interested in experimenting with other crops.

But in the 16th century, hemp became a vital part of the growth of Tudor England. In 1533, Henry VIII issued a mandate that all landowners grow hemp as a means of furnishing the English Navy with the ropes it needed for its ever-growing fleet of ships.

The most famous of these must surely be the Mary Rose, the pride of England's fleet that sank on 19th July 1545. Now the Mary Rose and I have had a life-long love affair, and a very colourful past. As a kid, I was so square. I was always at school when I was supposed to be (except when we did General Studies in the sixth form – what a waste of time, that was – and I took to oscillating on the local playground swings on Thursday mornings instead!).

But...

On one particular cold miserable day in October 1982, I took myself off to the sickbay to get out of PE. I put my fingers down my throat and made myself sick. I got myself a lift home so I could watch the raising of the Tudor warship on TV. There was absolutely nothing wrong with me, of course, apart from a love of old things! The ship had been discovered in the Solent six weeks before I was born and it had been something of an obsession since I was about six. There was absolutely no way I was going to play netball when that was going on!

Five hundred people died on the ship on that fateful day, after a skirmish with the French in 1545. Only 35 people managed to swim to safety. Two hundred tons of hemp rope in rigging, sails and various steering accoutrements went into the sea that day.

When Henry had taken the throne, he had inherited five war ships. By the time of his death, he had built 40 more. Edward VI and Mary both continued to build. When Elizabeth I ascended to the throne, a fleet review showed 39 ships in service with plans to build another thirty. She continued to add to the fleet at a steady pace throughout her reign.

Two hundred tons of hemp on each ship and a requirement to renew it every two years, the demand for hemp was extraordinary and was one of the driving forces behind England's interest in conquering the colonies (where hemp grew exceedingly healthily!). Add to that the numbers of ships required to transport hemp backwards and forwards, as well as guarding the colonies, one can see how cannabis became its own self-perpetuating industry.

By 1563 Elizabeth I had declared that any landowner with 60 acres or more would face a fine of £5 if they did not grow cannabis (two hundred years later this sentiment would be echoed in America, when the Founding Fathers recognised that if the country were to truly be independent from the bullish British then they must grow their own hemp and provide their own fabric, ropes, and economic stability).

So, this complete faith in the plant gives some context to our first herbal reference to hemp in 1538. It comes from William Turner, where he writes in his book *The New Herball*:

"Of hempe: cannabis named by both the Grecians and the Latines, is called in English, hempe in dutch hanffe, in French chanure."

Gerard and Parkinson both wrote of hemp but because most of the herbals of the time are re-hashes (see what I did there?) of the same hemp data that Pliny and Galen had written, we will skip forward a few years to the seventeenth century where a young man called Nicolas Culpepper, a fully apprenticed apothecary, can be seen walking the countryside collecting specimens. He is an odd so-and-so, disliked by many of his peers, mainly because he has a massive chip on his shoulder about his natural medicines being better than those "un-natural" ones of other doctors.

Not that I am one to gossip, as you know... and this has nothing to with cannabis at all, but since Nicolas Culpepper is such an important authority, I thought I'd provide a juicy bit of context...

The Culpepper family had probably become very used to being talked about, since grandfather Thomas made a fundamental error of cavorting with a rather ill-advised lover a century previously. In 1541, as we have seen, Henry VIII was somewhat distracted by his maritime endeavours, and just for a moment he averted his eyes from the marital bed. As the king focused on conquering the seas, there were whispers about conquests of another sort, of Thomas Culpepper and Catherine Howard. Thomas Cranmer, the archbishop of Canterbury, came to hear rumours of indiscretions and when later a letter to Culpepper came to light, signed off *"yours as long as life endures"* by the queen (Henry's wife number 5), rumours could no longer be ignored.

The king issued orders to arrest Culpeper and, in December 1541, they tried him for adultery next to another man, Francis Dereham, separately accused of liaisons with the queen. In Katherine's defence, her dalliance with Dereham had happened before she had been married to Henry, but that didn't seem to matter. Now the problem was that Catherine had been a little too open about her relationship with Culpeper with members of her household, and those members felt compelled to testify against her to protect themselves.

Now if you thought chivalry was now dead, listen to this. Culpepper is an unparalleled cad and a bounder! He blamed Howard, saying that she had enlisted one of her ladies in waiting to act as "agent provocateur" and engineered their trysts. He claimed he tried to end it, but that she was "dying of love for him."

Stories tell of how the queen seduced Culpeper at Chenies Palace in Buckinghamshire and private meetings at Hatfield House in Hertfordshire. It seems very likely though, from court testimony, that Culpeper had been instigator for some reason of political intrigue. It is still unclear whether Catherine did in fact take him to bed. Most evidence seems to point to nothing more than ardent meetings on the back stairs. However, Henry tortures him and eventually he surrenders the confession that they *had* been adulterous for many months. Both Culpeper and Dereham were found guilty and sentenced to death.

The verdict was both men should be hung, drawn, and quartered on account of their crimes of treason. Both plea for mercy; Culpeper, perhaps because of his close history of friendship with the King, had his sentence commuted to a simple beheading. Poor old Dereham received no such mercy. He swings from the hemp noose and then all manner of nasties await him.

Culpeper is executed along with Dereham on 10 December 1541. Their heads are grimly displayed, as traitors, on London Bridge. Queen Catherine is held under arrest at Sion Park and eventually in February 1542 she's taken by boat to the Tower of London and two days later on the 13th she, too, is beheaded.

So, that's enough about Thomas and his philandering britches, let's think about his grandson for a while. He was a youngster really, then. Arrogant and driven. He had a good upbringing, son of a clergyman and educated at Cambridge, and fascinated by plants, he took up an apprenticeship with an Apothecary where he served seven years training.

Then things began to go pear-shaped.

When he was training as an apothecary, his mentor famously absconded with the money paid for his apprenticeship and so poor Nicolas was left high and dry. Then his mum died suddenly and things did not look good for him. Luckily, he fell in love with a wealthy landowner's daughter, and her dowry allowed him to set up a little practice in Spitalfields in London where medicine was, back then, in a very poor and corrupt state.

His practice fell just outside of London and its economic restrictions, so Culpepper would collect herbs and plants from the countryside, expending no overheads and thus was able to offer many of his services for free, insisting *"no man deserved to starve to pay an insulting, insolent physician."* He was a busy man too, seeing up to forty patients some mornings.

As you know, much of his understanding of disease involved astrology, and he would prefer to treat the person holistically rather than taking the urine samples his colleagues were so fond of. Scornfully, he announced in his opinion *"as much piss as the Thames might hold",* would not help them to diagnose.

It never ceases to amaze me how medicine changes so much and yet it changes so little. In the context of this book, we see a radical outsider using hemp for people who cannot afford to be treated by the government!

Skipping forward a few years, Civil War breaks out and our Nic still had not really managed to make any friends, and eventually he was completely ostracised and accused of witchcraft. In answer, he ran off to join the rebellion against Charles I. On the battlefield, he became indispensable, treating musket shots and infected feet, then progressed to battlefield surgery.

Eventually he, too, sustained a chest wound and was discharged back to London. His breathing never really recovered and at just 37 years old he died of tuberculosis.

His famous book was published a year prior to his death.

So, let's have a look at what he says about the plant that would have been growing everywhere around him, and could have helped so many of those ailing people in the dirty London streets.

"This is so well known to every good housewife in the country that I shall not need to write any description of it.

"Time. It is sown in the very end of March, or beginning of April, and is ripe in August or September."

Government and virtues. *"It is a plant of Saturn."*

He continues: *"and good for something else, you see, than to make halters only."*

Eh? Off to the dictionary I goes! "Halters - a horse bridle made of rope!"

Aha! That makes the most delicious sense!

What else does he have to say?

"The seed of Hemp consumes wind, and by too much use thereof disperses it so much that it dries up the natural seed for procreation; yet, being boiled in milk and taken, helps such as have a hot dry cough."

So, it stops you farting, but it also renders a man sterile.

*"The Dutch make an emulsion out of the seed, and give it with good success to those that have the jaundice, especially in the beginning of the disease, if there be no **ague** accompanying it, for it opens obstructions of the gall, and causes digestion of choler."*

Ague, there's a word I haven't heard for years! It means fever or shivering.

So, choler is going back to the popular idea of the four humours at the time. It pertains to yellow bile but also anger, wrath, and irascibility. Just like Ayurveda and TCM, bile has elements and properties attached to it so we can say that yellow bile:

- Season is summer
- Age is youth
- Element is fire
- Organ is spleen
- Qualities are warm and dry
- Temperament is choleric, which we have already established is angry.

So yes, that fits in context. That the **seed**, not the plant here, is good for anyone presenting with early signs of jaundice, particularly if there is no fever. It unblocks the gall bladder and calms angry young souls.

He continues:

"The emulsion or decoction of the seed stays lasks and continual fluxes, eases the colic, and allays the troublesome humours in the bowels."

Lasks - now only used in veterinary medicine, but this is an old English word from the French meaning **diarrhoea**.

So, if you boil the seeds it stops the runs, and fluxes are the same really. Colic we know, and so where Culpepper had troublesome humours in his bowels we have grumbly tummies!

"...and stays bleeding at the mouth, nose, or other places, some of the leaves, being fried with the blood of them that bleed, and so given them to eat.

"It is held very good to kill the worms in men or beasts; and the juice dropped into the ears kills worms in them; and draws forth earwigs, or other living creatures gotten into them. The decoction of the root allays inflammations of the head, or any other parts: the herb itself, or the distilled water thereof doth the like. The decoction of the root eases the pains of the gout, the hard humours of knots in the joints, the pains and shrinking of the sinews, and the pains of the hips. The fresh juice mixed with a little oil and butter, is good for any place that hath been burnt with fire, being thereto applied."

So:

- Styptic
- Vulnerary
- Juice in the ear gets rids of earwigs or anything that has stolen into the ear canal (*ew, EW, **EW**...doesn't bear thinking about!*)
- Boil the root for headaches, or in fact any other part or preparation of the plant
- Decoction of the root for joint pain
- Juice in butter for burns

Now my immediate response to Culpepper's recommendation of using it in butter was surely it would fry? I don't feel at all right about it, but it is the butter that gives me pause rather than the hemp, and in 1698 the French chemist Nicolas Lémery described:

"Hemp contains much oil, little salt, it is specific for burns, for roaring in the ears and to kill worms." This is a re-iteration of the German botanist Leonard Fuchs who had said back at the beginning of the 16th century that *"the root pounded and wrapped is good for a burn."* Indeed, John Parkinson had also advised: *"Hemp is good to be used for any place burnt by fire, if the fresh juice be mixed with oyle or butter."*

Well, if it is good enough for JP, it is good enough for me.

We can see, though, that the extent of hemp medicine in England is for burns and trumping bums. Certainly, there seems to be no sense of the psycho-activity and it isn't really a medicine as such, it is a rope.

So how did we get from ropes and halters to the enormous accolades we give to cannabis today? Well, that is owed to the superlative work done by Sir William Brook O'Shaughnessy whilst working for the East India Company.

Born in Limerick in 1809, O'Shaughnessy had been a bright and brilliant kid, and by the age of 18 had secured himself a place at one of the best medical schools in the world at the University of Edinburgh. There, he worked hard studying anatomy and physiology (and experimenting on cadavers stolen by the infamous grave robbers Burke and Hare). Graduating in 1829, he moved to London and taught medicine for a year or so, and then opened his own forensic toxicology lab because he was not qualified to teach medicine in London.

It was working in his lab that he started to encounter blood specimens of cholera victims. Studying them, he made connections and in 1831 he wrote a short concise note that would be instrumental in saving thousands of lives.

"The copious diarrhoea of cholera leads to dehydration, electrolytic depletion, acidosis, and nitrogen retention. Treatment must depend on intravenous replacement of deficient salt and water." Incredibly, even though at this point in history they had no idea what was causing the cholera (for more history about this, see the Spikenard book), O'Shaughnessy had created the medical intervention that is still used today.

Two years later, he was to encounter a certain William Russell MD, who had just returned to London from Calcutta to form a cholera commission. Russell was so impressed with him that O'Shaughnessy secured himself a commission as assistant surgeon in the East India Company. In 1833, O'Shaughnessy himself landed in Calcutta.

His postings with the Bengal army meant he moved from place to place. The barriers of the three hundred or so languages of India seemed to dissolve, as he began to learn smatterings of phrases here and there. Soon, he had made friends with several Ayurvedic and Persian doctors. His work led him to be part of the founding of the Calcutta Medical College and there he was appointed Professor of Chemistry and Materia Medica.

He was made Chemical Examiner for the Raj in 1836. He married and asked for his cousin Richard to join him in Calcutta. Life was going well and he was working hard, teaching students at the college and creating spectacularly detailed textbooks for them. Even by today's standards, these works are exemplary scholarship specifically designed for students with English as their second language.

When he stood before his lecture theatre in 1839 and began to read a paper he had written about cannabis, the hairs must have stood up on the backs of people's necks because they were most certainly in the company of greatness. O'Shaughnessy had painstakingly collated and reviewed works of Ayurvedic and Unani practitioners, some of whom were undoubtedly listening there that day, and then he had created experiments of his own. The forty pages of research contained case history after case history that he had made.

The first experiments were carried out on rats, mice, cats, dogs, and rabbits, then over time he developed them, making extracts and titrations and using them on patients he had seen.

Amongst them were sufferers of rheumatism, hydrophobia (what we now call rabies), cholera, and tetanus. He even gave details of how a baby, less than six weeks old, was treated for convulsions, and he says: *"leaping from near death to the enjoyment of robust health"* in a few days. He declares that his research had *"led me to the belief that in hemp the profession has gained an anti-convulsive remedy of the greatest value."*

Despite his lauding of cannabis, he warns that a *"peculiar form of delirium may be occasioned by continual hemp inebriation"* and cautions doctors to start with low doses.

In 1841 his *Bengal Dispensary* is published, followed by *Bengal Pharmacopoeia* in 1844. Exhausted by the work on these three large works, O'Shaughnessy decides to come back to England but he brings with him samples of Hemp and nux vomica (about which he had written at length in 1837) to be added to the botanical collection at Kew Gardens. He secures a reprint of his cannabis article in the Principal Medical Journal in 1841, and suddenly English medicine's eyes open. Chemists all over the British Isles began to fervently try to isolate the active components that might create the magic in hemp, but that would take 120 years to achieve by a team in Israel.

The paper had blown hemp medicine wide open. Between 1839 and 1900, over a hundred papers were published, describing ever more medicinal properties of the plant. It is believed that even Queen Victoria's physician, J Russell Reynold, was now recommending his patients to take cannabis for their periods.

In a strange twist of fate, O'Shaughnessy returned to India in 1844 and completely changed careers, inventing a telegraph system. The copper wires we had in England would not stand the Indian scorching heat so he devised an entirely new system. It was his work on the telegraph that eventually led to him being knighted, not the work on cannabis or the lives he saved from cholera (although doubtless Her Majesty was thankful to him for his part in managing her menses. A girl does not forget those kinds of things!)

The official journal of research into cannabis pays homage to William, bearing the name *O'Shaughnessy's*.

Chapter 3 The Endocannabinoid System

Welcome to the world of words you can't pronounce! It's the most fascinating physiology I've ever studied, but nothing I've learned before has come close to being so exciting or so utterly infuriating.

It's still a very new area, so research is in its infancy and yet is extensive thus far. If the hundred papers written about cannabis between 1839 and 1900 seemed a lot, consider that by 2008 there were over 2000 papers on cannabis and 1500 experiments into the endocannabinoid system. Had I found *those* nuggets of data earlier, I'd have abandoned this book immediately and you would now be reading about violets!

But I didn't.

And I'm glad I didn't, because plant medicine never looked so good.

Buckle yourself in. We have a long ride.

First things first.

We are going to abbreviate wherever possible.

It will become increasingly obvious why. So, your first abbreviation is:

eCS – Endocannabinoid System.

Functions of the eCS

Discovered in 1988, this is an *endocrine* system. No, that's selling it short. Potentially, scientists suspect this may be our **primary** endocrine system. Its function is to modulate our hormones to ensure we maintain homeostasis. Composed of receptor sites and endogenous *endo*cannabinoids (ones we create naturally), the eCS runs throughout the entirety of the body. It is widespread, found in the brain, organs, glands, connective tissues, and immune cells. It regulates an inordinate number of processes, including the sensation of pain, our moods, and how good our appetite and memory are.

It forms the most intricate and dynamic communication network between different cells. Regulating and stabilising hormones and neurotransmitters, it functions as a protective network for the body. The more we learn, the more types of disease we discover it controls. Modulating the cardio-vascular system; digestive; respiratory; genito-urinary; reproductive; muscular; skeletal; immunity, connected with processes such as neural development; immune function; inflammation; appetite; reproduction and metabolism, research suggests it could be implicated in virtually every possible type of disease.

Never heard of it?

No, neither had I, but let me clarify, it's only recently been discovered, but that doesn't mean it's a new system or that it is unique to humans. This primitive messaging system is believed to date back as many as 600 million years and is found in every group of creatures except for insects.

We can break the system down into three main groups:

- Endocannabinoids – endo- meaning found naturally in the body.
- Cannabinoid receptors
- Enzymes that both synthesize and degrade endocannabinoids

Don't worry, we are going to cover each section in turn.

It's a very efficient system, taking the body an inordinately small amount of energy to run it. The body holds the system perpetually in standby mode, and for a long time it was thought endocannabinoids were manufactured **on demand**, since the system didn't seem to have a storage facility. It's now understood that endocannabinoids rest in intracellular stores known as ***adiposomes*** until they are required. When they are finally called up for action they travel merrily backwards and forwards across the cell membrane. They do this with help from certain fatty acids and proteins known as transporters.

That is of course, if our bodies have had enough of them. Problems arise when we don't make enough, or an imbalance develops between how many endocannabinoids we have and how many receptors they can couple with. Then, we see all manner of diseases and conditions, from anxiety and depression to diabetes and metabolic syndrome. It's a sad, sick story.

Now, endocannabinoids are determined by many things: lifestyle, meditation, and exercise, but particularly nutrition. More specifically, levels of fish oils and some vegetable oils can have a very large impact. If, for example, there is a deficiency of Omega 3 in your diet, levels of manufactured endocannabinoids organically drop. It's complex, but as we continue the problems and solutions become clearer.

In times of endocannabinoid deficiency, our bodies happily welcome supplementation found in nature, ***phytocannabinoids***. Phytocannabinoids can only be found in cannabis, but they are not our only tool. Other plants provide chemicals that act in a similar way, but coming from any other plant than cannabis we call those *cannabinoid-like* plant constituents or *cannabinomimetics*. We'll look at these in more detail in Chapter 9.

Receptors

Two G Protein receptors predominately control the endocannabinoid system. These are activated by ligands that act almost like keys fitting into, and opening and closing locks (the receptor). Receptors are:

- Stimulated or switched on when the ligand is working as an *agonist*
- Blocked when the ligand operates as *antagonist*

The two types of receptors we need to get to grips with are known as cannabinoid receptor 1 (CB_1) and cannabinoid receptor 2 (CB_2). Discovered in 2003, they have many functions.

CB_1

CB_1 is the most abundant receptor in the brain. Found on other body parts and organs, albeit in far smaller numbers than in the brain, it controls short-term memory, pain, emotion, and hunger.

Abundant in the cerebellum, cortex, amygdala, hippocampus, and the outflow tracts of the basal ganglia, CB_1 receptors can be activated by our native endocannabinoids *anadamide* and 2-AG, and also by the phytocannabinoid THC.

As the science becomes more complex, we'll talk about certain receptors in different parts of the brain, so it helps to have a cursory understanding of which part of brain does what, and thus, how the receptors can influence that, so here goes:

Basal ganglia

Most of what scientists know about this part of the brain comes from studies about Parkinson's and Huntington's diseases. Both affect the motor control areas of the brain. The basal ganglia assists the body with movement and cognitive processing. Anyone with a problem with this part of the brain will struggle with their memory and movement.

Hippocampus

Regular readers should now understand the hippocampus to a certain extent. We talked about it in the *Rose* and *Helichrysum* books. It's a very important part of the limbic system because it's the region that regulates emotions. Quintessentially associated with memory (in particular with *long*-term memory), it also plays an important part in spatial memory.

Cerebral Cortex

Or as its sometimes known as the cerebrum, the cerebral cortex is the largest part of the human brain. We associate it with *higher* brain function such as thoughts and actions. Divided into four sections we call *lobes* you will likely have heard of the frontal lobe, the temporal lobe, the occipital lobe, and the parietal lobe.

- **The temporal lobe** is associated with *perception* and *being able to recognise sounds*. It controls *memory and speech*.
- As you might imagine, the **occipital lobe** is associated with *visual processing*.
- The **parietal lobe** controls *orientation and relaying that into movement*. It controls *recognition* and *perception of stimuli*.

- **Cerebellum**

Associated with **regulation and coordination of movement**, this part of the brain controls **posture** and **helps you to balance**.

Finally, the....

- **Amygdaloid nucleus.**

Contained within the temporal lobe, this is closely associated to the hypothalamus, the hippocampus, and the cingulate gyrus. Its role in the limbic system is fundamental, because it influences the sense of smell. Psychologically it affects motivation and many different emotions. It's an aromatherapist's best friend.

Now, it is so easy to get bogged down by the science, and since one of the fundamental lessons cannabis was sent to teach us was compassion and a sense of us all being one, let's try to be mindful of the struggles that the patients we aim to treat here might be having. For a moment, try to perceive how the fragrance of a rose would trigger in your parietal lobe. Visualise the struggle you would have if you wanted to pick it. Now imagine you wanted to communicate how lovely the flower was to someone, but found it difficult because of problems in the frontal lobe.

So, if we picture these different parts of the brain as each having little locks that we can put keys into, we can see how the endocannabinoid system can be switched up or switched down. Thus, we can see how we might be able to improve function throughout the body. For example, when CB_1 receptors are activated in hypothalamic nuclei and in the limbic system, changes take place in feeding behaviour. We feel hungrier, the sweetness is more intense and we enjoy a more rewarding relationship with the food. We'll explore this more deeply when we look at the clinical evidence for anorexia, obesity, and diabetes.

Other CB_1 agonists affect:

- Memory
- Emotion
- Cognition

- Motor function
- Pain
- Itchiness
- Muscle tone

The endocannabinoid system also gets its hands mucky in the gastrointestinal tract. Specifically, here, CB_1 receptors look after propulsion and secretion. Propulsion in the digestive system is how food travels through the alimentary canal; so, this includes both swallowing and peristalsis where the digestive system pushes your chocolate cake though your body using alternating waves of relaxation and muscle contractions. If CB_1 signalling flounders, digestive problems ensue.

The endocannabinoid system has vital physiological functions outside of the central nervous system in peripheral tissues (that's anything outside of the brain basically!).

In the periphery, cannabinoid receptors can also be found on adipocytes (fat cells), skeletal muscle, in the gastrointestinal tract, and in the liver. Together they modulate how effectively we metabolise energy. Later we'll see that CB_1, incorrectly regulated, leads to obesity.

Before we move onto CB_2, here is an interesting little fact:**There are no CB_1 receptors in the brain stem.**

One of the jobs that the brain stem does is modulating respiration. This area of the brain is heavily laden with *opiate* receptors, but conversely, no cannabinoid receptors. Overdoses of cocaine or heroin are common, because opiate receptors affect breathing. No deaths from cannabis overdose have been recorded since the respiratory system is unaffected.

CB_2

The CB_2 receptor is molecularly similar to CB_1. It is smaller, made up of 360 amino acids where the CB_1 has a longer chain of 473. Where CB_1 is predominately found in the brain, CB_2 is far more widespread. Its expression in the central nervous system is rather limited, since most CB_2 receptors are found in the peripheral tissues linked with blood and immunity.

We find CB_2 receptors on:

- Lymph nodes
- Bone marrow
- Tonsils
- White blood cells

- Splenic tissue

They can also be found in fewer numbers in the brain, liver, and pancreas.

CB_2 receptors are activated by the endocannabinoids anandamide and 2-AG. They can also be triggered using phytocannabinoids, cannabinomimetics, and the plant-derived terpene beta caryophyllene found in large amounts in hemp essential oil.

Being able to activate CB_2 receptors is extremely useful, since there is no psycho-activity attached to them. What they *do* do though, is bring about **tremendous reduction in inflammation.**

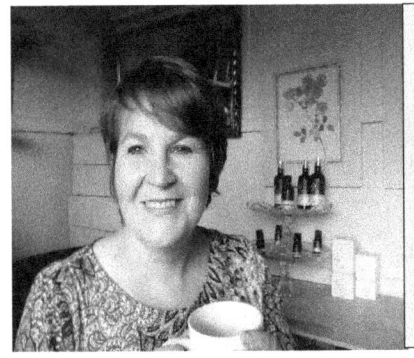

Would you like to understand receptors on a deeper level? It took me weeks to get my head round them. I made a video of my notes. Feel free to access it. You will get more from the science later, if you do. You can find it at:

https://buildyourownreality.lpages.co/receptors-

Endocannabinoids

Endocannabinoids are the ligands that activate the receptors. It might be useful to have a little bit of context here before we go too deep.

Let's begin with morphine, the psychoactive component of the poppy. First isolated in 1805 by Friedrich Sertürner, it's generally believed this might have been the first isolation of *any* active plant ingredient. Morphine is an opiate, as is codeine (discovered by Pierre Jean Robiquet in 1832), which we use today in everyday painkillers. Morphine is a ligand of the opiate receptor.

It took nearly 150 years for somebody to isolate which part of cannabis was psychoactive.

That discovery was made by a team of researchers working in the laboratory of Professor Raphael Mechoulam *at the Weizmann Institute of Science* in Rehovot, Israel. Bulgarian born Mechoulam had somehow very easily obtained hashish from the head of Israel's investigative branch of the national police. In 1963, his group determined the structure of one of cannabis's most important phytocannabinoids: CBD (cannabidiol).

By 1964 they had also isolated THC (9 delta-tetrahydrocannabinol) as the part that made the mind trippy.

There's a lovely video on YouTube where Mechoulam reminisces to a group of American researchers about how easily he had obtained the hashish and then all the trouble both he and the police chief subsequently got into when the Ministry of Health found out about the exchange. Flabbergasted by the deal that went down, they created a procurement structure. Since then, all source material has mandatorily been obtained from them! One wonders how much of the cannabis research would have been possible had that original naiveté not taken place.

But the discovery of a receptor that generated a psychoactive effect opened a whole new set of questions. Why would the body have a receptor for a plant constituent? It didn't make sense. It's simply not how we are made. So, within the human body, there must have been something else - that the body manufactured itself – something that bound to this receptor.

We now know that there are at least two ligands endogenous to the human body. Since they work like the ligands from the cannabis plant, they are also called cannabinoids, but these are endogenous – meaning *natural in the body,* so these are called endo-cannabinoids. The primary endocannabinoids are:

- *N -arachydonylethanolamide* **(AEA)** - also known as ***anandamide.***
- ***2-arachidonylglycerol (2-AG)***

Anandamide

Mechoulam's team toiled for three long decades after they discovered THC. Given the complexity of cannabis, it's virtually impossible to understand what each component does in situ because compounds skew results. Far simpler to study a solitary component in isolation; a synthesised version of THC became vital. They identified its structure, and then set about elucidating it.

The diligent years of studying receptors paid dividends, and in 1995 the team discovered the endocannabinoid **anandamide**. A neurotransmitter, anandamide has a molecular structure very similar, but not identical, to THC. Often referred to as the Bliss Molecule, Mechoulam named it after the Sanskrit word Ananda, meaning *bliss* or *joy* - an indication not only of its action of making us feel happy but also the sheer elation of hard work paying off.

The molecule mimics THC.

Or one might say that...

THC mimics Anandamide.

Anandamide does the same as THC but on a much smaller scale. It plays an active part in pain, depression, fertility, and memory. I am glad to say that every one of us will have experienced its affect at least to some degree because research demonstrates it being released into the brain when we meditate and it is also found in chocolate.

Anandamide is quintessential to the eCS. Indeed, had it not been discovered, scientists would still be blissfully unaware of the existence of the system.

2-AG

Now, after doing such a romantic job in naming anandamide, Mechoulam gave up and took to concentrating on science. No more descriptive molecule monikers from here on in. Now, they all have complicated or very boring names.

Here's the first. **2-Arachidonoylglycerol**. Perhaps we should change it to Burt? No? Trevor then? Are you sure? You might regret sticking to the real names…

No? Gosh you're grown up and boring.

Okay, have it your way.

2-Arachidonoylglycerol (forever more referred to as 2-AG) is the endogenous ligand activating both the CB_1 and CB_2 receptors. For those interested in essential oil chemistry, it is an ester. It forms from the omega 6 fatty acid called arachidonic acid and from glycerol, or two other essential fatty acids EPA (eicosapentaenoic acid) and DGLA (Dihomo-γ-linolenic acid).

Found in high levels in the central nervous system, it seems to modulate the system's activity. It is vital to immunity, inflammation, and pain management: it stimulates the immune system and balances appetite. A nice example of the majesty of the eCS: 2-AG is found in breast milk, and its co-ordinating receptors are found in babies' mouths, encouraging them to suckle, eat, and thrive. Anyone who recognises getting the munchies when high is experiencing the same biological reaction as THC mimics 2-AG interacting with the CB_1 receptors.

Most endocannabinoids prefer to interact with the CB_1 receptor but will also stimulate CB_2 to a lesser degree. 2-AG is unusual, activating both CB_1 & Cb_2 receptors to an equal potency.

The Other Players

AEA (anandamide) and 2-AG are superstars of a larger company of endocannabinoids. Three other molecules are suspected to be endocannabinoids:

- *2-Arachydonyl glycerol ether* **(2-AGE)** reduces blood pressure.
- *o-arachidonyl ethanolamine* or **virodhamine** - a vaso-relaxant.
- *N- arachidonyl dopamine* or **NADA** involved in hypothermia, hypo-locomotion, analgesia as well as cataplexy, a strange phenomenon where muscles lose power because someone is laughing too much. Contracting smooth muscles and relaxing blood vessels, NADA has both neuroprotectant and antioxidant properties, regulating both the peripheral and central nervous systems.

There is a theory **lysophosphatidylinositol** may also be an endocannabinoid, interacting with a receptor that has yet to be elucidated. It seems, however, to interact with the receptor, GPR 55 when mediating ovarian cancer.

Degradative Enzymes

At the beginning of this section I said that the eCS was made up of receptors, the endogenous ligand (endocannabinoids), and the enzymes that synthesized and degraded them. These enzymes decide whether endocannabinoid levels remain high enough by producing or breaking down AEA and 2- AG.

The main ones we are concerned with are:

- Fatty Acid Amide Hydrolase - FAAH
- Diacylglycerol Lipase - DAGL
- Monoacylglycerol - MAGL

FAAH

This is a specific type of enzyme called a serine hydrolase, whose job is to break down anandamide (as well as oleamide and myristic amide) when the body is finished with them.

DAGL & MAGL

They might sound like investment brokers but these, too, are serine hydrolases. More importantly, they are precursors to the endocannabinoid 2-AG. More than 80% of 2-AG's hydrolytic activity in the brain can be attributed to MAGL.

So later, when you see that "it inhibited MAGL", which you will... It means the body couldn't make as much 2-AG, so therefore binding to the CB_1 or CB_2 receptors was reduced too, thus bringing about a physiological change in the brain.

ECLs

In addition to the ECs, there are also a number of **endocannabinoid-like ligands,** ECLs. These include *N-oleoylethanolamine* (OEA) and *N-palmitoylethanolamine* (PEA)

Forming the substrates for the same enzymes as endocannabinoids use, ECLs are thought to enable and protect any activities Anandamide or 2-AG need to carry out, also possessing their own biological functions. PEA is involved in regulating pain and inflammation, and has anti-convulsant abilities. *N-oleoylethanolamine* is connected to preserving body weight.

To clarify...

ECLs are *not* endocannabinoids, but they work in a very similar way, locking/unlocking and thus controlling receptors in much the same way. In particular, they lock to either or both of two receptors that we will meet later: GPR19 and GPR55.

Transport Proteins

So, you may wonder how cannabinoids cross through cell membranes.

No?

Not considered that?

Neither had I, until I stumbled across the research after writing 258 pages.

But…it is very, very interesting.

Here's the quandary…

On entering the cell, eCBs encounter cytoplasm. Cytoplasm is aqueous, and endocannabinoids, like cannabinoids, are fatty. More specifically, they are non-charged lipids. Either way, they don't mix well with water. Despite that, they can pass readily through the lipid membrane… But then, when they get there, how do they manage to interact and operate in such a hostile environment?

The clue lies in neurotransmitters… Most of *those* are also water soluble. *They* use transmembrane proteins to carry them across the membrane. Endocannabinoids appear to do the same. Intracellular binding proteins ferry them around, in particular, fatty acid proteins, albumin, and heat shock protein 70.

FABPs are Fatty Acid Binding Proteins which bind with anandamide to transport it. Cell culture experiments demonstrate that FABP inhibitors reduce the breakdown of endocannabinoids by FAAH. So, it is likely FABPs are employed as part of FAAHs demolition team, clearing up endocannabinoids after their work is over.

An interesting point is one of the inhibitors researchers used in these experiments was SB-FI-26. It comes from a virtual library of millions of compounds and belongs to a class called Truxilloids. Now, truxilloids come from a pretty plant, *Incarvillateine incarvillea sinensis,* which is used extensively in Chinese Medicine to treat rheumatism and pain. As a constituent, we know that truxilloids exert anti-nociceptive (pain killing) and anti- inflammatory effects when they are used in animal experiments on mice.

It's possible the anti-pain effects are modulated through the truxilloids blockading anandamide, so it can no longer interact with the CB_1 receptor in the same way.

Confused? Yep, the head spins with all the links and interactions, doesn't it?

Go and grab a cuppa and we'll take a break from the body for a while and get to know cannabis a bit better.

Chapter 4 Hemp's Healing Components

Unbelievable! We're over a hundred pages in, and only just approaching the medicine. We finally made it. Well done for hanging in there.

It was a deliberate decision for us to wander a winding road to get here, because I wanted to ensure we avoided a common misconception. It's so tempting to fall into the trap of imagining that our bodies have evolved some mystical link with cannabis, but from an evolutionary point of view that's impossible.

Evidence demonstrates the endocannabinoid system existed in the mammalian organism as far back as 600 million years ago. The earliest evidence of a cannabis plant is over 500 million years later, dating to about 25 million years ago. We lasted a long time without it.

Having said that, I do keep pondering the strange coincidence of hemp being one of our original agricultural crops. Later in the book, you'll find that cannabis solves very real problems perpetuated by newer cereals that took its place. Those caused by gluten, in particular.

There's no doubt Mother Nature is a wise and whimsical gal.

Likewise, understand that whilst the cannabinoids are interesting and form an enormous part of this book, they are a such a small part of the cannabis picture. Its plant chemistry is majestically complex, comprising around 480 compounds in total.

This constitutes:

- 100 or so cannabinoids
- 120 terpenes
- Amino acids
- Proteins
- Enzymes
- Ketones
- Fatty Acids
- Steroids
- Flavonoids
- Vitamins

... To name but a few!

Depending on the method of extraction, and whether the cannabis is raw or prepared, that cocktail can change in many ways.

Further, there is an elegant interdependency between the components: serendipity for the holistic therapist, but a nightmare for drug companies. In cannabis more than any other, synthesizing components completely compromises the integrity of the medicine. Later, we will learn how different components modulate and enhance the effects of others. It's the wholeness of the plant that brings about the healing. Its actions take place through an "**Entourage Effect**", canna-speak for how we would use the term **synergistic** in aromatherapy.

In this section, we'll focus on aromatherapy's newly discovered components - the phytocannabinoids. We'll look at the terpenes and flavonoids later.

Phytocannabinoids

Cannabinoids are lipophilic components. That is, they dissolve readily into fat but not into water. They are _hydrophobic._ That means they can't pass through distillation into the hemp essential oil. However, readily extracted by CO_2, this has now become the preferred method of extraction, for the most part replacing the ground-breaking method pioneered by Rick Simpson. High CBD hemp oil is one of these, a CO_2 extraction.

Just as an assurance, the essential oil is magical in its own way and we will cover it at length later.

But just to clarify:

There are **no cannabinoids in hemp essential oil or in hemp _seed_ oil.** As its name would suggest, however, **they are plentiful in the CBD-rich hemp oil.**

THC - Delta 9-tetrahydrocannabinol

The most abundant and widely recognised cannabinoid in cannabis. The psychoactive component mimics the actions of the body's native neurotransmitters, anandamide and 2-arachidonoylglycerol.

Psychoactive... Too clinical a term...

You might prefer blissful euphoria, or warmth and wellbeing, and endless time seemingly going on forever.

My words are meaningless here. Let's drift on some of the Sanskrit descriptions of the herb.

ananda - the joyful, joyous, laughter-moving bliss

bahuvadini - causing excessive garrulousness

capta - light-hearted

chapala - causer of reeling gait, causer of vacillation

cidalhada - gives happiness to the mind

harshini - the exciter of sexual desire, the rejoicer, delight-giver, causer of elation

The effects associated with cannabis take place as THC binds to the CB_1 receptors in the brain and in the body.

The ***International Non-proprietary Name***, or ***INN*** is the official name given to a pharmaceutical drug or an active ingredient.

There is a pure isomer of THC by the INN of Dronabinol. A synthesised version of THC, Dronabinol is used to treat anorexia in sufferers of HIV and AIDS. Given to people struggling with nausea and vomiting, THC has been available on prescription to people undergoing chemotherapy since the 1980s.

The first synthetically engineered Dronabinol-based medication to be approved by the FDA was a drug called ***Marinol*** in 1985. Subsequently, several other THC pills were developed, including a pill called ***Cesamet***, again regularly prescribed to boost appetite in HIV and cancer patients. Research into Marinol also suggests the THC mimicry goes further than making people hungrier: it actually *stimulates* the body into gaining weight. A mouth spray, ***nabiximols***, approved here in the UK in 2010, is a Dronabinol-based medication prescribed to MS patients. It soothes neuropathic pain, reduces spasticity, and relieves the burden of an overactive bladder and other associated symptoms.

Pain relief might possibly be the most important aspect of THC. Studies reveal it activates pathways in the CNS, placing obstacles in the pathways of pain signals being sent to the brain. It is a powerful weapon against both neuropathic and nociceptive pain.

It's also very useful in the treatment of memory, in particular PTSD. Bizarrely, it is suspected the high that you get from THC may be associated with experiencing temporary memory loss. We investigate CBD's effects on PTSD in clinical studies, but recent research shows that an oral dose of THC can bring relief to all manner of PTSD-related symptoms, including flashback nightmares and agitation.

Studies from the 1970s show marijuana eases glaucoma symptoms. But, since the preferred medium would be through smoking, to some extent the risks to the lungs out-weighed the potential benefits to the eyes. An attempt was then made to design an eyedrop, but...

You tell me... Why might that not work?

Cannabinoids don't like water, do they?

Right!

So, since THC isn't water soluble, back to the drawing board they had to go.

But, while millions of glaucoma patients feel smoking medical marijuana helps their condition, the American Glaucoma Society insist the effects of the drug are far too short-lived to be considered a viable treatment option, only lasting between 3 to 4 hours.

THC is also proven to help asthma, although as yet no pharmaceutical avenues have been successful in finding ways to exploit this.

Lastly, given the irresistible laziness weed induces, it's not surprising that research shows THC is largely responsible for cannabis's effect on sleep. Trials pay testament to oral doses of THC helping people fall asleep faster, improving night time breathing, and reducing intrusions from sleep apnoea. Interestingly though, as we will learn later, CBD does the opposite - it wakes you up!

No fatalities have ever been recorded from overuse of THC, but many reports suggest it might pose an increased risk of heart attack if you smoke too much for too long. It's not suspected this danger would apply if you were taking it orally, but THC's toxicology data is mainly drawn from animal studies. No human studies exist to compare, and so as such whether we can depend upon this data is uncertain.

CBD - Cannabidiol

The most important constituent of CBD-rich hemp oil.

First isolated by American organic chemist Robert Adams around the time of the Second World War, the structure of CBD was elucidated in 1963 by Mechoulam. Since it has no psychotropic effects it offers huge therapeutic potential as it's:

- Anti-inflammatory
- Anti-nausea
- Anti-emetic
- Anti-oxidant
- A neuro-protectant

Despite the absence of psycho-activity, several other neurological effects still take place as CBD interacts with a variety of signalling pathways and receptors.

Its interplay with both CB_1 and CB_2 receptors is weak, but nevertheless still provides potent anti-inflammatory effects. Exerting protective effects on the liver, brain, and immune system, it modulates several bodily mechanisms outside of the endocannabinoid system, which again we'll cover in more detail later. Its greatest biochemical affects, though, occur through changes it makes to gene transcription.

Some endocannabinoids appear not to do much when tested alone, but when combined with AEA (anandamide) and 2-AG, experiments often reveal these entourage compounds strengthening the analgesic, anti-inflammatory, or other functions of their molecular colleagues to a considerable degree. The same thing happens with phytocannabinoids. CBD drastically determines the way THC will work. THC, an agonist of both CB_1 and CB_2 receptors, shows preference for CB_1, so this is where it exerts its most dominant action. But, when CBD also participates, it nudges THC's action over from the CB_1 receptor to CB_2. There, THC provides a vastly improved immune and anti-inflammatory response than it would have, had it worked alone.

This partnership has already been exploited pharmaceutically. Sativex, a medicine of 1:1 ratio of CBD: THC made by British company G W Pharmaceuticals, is used to treat spasticity in multiple sclerosis and scientists anticipate it may eventually help to slow progression of Huntington's disease. Hopefully treatment may also be possible for Seronegative Stiff-Person Syndrome, a very rare and poorly treated disease presenting, again, with muscle rigidity and spasm.

Right, now...

I'd like to introduce you to a very clever molecule with the Star-Wars-sounding name: CP55940.

Created in the early 1970s, it mimics the effects of THC and is used as a means of studying endocannabinoid activity.

A quick recap to stop you spinning.

THC binds to CB_1 receptors, which anandamide also does, although to a much weaker degree.

CP55940 does the same job. So, by watching what it does, we can see what both the endo and phytocannabinoids could do in its place. We also gain an opportunity to see how other compounds interact with it.

Here's the thing...

CBD displaces CP55940.

That means it prevents it from binding to the receptor. This is partly how we know that CBD is what calms down the psycho-activity of THC, and why there are so many side effects with the synthetic versions of THC...because CBD is no longer there, providing the muscle and keeping it in check. The hedge witch inside of me suspects there will be other components in the complex helping in other ways too.

In *some* test tube tests, CBD has also been shown to be a low potency CB_1 receptor reverse agonist.

I know...

Double Dutch!

Just stop for a second and think that one through, because it seems to be deliberately confusing.

Agonist - switches it *on*

Antagonist – switches it *off*

So, a reverse agonist does not switch it off... It makes the action the *opposite* to what it would normally be.

Now, remember Gi is an **inhibitory** G-protein receptor.

G_s is a stimulatory (or **excitory**) one.

So, CBD calms a G_s receptor down, or revs a G_i receptor *up*. It makes it work the opposite way.

Working synergistically with THC, CBD complements THC's capacity to treat pain but is a spectacular anti-inflammatory agent in its own right. Compare CBD with side effects we've come to expect from the doctor's allopathic, non-steroidal anti-inflammatory drugs – the increased risk of heart attack or stroke, for example - existing without these, cannabidiol pretty much provides a get-out-of-hospital-free card.

In "Whole cannabis" for want of a better term, cannabidiol also counteracts some effects that aren't as nice from THC, like its tendency to produce anxiety and make your heart race. More importantly, cannabidiol has its own magical medicine that THC doesn't possess. It's a blissful anti-anxiety angel, as well as being anti-psychotic.

Another spectacular area for CBD is epilepsy. Anti-convulsant, it has a broad spectrum of activity. Alleviating many types of seizures, it exerts this tonic action on the brain without causing hallucinations.

Essentially, cannabidiol stabilises the endocannabinoid system. When systemic tone plummets and homeostasis becomes threatened, the outcome is hideously chronic illness. Cannabidiol strengthens and tones the endocannabinoid system in its entirety, returning it to balance and health.

But, despite these extensive properties, CBD's binding affinity to endocannabinoid receptors is mild: its action upon them is comparatively weak.

Clearly then, something else is going on.

Most of CBD's magic doesn't even come from the endocannabinoid system at all. Instead it does *even more stuff!* We'll get to that in the next chapter, but first I want to introduce you to some of the other cannabinoids present in the plant. I say some, because research has hardly started yet. We wait with bated breath.

Cannabis molecules move together in a gloriously enigmatic dance. Phytochemistry changes as plants age. Flavonoids, terpenes, and phenols join cannabinoids to create an even more impressive healing troupe. Our bodies then metabolise components at the liver, birthing even more new chemicals therefrom. Components intimately react, modulating each other's effects mysteriously.

CBN – Cannabinol

Not to be confused with cannabi*diol*, a different one.

There is very little CBN in fresh cannabis. It derives from the degradation of THCA and thus is mildly psychoactive. Historically, it had a bad reputation because it occurs in large amounts when old marijuana buds become oxidised if they've not been stored properly. Now, CBN is a hot potato that all the scientists want to research. It has been found to be involved in cannabis's effects on pain relief, appetite, anti-bacterial properties, anti-inflammatory and anti-convulsive effects, and insomnia. By far its strongest action, though, is as a sedative.

CBC - Cannabichromene

Cannabichromene is structurally similar to other natural cannabinoids including cannabidiol, cannabinol, and tetrahydrocannabinol.

It's likely we'll find CBC makes a far larger contribution to the overall analgesic effects of cannabis than we can yet imagine. A 2010 study showed CBC working closely with CBD and THC to bring about antidepressant effects. A 2013 paper then proved it promotes neurogenesis, encouraging neural stem cells to become neurons.

Preliminary evidence suggests Cannabichromene probably plays valuable roles in anti-inflammatory, antiviral, and anti-fungal properties of the plant.

CBG - Cannabigerol

You find higher levels of **Cannabigerol** in hemp than you do in cannabis cultivated for high levels of THC. It relieves pressure in the eye and is thought it might be of benefit to people with glaucoma. Mice experiments also show an improvement in inflammatory bowel disease. CBG inhibits uptake of the neurotransmitter, GABA, in the brain, decreasing anxiety and relieving muscle tension.

THCV - Tetrahydrocannabivarin

Depending on where this grows in the world, the cannabis bush might produce far higher levels of THCV. Plants grown in China, India, Nepal, Thailand, Afghanistan, and Pakistan, as well as Southern and Western Africa, all produce far higher levels of this cannabinoid. It switches on CB_2 receptors and switches off CB_1.

Trials are underway, studying plant-derived THCV in conjunction with metformin to reduce blood sugar and insulin resistance in type 2 diabetes, as well as reducing appetite.

CBDv - Cannabidivarin

Structurally similar to cannabidiol, **CBDv** has been proven effective in treating neurological disorders such as Parkinson's disease and intractable childhood epilepsy. Like THC, CBDv is also good at reducing sickness and vomiting induced by pharmaceutical drugs and chemotherapy.

Myriad cannabinoids have yet to be researched, promising to keep laboratories busy for decades to come. These include:

CBL - Cannabicyclol

CBV - Cannabivarin

CBGV - Cannabigerovarin

CBNV - Cannabinchromevarin

CBND - Cannabinodiol

CBT - Cannabicitran

CBE - Cannabielsoin

CBCN - Cannabichromanon

CBLV - Cannabifuran

CBR - Cannabiripsol

On the surface, it might seem like the magic of cannabis crackles solely in the cannabinoids, but this is absolutely not the case. Problems arising from synthesizing components come from each component supporting and interacting with another. Just as we saw with CBD modulating the psychoactive THC, when one constituent is removed a component works in an entirely different way.

Terpenes

Moreover, as aromatherapists we expect many of the effects naturally come from terpenes in the plant.

B-Caryophyllene

So, if the essential oil does not contain cannabinoids, that means it doesn't interact with the endocannabinoid system.

Right?

You'd have thought so, wouldn't you?

But no. Wrong!

Research demonstrated that *C. sativa* essential oil displaced CP55940 from the CB_2 receptors. It was the beta caryophyllene binding and interacting with the CB_2 receptor. Thus, as you start to understand the science more fully, you will realise that if a condition is derived from poor mechanics of the CB_2 receptor then the essential oil may potentially also help.

If you can get your hands on a gas chromatography report for your essential oil, as ever it will tell you a great deal about our hemp oil. Terpenes have become big business in the cannabis industry because it really influences how the marijuana will taste and smell. Clearly, if you can find a plant that will retain its terpenes longer, then you are onto a winner. But the terpenes don't only influence the senses, of course. They will also dictate the predominate actions.

Strains of marijuana like Green-O-Matic and Diamond Girl all have high levels of the constituent Borneol, very popular in Chinese Medicine for treating stress. Its sedative and calming vibration comes from borneols' clinically spicy but menthol note.

Where the body is struggling to cope with moisture from heavy periods, streaming hay fever, or grief that holds you in a perpetual stream of tears, strains that smell of pungent cedarwood after rain, because of the terpene Carene, are best suited.

Bubba Kush and Kings Kush both boast high levels of eucalyptol, making them helpful for suppressing coughs. Diamond Girl and Jack the Ripper offer a more exuberant mood through the citrusy limonene top note.

I'd suspect strains such as LA Confidential and Amnesia Haze to give above average relief to fibromyalgia sufferers since they have such high levels of linalool. If you were to find an oil made from these strains, blend it with Basil Linalool to add to the richness of the sweet candylike note.

A tiny list of a massive menu of constituents, all elegantly wrapped into a drop of essential oil, or with cannabinoids in a smudge of extract no bigger than a grain of rice.

Chapter 5 Properties and Interactions of CBD

This is a long and difficult chapter, with moments which I have clearly written when I was having a bit of a "different" day in a bid to make the medicine lighter. Goddess knows the science could do with that. I have added in a couple of videos to take the sting out too.

A quick recap then: the endocannabinoid system comprises of CB_1 and CB_2 receptors. However, cannabidiol is a weak agonist of both. To understand the medicine in the clinical evidence we need to make ourselves aware of other systems in the body effects.

We'll look at each section in turn.

- The orphan receptors GCPRs 55, 18, 119
- The signalling protocols of the system
- Gene transcription and how CBD's effects on that influences healing
- The MAP/ERK Pathway
- The PPAR System
- The COX Pathways
- TRPV Channels

Babble, right? Completely white noise! Don't worry. It becomes clearer.

If you do lose track, just think to yourself... *CBD affects this* and you'll be back.

Orphan Receptors

These are receptors suspected to operate within the endocannabinoid system, but as yet their endogenous ligands have not been discovered. In other words, we know something in cannabis activates them, that has been proven, but scientists still don't know what we naturally produce ourselves to do the same.

GCPR55

GCPR55 is implicated in inflammatory pain, neuropathic pain, metabolic disorder, bone development, and cancer. CBD blocks its signalling.

It is now classed as a *de*-orphanised receptor, because scientists suspect they may have found its partnering. Nevertheless, it must go somewhere, so here is as good a place as any!

Unlike the other CB receptors, its agonists still, for the main part, remain elusive to researchers. AM251, an enzyme, is a selective CB_1 antagonist that also seems to activate GCPR55, as does lysophosphatidylinositol. You might recall I said they can't decide if this was cannabinoid or not. This is one of the reasons why.

Cloned almost a decade ago, the receptor is found in both brain and peripheral tissues, but we still don't have comprehensive understanding of its complete distribution. GCPR55 is found widely inside the brain, especially in the cerebellum, and is linked to modulation of bone density and to blood pressure, as well as with cancer cell proliferation. Anandamide also binds to it and helps it to produce GTP as a vital part of enabling cells to divide and multiply.

In 2008, Waldeck-Weiermair *et al* discovered a vital interaction between GCPR55 and CB_1. They described how joint signalling of the two receptors caused a clustering of a family of receptors, integrins. Living on the surface of a cell they mediate the communication of cells with the extracellular matrix (ECM). This collection of extracellular molecules secreted by cells provide surrounding cells with structural and biochemical support and largely determine how a tissue will look and function. It is made up of water, minerals, fibrous proteins, and proteoglycans (a protein compound found in connective tissue).

Integrins act as a bridge between the components of the matrix, the cytoskeleton and other proteins, regulating:

- survival of cells
- proliferation (how the numbers of a cell grow by division, taking into account cell deaths)
- differentiation (where the cell becomes more brainy or specialised)
- migration (like the swallows!)

If integrins *un*cluster, the CB_1 receptor activates *spleen tyrosine kinase* (Syk), an inhibitor of *PI3K*. We don't need to understand what these are, simply that GPR55 signalling can only work effectively if PI3K works properly and activation of CB_1 receptors will prevent that. So then, GPR55 signalling will *always* be inhibited when CB_1 receptors are activated. When integrins are induced, they form clusters, dissociate from the CB_1 receptor, and GPR55 can get to work again.

In the same way, cannabidiol blocks GCPR55 signalling and how the body creates inflammatory pain, neuropathic pain, metabolic disorder, problems with bone development, and cancer.

So GCPR55 is a bad guy, right?

It certainly seems like it, and CB_1 keeps him in check.

But when he works with CB_2, he is still in permanent conflict, but thanks to a 2011 study by Balenga *et al* we know GCPR55 works in tandem with CB_2 to fight inflammation.

Our first line of defence against infections is our innate immune system, consisting of macrophages and granulocytes. Macrophages, regular readers will know, are my beloved warrior cells surrounding and overpowering infection like gladiators in an arena (be warned, I do tend to get rather excited about these *warrior immune cells*. It's the armour glinting in the sun that does it for me, I think!). Every time one of these Russell Crowe white blood cells enters the arena a tiny battle cry sounds out across the body.

"I am Macrophagius Decimus Meridius, father to a murdered son, husband to a murdered wife. **I** will have my vengeance, in this life or the next."

Damn right he will, and we'll see how in a second, but...

Granulocytes, perhaps you don't know, these too are white blood cells that have small granules or particles containing proteins to help the immune system to fight off viruses and bacteria. They form and mature in bone marrow.

There are three types of granulocytes:

- Neutrophils
- Eosinophils
- Basophils

When a new site of inflammation appears, neutrophils are the first granulocytes recruited to the scene. Their mission is simple: locate bacteria, recognising it as enemy, and destroy it. Maturing speedily, they gain special capabilities as they grow.

Where macrophages are gladiators, I like to think of granulocytes as superheroes.

Their powers are as follows:

- Enormous potential for efficient migration, super-scooting at top speed
- Phagocytosis – Phago is Greek for devour, they ingest bacteria. Effectively they become Pac-Man
- Production of reactive oxygen species (ROS), as well as enzyme-rich granules.

Now, injured tissues are noisy, messy creatures sending out all manner of mediators to garner an army to their cause. The warrior cells, macrophages, start banging on their drums too, summoning:

- Complement factor 5a (C5a) - contributes to the pathogenesis of inflammatory diseases
- Interleukin 8 (IL-8), effectively the chief chariot driver. Inducing chemotaxis in cell targets, it directs the battalion toward the site of infection. Its army will predominately be made up of neutrophils, but it might be other granulocytes too.
- Endocannabinoids – you might have heard of these.

Now here, interestingly, macrophages *produce* the endocannabinoids anandamide and 2-arachidonoylglycerol (2-AG).

(Didn't I tell you these were great...love macrophages... Look at me, I'm positively bursting with pride. Such a groupie. I feel quite emotional. Here, hold my camera. I'm gonna throw my knickers!).

This migration of the neutrophils towards inflammatory mediators, via the chemokines and cannabinoids, happens through the activation G protein coupled receptors. It's a really organised process.

Controlling this neutrophilic migration is one of the most crucial roles for our mate, the CB_2 receptor, but it always seemed likely to scientists there must also be other sites modulating it too. Recently found evidence shows GPR55 potently modulating CB_2 receptor's responses. It is the gear-lever, if you will. GPR55 is *expressed* in human blood neutrophils and when activated it opens the gateway for 2-AG, the agonist of CB_2.

GPR55 and CB_2 consistently interfere with each other's signalling pathways via tiny GTPases (enzymes that bind to GTP), bickering like seven-year-old friends in the playground. It's like a tiny tug of war over Sylvanian families. Together, their pushing and pulling leads to cellular polarization, where the chemicals feed in and out of the cell effectively. So now, we have efficient migration of the neutrophils, but now there is a compromise. Degranulation is cancelled as release of cytotoxic molecules is diminished, as is formation of ROS. In this way, GPR55 limits inflammatory responses that cause injury to tissue by the CB_2 receptor, but it also plays nicely with it, recruiting neutrophils to their gang at sites of inflammation.

Anandamide also binds to GCPR55 and helps with production of GTP. When it does, an increase of intracellular calcium floods certain immune cells.

Interestingly, THC shows a greater affinity to GPR55 than it does to either CB_1 or CB_2.

GPCR 18

It was recently suggested that GPR18 might well be a potential fourth receptor and research supports the hypothesis that GPR18 might be an abnormal cannabidiol receptor.

Activated by a metabolite of anandamide, *N-arachidonoylglycine* (NAGly) GPR18 is expressed in immune and gastrointestinal tissues, and those of the testes. Found in large populations in the brain stem, striatum, and cerebellum, GPR19 regulates how microglia migrate to sites of inflammation or damage to the central nervous system.

Resolvin, a metabolite of the omega-3 fatty acid, docosahexaenoic acid (DHA) is a ligand for GPR18. It's thought the many benefits of eating an omega-3-rich diet are accumulated thanks to GPR18. In animal trials, its stimulation seems to begin to remedy of inflammation and it is expected the same would happen in humans.

GPR119

GPR119 is mainly expressed in the gastrointestinal tract and the pancreas. Rat trials show our rodent friends eating less and gaining less body weight when GPR119 is activated. It regulates incretin, the hormone that tells the body to secrete insulin after meals, so as you might imagine, scientists are busy torturing some wee creature as we speak in a bid to use it to design new design treatments for obesity and diabetes.

Several endogenous and synthetic ligands for this receptor have been identified that interact with this receptor, including Anandamide.

NSAIDs, like aspirin, also exert some of their painkilling ability through acting on this receptor.

So, we understand the receptors, but what are they for?

The endocannabinoid system forms the most elaborate communications network you could ever imagine.

Signalling Protocols

A four-directional cross communications web brings all of the body's functions together.

- Presynaptic signalling
- Postsynaptic signalling
- Orthosteric and allosteric influence
- Tonic and phasic signalling

Presynaptic Signalling

This is the normal signalling we expect to see day to day. A neuron (nerve cell) wants to send a message to another neuron. It uses chemicals and neurotransmitters to signal across the gap between them, the synapse.

So, example…hmm, dunno, let's see…

My neuron wants to alert his neighbour that I've seen a slice of lemon cake and he wasn't to tell it: "Expect what's coming next to be fantastic", so he despatches dopamine to get my mouth watering and to move my arm to shove it in my face (because, clearly, neuroscience is that simple!).

The dopamine goes from the **presynaptic** neuron to the **postsynaptic**.

Postsynaptic Signalling

The endocannabinoid system communicates messages differently. It sends instructions "backwards." So, as soon as the postsynaptic neuron is triggered, cannabinoids are despatched from its fat cells. They release from the postsynaptic terminals to travel *back,* to the number one neuron, attaching to its cannabinoid receptors.

CB_1 receptors are found on the presynaptic membrane, so when cannabinoids activate these *pre*synaptic cells, they now have dynamic information to control how much hormone will be expressed and is next activated (*don't send any more, we have enough).* They perpetually act like volume controls for presynaptic neurons, suppressing or increasing how much of each neurotransmitter is released in the next burst.

Can you see how its dysfunction can lead to so many problems? If the eCS doesn't work properly, the body has no idea when to stop sending out more hormones or neurotransmitters. It's a hideous assault on the system.

Fundamentally, the endocannabinoid is the OFF Switch.

Orthosteric and Allosteric Sites

Now, you'd expect CBD and THC to interact with receptors similarly, wouldn't you? But they don't.

As you get to know CBD better, you'll realise she is a dreadful busy body, always putting her nose into other cannabinoids' business. She mean's well though, and admittedly she does have very good instincts. I'm sure she won't mind me telling you that she is a back door kinda gal. No hammering at the front door to complain about THC's rather erratic behaviour - she is more discrete. Wandering up the garden and knocking on the back door, she likes to conduct her business where no-one else can see.

THC comes in the front door of the cell at the ***orthosteric*** site. CBD binds to another site on the receptor, the **_allosteric_** site. This clever mechanism is how she can slip in and alters the binding of not only THC, but endocannabinoids too.

So basically if THC is present, CBD gets involved like a clucking mother hen and interferes with the big plan. Just as I can hear myself wading into the kid's games, spoiling all their fun and haughtily waving some offending toy in the air declaring "It's for your own good," CBD recognises and admires THC skills but knows he can be a bit full on, so she does the same.

She impedes the trippiness (impedes, not stops) and all of THC's other activities too, like anti-nausea, for example. Helpfully, she also interferes with the bad stuff too, dimming the lights on anxiety and settling heart rate.

The grownup term for cannabidiol's interfering action is ***negative allosteric modulation***. CBD is the negative allosteric modulator for CB_1 receptors.

Read that again. Now repeat it to yourself. And again.

It's very easy when you are reading the clinical evidence to dismiss actions of the CB_1 receptor, thinking CBD doesn't affect it. That's wrong. It does.

The most interesting thing is that, unlike most essential oil components we might normally use, it might have a sedating or stimulating effect on...well, any system, really - cannabidiol has a **buffering** effect. A bit like the buffers you put up when the kids (or – ahem - essential oil researchers) go bowling. If the ball goes too far left, the buffer puts it back to centre and the same will happen if it goes too far right. So, cannabidiol works in the same way. If the system has problems with excess in the receptor signalling it will calm it, just as it will also boost any deficiencies, bringing the entire system into balance.

Tonic and Phasic Signalling

So, the network is already looking pretty impressive, isn't it? But another layer is now laid over the top, because signals are sent between the nerves by one of two different signalling methods. They might be fast signals or slower and steadier ones.

- Tonic – slow and constant
- Phasic - sudden and more sporadic

We will meet tonic and phasic signalling many times on a CBD journey through the brain. It especially applies in issues like autism and epilepsy.

Tonic activity is often characterized by a **steady** firing of signals at a **constant frequency**. Clearly, here it applies to neurological signalling, but this signalling can be involved in anything physiological, so it might be signals to muscles, for example.

Let's put this into some easier context.

You've got one of those infuriating twitchy eyes and you can feel it flick, flick flicking, and there's nothing you can do about it. As fast as it comes, it is gone. A very strange thing! Twitching is an immaculate personification of phasic signalling. Phasic firing to takes place when a neuron activates **in response to presynaptic activity**. Usually, this will be just one, or at most a few, short bursts of action potential before the activity hastily returns to a resting state again. The twitching stops.

But tonic activity, however, doesn't really need any stimulus at all and its more controlled, like crossing and uncrossing your legs if you like.

Imbalance

We now recognise the receptors. We also recognise the endogenous ligands, anandamide and 2-AG. If they are both in the body, then everything should be tickety-boo, right?

Well, yes, as long as there is enough.

Consider I have now eaten the lemon cake and I now notice there is an éclair on the cake stand too. The CB_1 receptors want to say, *"Enough already, you greedy pig"* and the anandamide comes to do its job.

But it's a chocolate éclair. And it's oozing cream, and there is a veritable dopamine flood heading their way. The anandamide molecules look left and then right and realise there simply aren't enough of them. So, the CB_1 receptors cry, *"leave it to us"* and multiply in a bid to link to more anandamide and make a fence to contain the dopa-flood. But since I have eaten more tarts than trout, there hasn't been enough omega-3 to make enough anandamide to go around… Dopamine surges right though, and now I have crème pâtissière all over my chin.

As the second bite is being raised to my mouth you can hear the inadequate army of anandamide sob *"I just can't cope"* and that's exactly the words you'll hear coming out of a patient's mouth. Later, in the PTSD section, you'll see an interesting study of survivors from Ground Zero on 9/11. They have just this thing…very low levels of anandamide and a vast surplus of receptors as the brain has tried and tried to sort the mess out. It's a very good predictor of anxiety.

So that's signalling, but what does that signalling lead to? Well, all sorts of things, but here we'll focus on how CBD affects signalling that leads to gene expression and the effects that can have on health.

Gene Transcription

Have you ever wondered how cells move about the body and change? I'll be honest, when I suffered a blood clot in my lungs in 2008, I felt so poorly for over a year that anyone in close proximity to my bedroom door would have heard me sobbing *"why me?"* many, many times. And many people answered, *"It's just one of those things"*, which helped a little, I suppose.

I now know it was down to gene expression of a blighter called interferon, whom you will meet more in depth in the inflammation section of the clinical evidence. If its gene expression hadn't gone haywire, my blood would not have got sticky and I'd have had a lot healthier pregnancy.

Cells replicate, carrying the genetic code, the DNA, through to the next cell via a process of gene transcription. When expression of certain inflammatory genes is upregulated for example, they bind to co-activator molecules and accumulate chronic inflammation. Expression is the interface between genes and environment. It dictates everything, from plasticity developing in the brain, enabling us to learn, remember or indeed, forget, to how our body deals with insulin in diabetes.

Uncontrolled cell growth and proliferation is characterised by cancer. Cancers grow when the regulatory mechanism breaks down. As cells divide and multiply, messenger RNA – the coding that crosses to the new cell - contains identical mutations, spreading the anomalies across every cancerous cell, which then divides, multiplies, and spreads it exponentially.

MAP/ERK Pathway

MAP/ERK is a chain of proteins in a cell that control the cell's growth.

Uncontrolled growth is a necessary step for the development of cancer. Communicating signals from the receptor onto the surface of the cell, then into the DNA in the nucleus of the cell, the MAP/ ERK pathway perpetuates cancers such as melanoma, for example, when it goes awry. Pathway defects trigger this mechanism of uncontrolled growth. Many compounds have been identified to inhibit this and may lead to novel treatments for cancer. The phytocannabinoids THC and CBD are just two of these compounds.

In a 2012 study by the University of Tel Aviv, scientists compared how THC and CBD affected gene expression in glial cells.

- THC upregulated 36 genes and downregulated 29.
- But CBD upregulated 658 genes and downregulated 517.

Downregulation is where a cell switches down how much there is of a certain cellular component. The complementary process, upregulation, is an increase in components.

One of the key modulators of gene transcription is:

PPAR System

These are ***Peroxisome Proliferator Activated Receptors***.

There. You're clearer now, aren't you?

Let's take it slowly.

Peroxisomes

- These are small, membrane-enclosed organelles (tiny part of cells) containing enzymes involved in a variety of different metabolic reactions.
- Their job is to break down nutrients the cell has acquired and used.
- They absorb fatty acids (this will become important to know later).

- They also absorb ethanol and alcohols so, as you would imagine, you find them in large concentrations in the liver cells.
- They are involved in the synthesis of cholesterol and how effectively you digest amino acids.

PPARs regulate genes and many of the genes they regulate are involved in:

- Energy homeostasis
- Uptake of lipids (for those unsure, '**Lipid**' is just medical jargon for fat, but the word is usually used more in the context of fat within the blood stream).
- Insulin sensitivity
- Metabolism and other metabolic functions

Naturally, we have endogenous ligands for these – the peroxisomes – that fit the receptor keyhole, but CBD will also act as a key instead.

These are ***nuclear receptors***.

Nuclear hormone receptor proteins belong to a class of ligand activated proteins. Binding to specific sequences of DNA, they act like on-off switches for transcription within the cell nucleus, the process where the information in a strand of DNA is copied into a new molecule of messenger RNA (mRNA). DNA then safely and stably stores the genetic material in the nuclei of cells to act as a reference, or a template.

Triggered by hormones, steroids, fatty acids, and nutritional compounds, these switches control development and differentiation of skin, bone, and behavioural centres in the brain and continually regulate reproductive tissues.

PPARs bind to segments of DNA, to either promote or prevent transcriptions of specific genes.

PPARs are a group of three types of nuclear receptors

- PPAR Alpha
- PPAR Gamma
- PPAR Delta

PPAR Alpha

PPAR α regulates lipids in the liver. Activated when the body is deprived of energy, it is necessary for ketogenesis, an important adaptive response to fasting (you might want to cross reference this in the rose book under epilepsy. We talk about ketogenesis there).

PPAR Delta

Its role of this receptor is still unclear. PPAR β seems to be implicated in chronic diseases including diabetes, obesity, atherosclerosis, and cancer. There has been a great deal of research to determine how it affects cancer but results are always contradictory. There is no consensus as to whether it prevents or promotes cancer formation.

PPAR Gamma

PPARy regulates glucose metabolism and storage of fatty acids. Any genes activated by PPARy stimulate production of new fat cells and regulate how much lipid those cells will take in. If a mouse has this receptor removed, and is stuffed with high fat food, it still won't generate any adipose tissue (I'm thinking of seeing if they can fit me in to get mine removed on Thursday!). Many diabetic drugs use PPARy as a way to lower blood glucose without further raising insulin.

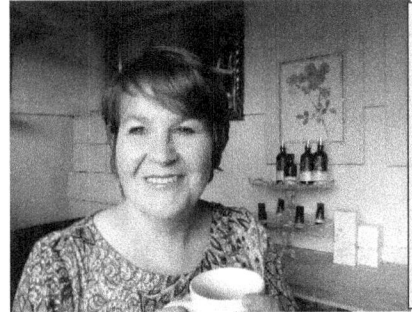

https://buildyourownreality.lpages.co/gene-transcription-video-optin/

CBD also enjoys a very happy friendship with the COX Pathways.

COX Pathways

Cyclooxygenase (COX), or **prostaglandin-endoperoxide synthase** (PTGS), is an enzyme responsible for making prostaglandins and prostanoids implicated in inflammation. The body manufactures prostaglandins, hormone-like lipids, at injuries of inflammation to try to speed the healing process. Modulatory compounds, they exert a variety of functions, dilating, constricting, contracting, and relaxing in many functions, including blood pressure and inflammation. They also enable us to give birth. I can remember the midwife telling me to use evening primrose in a bid to get the prostaglandins going, to trigger contractions and speed along a tardy baby. They are healthy and useful things.

Like everything else, levels can wander off balance, leading to excess inflammation or retarded wound healing. These problems are manufactured by the cyclooxygenases. Later, you will see that many of CBD's healing actions are thought to be executed through the COX pathways, inhibiting pain and soothing inflammation. But this is not new territory. Both aspirin and ibuprofen use the COX pathways to heal.

It's thought the degradative pathways for anandamide and 2-AG both involve COX pathways. By inhibiting the pathways, CBD maintains the elevated levels required to sooth pain.

TRPV

Together with NADA (one of the guys with the long names they think might be an endocannabinoid), 2-AG has an interesting relationship with the receptor **TRPV1**. This is **Transient Receptive Protein Vanilloid Type 1**. I felt mine kick in yesterday when I went out to collect logs for the fire and my hands were super-painful from the cold. TRPV1 provides the sensations of heat and pain, and regulates body temperature.

Activation of TRPV1 regulates synthesis of anandamide.

CBD activates *Transient Receptor Potential Vanilloid type 1.*

What's a vanilloid?

Vanillyls are a functional organic chemistry group and a vanilloid is a vanillyl!

Well, that's clear then!

Don't get your head involved in it.

It's what TRPV does that is important.

It is responsible for two of our most primordial survival mechanisms. These are temperature and pain.

So, it's because of these we feel extreme heat, but also varying levels of pain.

The scientific terms for:

Perception of **pain** – Nociception

Perception of **heat** - Thermoception

TRPV receptors are found in membranes of every cell. There are literally millions of them all over the body. They interact closely with anandamide and when they encounter heat, they change shape.

Imagine, for a moment, putting your hands onto a hot stove. It's weird, isn't it, because you move your hand before you even realise you have done it. That's because nerves sending messages from the cells, comprise three different fibres, all transmitting data at different speeds.

Alpha β (Beta) are big. They are wide and surrounded by stacks of myelin. Myelin is a speedy insulator, but because the cell is wider, there's also less resistance as the message flies to the brain. These fibres hastily carry the message to SHIFT THAT HAND before any damage can be incurred.

Since Alpha Delta have less myelin, they are smaller in diameter. It follows, then, that they are not such fast conductors either. These are the ones that mock you in that split second afterwards – "You silly cow! That's hot!"

The slow ones are even thinner, having no myelin at all. Since the message isn't well insulated, it encounters tons of resistance and its journey takes longer still. This is the lingering throb that says...pain, pain, agony pain. Are you remembering the stove's hot yet Einstein?!

This pleases me.

In the land of TRPV, the fat ones are the superheroes that save the day and the skinny ones just sit about and moan.

Not often we see that happen. Vive la révolution!

Now, we've talked about phytocannabinoids affecting the same receptors as endocannabinoids. Here we see it again, a plant molecule interacting as ligand to receptor. Another plant molecule that activates TRPV is called capsaicin and you'll find it in chilli peppers.

So, when you eat a chilli, what happens to you physiologically?

You get hot; you start sweating. If you haven't adequately rinsed your hands and then go to the toilet...there is burning! All these responses derive from capsaicin acting as a ligand on the TRPV1 responses, thereby expressing the heat/pain sensations.

Six different TRPV pathways exist in total, and in recent years it has become apparent that this channel holds vital clues to how pain emanates in fibromyalgia. In 2015, researchers at Kyoto University in Japan experimented, placing miniscule gold nanorods coated in lipids into the TRPV channel, and then exposed them to near infrared light. Prolonged activation of the TRPV channel, as the rods heated, brought about relief from the fibromyalgic pain. Sadly, if continuously stimulated, this receptor is subject to desensitization. The pathway slows down and in extreme cases will even stop. There's a little way to go with that experiment. It's a shame we can't find another molecule that might be able to modulate TRPV...

Endogenously, it's anandamide's job to activate these receptors, but strangely it appears THC doesn't bother. It's cannabidiol that interacts, but for we aromatherapists the exciting thing is it's not alone in this ability. You might remember from the rose book, that citronellol can do it too, as can geraniol.

Apart from on human sensory neurons, TRPV channels are found on skin keratinocytes and hair follicles. So, activating the TRPV1 receptor might be a valuable way for CBD to treat skin conditions too, and it raises therapeutic possibilities for certain kinds of neuropathic pain.

For fear of making it sound like CBD is the only part of cannabis that does any heavy lifting, clearly that's not going to be the case. Often, it's laziness on my part that prevents me from following the research pathways of other cannabinoids, or other times perhaps the data simply does not exist (more likely the former though, if I am brutally honest!). Sometimes though, it falls in your lap!

A 2011 study by the Endocannabinoid Research Group at the Institute of Cybernetics, CNR, Pozzuoli (NA), Italy, were kind enough to do the work for me.

They reported seeing CBD, CBG, CBGV, and THCV all stimulating and desensitizing TRPV1 channels in humans.

In rat experiments, they witnessed CBC, CBD, and CBN all potently working as both agonists and desensitizers of the TRPV1 (implicated in pain, itching, and respiratory disorders). One of the precursors to THC, Tetrahydrocannabivarin (THCV), had been the most potent compound here.

Of the receptors that mediates cold and binds to menthol TRPM8, CBG and THCV were the most potent antagonists. Only CBC and CBN of non-acid cannabinoids had failed to strongly activate or desensitize rat TRPV2, the channel that kicks in when exposed to extremely high temperatures.

Chapter 6 The Nervous System

To truly grasp the complexity and beauty of the endocannabinoid system and how *extraordinary* the research into it is, we need to go right back to **Nervous System 101**.

By the time you leave this book, my aim is that you fully understand:

- how the system works
- why it is so *magical*
- and to be able to evangelise to anyone who will listen that we should be able to get access to this plant.

Some of this you will already know, but I can guarantee you there will be gaps, so I suggest you take an hour or so to wade through it.

The Electrical Nervous System

The system has two main divisions. These are:

- The Central or Cerebrospinal Nervous System (CNS)
- The Autonomic System: broken down into **the sympathetic** and the **parasympathetic systems.**

The foundation of every nerve is a cell called a neuron. It's the body of the cell. Neurons have incredibly long, branch extensions, sometimes up to a metre long, and are referred to as nerve fibres. Neurons also have very specialised projections known as **dendrites and axons**.

Dendrites

Bring messages *to* the cell body.

Axons

Take messages *away* from it.

Neurons are protected and surrounded by a fatty sheath. The white nerve fibres are **medullated,** meaning their sheath comprises of a substance called myelin. **Grey nerve fibres** are **non-medullated,** thus it follows they have no myelin.

Myelin

Found only along the nerves of the Central Nervous System, it consists predominately of proteins and lipids. Its job is to insulate electrical impulses travelling along the axon. It works a bit like a rubber casing would, around a copper wire. One of the primary indicators of multiple sclerosis is damage to this myelin sheath. Doctors believe an unusual infection or attack might cause scarring, lesions, or bare spots in the sheath, which then in turn distort electrical messages to and from the brain.

If we had a scalpel and were to cut away at the spinal cord, we would see nerves are arranged in the shape of an H. The grey ones make up the letter's shape in the middle, and the white ones are placed in between.

Every one of the nerves of the body (except for the olfactory nerves which run through the sinus cavities) feeds through the spinal column. Take a moment to consider how much of the body's control centre is running between each vertebra. It's easy to imagine why damage to the back would be such a terrifying thing. Spinal damage leads to partial or complete paralysis *below* the injury. Brain injury (if it doesn't kill you) results in either physical or mental impairment.

Nervous tissue is made of uniquely structured cells called:

Neurones

There are three types of neurone. These are:

- **Sensory**

Conveys information about your surroundings to the brain about heat, pain, pressure, light, and sound etc. via the spinal cord.

- **Motor**

Transmits impulses to your muscles. A motor end plate is attached to the end of a motor neurone (anchored to a solitary muscle fibre). Messages travel along these from the brain and trigger movement.

- **Connector**

Also known as Relay, Transfer, or Immediate neurones. As the name suggests, these link to the actions of other neurones. There are literally thousands of millions of these in the spinal cord and the brain.

We call a connection between two or more neurons a synapse.

Synapses

To cross between two places – the neurons clearly need to have something to connect across the synaptic gap, and this is bridged by some familiar little chemicals called the neurotransmitters, which we'll come to in more depth in a moment.

Brain

The most important part of this system is the brain, so let's remind ourselves of its anatomy and get an idea of how things work.

It comprises three very differing structures:

- Cerebellum
- Cerebrum
- Medula Oblongata

As we saw in chapter 3, these are liberally scattered with CB_1 receptors.

Weighing a little over 1,360 grams, if you were to place it unsupported onto a hard surface it would slump like a blancmange because it's brimming with water.

A little quiz for you:

How many nerve cells, or neurons, do you think the brain contains?

An estimated **12 billion**.

How close did you get?

Glia

At every corner, cannabis turns anything you thought you knew on its head...about everything. Possibly, we see this to the greatest extent in glia.

As you know, I am proud of my aromatherapy heritage and the excellent training I received. At school, my affinity for medical sciences was completely lost because I had to choose between sciences and languages, and languages won. It was not a hard decision after I'd embarrassed my poor dad with a tremendous score of 18% in my chemistry exam! It was only when I started to study anatomy and physiology (A&P) for my diploma that I realised that everything everyone else found difficult was a cinch for me.

I especially loved learning about the nervous and endocrine systems, and I imagine you can tell that from reading. Try to visualise my horror, then, when cannabis led me to the discovery that everything I had learned about the brain and about hormones was not only woefully inept, but for the most part it was completely wrong. I feel sure that when you start to discover the new-found evidence you will question everything you have ever learned too.

I want to stress, at this point, that it is not the teacher's or even the governing board's fault; what they were teaching us was right...inasmuch as scientists construed it. Hell, this section even brings into question at least four Nobel Prizes won on research about the neurological system. Their research was right, at the time, but is now recognised as incomplete. It's radical science, and yet it is now deemed not only to be correct, but fundamental to your understanding of how cannabis works, as we soon head into the clinical evidence.

Welcome to the world of glia.

So, what are glia?

Well, do you remember as a child you were probably told that we only use 10% of our brains? That's because the brain is made up of around 10% of neurons and the rest is some kind of glue-y sticky stuff. It is the stuff we spoke of earlier that makes our brains seem like jelly. This jelly is called glia, and the word literally translates as "glue". It was called this because, historically, the scientific world accepted that glia held our brains together and that otherwise it had no real usage except to insulate and provide structure and protection to the neurons. That it was void space, and we could consider it to be the nuts and bolts of the scaffolding of the brain, if you like.

This is not only wrong, but it couldn't be further from the truth. In fact, we now know that, really, the science of the brain is probably incorrectly named – neuroscience – because the neurons are *secondary* in function to the far more powerful and important glia.

Currently, glia is one of the most highly researched areas in medicine. We know that healthy glial cells look very different to those found in pathological brains. We also know they age. It was recently revealed that if you study the brain post-mortem, the glia gives an almost perfect indication of how old a person is. Rather than the brain losing neurons as we age, we now understand that it is <u>numbers of glia that change</u>.

This interest in glia comes from three distinct areas:

- The way glia signal to each other **means they can store information.**
- Most brain tumours are gliomas. These are made up of glia.
- Researchers have now determined that glia are **adult stem cells**.

Now, that gave me pause because we hear the term stem cells all the time, don't we? Then I realised I had no idea what it really meant! So, a stem cell is one distinct cell that comes from a multicellular organism (that could be a human, cat, or plant...anything that has more than one cell). This cell can create indefinitely more of the same kind of cell, but it can also create other kinds of cells from it.

The "old brain dogma" – pre-glia - explained our brains developed in utero, and into early childhood. Then, they would stay that way until we died.

Current thought disagrees.

It says no, that's not true.

We regenerate brain cells in adulthood.

More... Glia are the stem cells that allow that regeneration to take place.

Not only that, but they can also regenerate neurons if they need to too.

So, that's exciting, isn't it?

It gets better.

What glia do, is they congregate and multiply in the part of the brain that you use the most. When Albert Einstein's brain was analysed (post-mortem) he was found to have significantly more glia in the part of the brain known as the left angular gyrus. Now this is mind-blowing (see what I did there?) because that's the area of the brain that scientists believe governs mathematical processing and language.

I like that!

So, can we say that glia equals intelligence?

Well, potentially, yes, we can. If we say that humans are the most highly evolved species, then if we compare the number of glia in lower species we should expect to see fewer. Right?

We do.

Begin with the lowly leech. For every one glia, he has 30 neurons. This single cell orchestrates every action a leech has to perform. I suspect that one might shout "blood!" but I can't be sure.

We move onto a rather well-researched worm. Elegant by name, elegant by nature, *Caenorhabditis elegans*. He's no Einstein, but he'd outwit the leech, bless him. Glia make up 16% of his nervous system. They make up 20% of a fruit fly's brain, 60% of a rodent's brain and 80% of a chimp's. We are the Master Race at 90% of our brains.

(Just remember that when you can't quite manage to swat that pesky fly!).

But, it is not only the number that's important...as every gal knows...size matters.

Human glia are 27 times bigger than a mouse's. A mouse has three astrocytes to every neuron, whereas a human has just 1.65. In other words, the impetus from a human glia is stronger than that of a mouse.

(Obviously, none of this applies to Brain out of Pinkie and the Brain. He is a glia-mungous, and that's why he's going to do the same thing they do every night, Pinky... Try to take over the WORLD!).

Ok, so the brain is like jelly, right? And it is wrinkly like a walnut too. Agreed?

The grown-up term for the walnut is the folded cortex. Actually, not all animals have folds, they only happen in higher level species like cats, dolphins, and primates. These folds happen to make more room for processing, because a bigger brain would be cumbersome and would not fit inside your pretty little skull. Humans have 35% more glia in their folded cortex than primates do (remember they do have a lot, because it makes up 80% of their brains).

Now, it has been suggested this massive excess of glia maybe the reason that we, as humans, see so much more degenerative disease in thought patterns than other species do. I had never considered it before, but you don't see sheep with Parkinson's or dogs with Alzheimer's; these are human diseases (although I am not sure I'd look for it in an addled sheep, I must confess).

We as aromatherapists have a rather unique experience of glia, because the place which enjoys the largest turnover of cells is the olfactory bulb. Since the body processes so many different scents all of the time, then cells wear out quickly and need to be replaced. One of the first symptoms of degenerative diseases is often the loss of the sense of smell, pointing to that regeneration of cells slowing down.

Actually, there are a whole host of different types of glia to love, and each do their own separate thing.

- Schwann cells
- Müller cells
- Ependymal cells
- Oligodendrocytes
- Tanycytes
- Microglia
- Astrocytes

You know what? These are interesting guys. I'm inviting them to dinner. Pop on a pretty frock and some lippy. Let me introduce you.

Schwann Cells

These live in the peripheral nervous system and support the neurons. They make up the olfactory unsheathing cells. Unique in their mastery, these are responsible for the successful regeneration of olfactory axons we spoke of earlier. They also make up the *enteric glia*, the vital components of the enteric nervous system (the nervous system connected to the gut). Forming an intricate network in the mucosa of the gastrointestinal tract, previously they were imagined to be nothing more than passive support cells. It's now clear they actively control motility and the function of epithelial barrier of things like the intestine. They do this by forming a sophisticated cellular and molecular bridge between enteric nerves, immune cells, and epithelial cells, as well as enteroendocrine cells found in the wall of the gut. These enteroendocrine cells then secrete hormones to regulate any number of processes in the body, including controlling glucose levels, food intake, and emptying your tummy!

Schwann cells are found at sensory nerve endings such as the Pacinian corpuscle, the nerve ending in the skin responsible for sensitivity to vibration and pressure.

Now, there are two different types of Schwann cells. These are:

- Myelinating
- Non-myelinating

Myelinating Schwann cells wrap around the axons of motor and sensory nerves to make a myelin sheath to insulate them.

There are three main diseases you may have heard of that affect these cells. In **Charcot-Marie-Tooth disease** the muscles of the foot, hand, and forearm all degenerate because of mutations in these glia.

In **Guillain-Barré syndrome,** the auto-immune system kicks into overdrive and the immune system uses the Schwann cells to attack the peripheral nervous system.

In **leprosy**, bacteria actively target Schwann cells to exploit their stem cell ability and spread disease throughout the body. The bacteria reprogram cells into their stem-like state. It switches off any genes associated with mature Schwann cells and then switches on ones used in embryonic and developmental stages. Then, these stem cells migrate to different parts of the body with the bacteria riding piggy back. Infected cells reach other tissues (skeletal muscle for example), merge with that tissue's cells, and spread the bacteria. The infected stem cells secrete chemokines to attract more immune cells to the party, allowing the bacteria to hitch a ride on these cells too.

We humans thought we were clever holding chicken pox parties…leprosy beat us to it by years.

Scary, isn't it?

What's that you say? You'd rather not be seated next to Schwann cell at the dinner table?

Hmm, yes, I can see how leprosy might put you off your dinner.

Come and meet Müller, instead. He's an eye specialist. See what you think of him.
Müller Cells

Glial cells of the retina, the jobs of the Müller cells are to support the neurons of the retina, to uptake neurotransmitters, to regulate the levels of potassium, to remove debris from the eye, and to store glycogen.

And yes, if you have the same strange quizzical mind as me, there *are* neurotransmitters in the eye. The retina expresses dopamine, serotonin, glutamate, and GABA.

Neuroepithelial Cells
Very quickly, these are the stem cells of the nervous system.

Ependymal Cells
These constitute a very thin epithelial lining for the spinal cord ventricular system. The four ventricles are full of cerebrospinal fluid to bathe and cushion the brain and spinal cord, to protect them from the sharp edges of the skull and spine. This cerebrospinal fluid is thought to be manufactured by the ependymal cells and might possibly be the reservoir of neuro-regeneration.

Oligodendrocytes
Now, I did learn about these guys in my diploma, because I can remember trying to learn how to spell them!

Remember myelin, the sheaths protecting the axons? Oligodendrocytes form that electrical sheathing if it wraps around axons in the *Central* Nervous System, where Schwann cells sheath the axons of the *peripheral* nervous system. This sheath constitutes 80% lipid and 20% protein. Now, where the Schwann cell, in effect, does the same wrapping job, it can only wrap *one* axon, whereas an oligodendrocyte can extend its processes to over 50.

Tanycytes
Remember ependymal cells live in the ventricular system? So, tanycytes are specialised ependymal cells that live in the third ventricle and on the floor of the fourth. Their processors reach right the way down into the hypothalamus. It is

not entirely clear what, exactly, they do, but it is likely they transfer signals from the cerebro-fluid to the central nervous system.

What we do know, however, is they are also involved in the manufacture of Gonadotrophin Release Hormones which we need for growth, sexual development, and reproductive function.

Okay, now in my opinion we are onto the two superstars.

Obviously, I get to sit by these guys because it is my party, but I will introduce you.

Pay close attention because these guys, the astrocytes and microglia, are show offs that you see everywhere in the clinical evidence.

Microglia

About 10-15% of all cells in the brain are microglia. They are the resident macrophage cells. So, these macrophages, the microglia, are distributed across the entire central nervous system and are the first line of defence against pathogens threatening the health of the CNS. They are never still, these little warriors. They are always on the scavenge, on the lookout for plaques, damaged or unnecessary neurons and synapses, and of course, any infectious agents.

Microglia are extremely sensitive to change. They need to be, to react speedily to any nasties that might have breached the blood brain barrier. It is this sensitivity that makes them so efficient and the skill comes from being able to detect minuscule changes in potassium channels (we'll talk about channels in a moment).

Astrocytes

Now, we briefly met astrocytes in the Spikenard book when we were talking about Alzheimer's. I told you these were the stars, and even their name means star because they are star-shaped. We find them in the spinal cord and the brain. They are tremendously abundant, comprising between 20-40% of your brain (depending on which scientific counting method you ascribe to), and they are the most abundant cell in the human cortex. Astrocytes have many functions, including making up the endothelial tissue of the blood brain barrier (BBB).

Imagine that the neurons make a highway, then astrocytes are little cities that are built up along the highway where all the storage happens but also all the cleaning and communications too.

I'll summarise the functions, because it will make it easier for you later. You might find you want to keep checking back on this one.

They:

- Make up the BBB
- Provide nutrients to nervous tissue
- Regulate the repair and scarring processes of the brain and spinal cord after someone has sustained a traumatic brain injury
- Release gliotransmitters in a calcium dependant manner.

(Bear with me, you'll get to understand this one a bit more as we go).

First of all, what's a gliotransmitter?

These facilitate communication between glial cells and the neurons. Microglia or oligodendrocytes can also release gliotransmitters, but usually, they are released from astrocytes.

Now, this star shape means they can hold hands with many other astrocytes at the same time and they can make contact with an unimaginable 10,000 synapses (actually, it is more correct to say they don't hold hands so much as they wrap their feet around each other). Since not only are they great communicators but also good listeners, they are able to absorb information from other astrocytes and neurons too. This is referred to as **bi-directional communication**.

Now, while astrocytes are very sociable beings, they are also incredibly self-sufficient. They self-replicate and an astrocyte will chat away to itself all day quite merrily. As it chunters on it also communicates with things around it. Now, this is a very important distinction because a mature neuron can't do anything without an astrocyte telling it to, but an astrocyte is utterly liberated, she really doesn't need the neuron. So, while a neuron might trigger your arm to move, it cannot do anything until the astrocyte gives it the idea and cracks the whip.

Neurons exist to *support* the astrocytes.

Now it has been found that the glia can communicate between themselves through electrical networks made up of calcium ion channels. Clearly, in order to receive sensory input from a neuron, they would need a receptor. So, what does our little glia do? Well, of course she makes her own.

Glia express receptors.

In the central nervous system, we predominately find cannabinoid type 1 receptors (CB_1) on neurons, and to a smaller degree on glial cells. How much the CB_1 receptors are expressed varies depending on what area of the brain it is and the different types of neurons. The expression of receptors on GABAergic cells is high in the hippocampus, but glutamatergic neurons have a much lower CB_1 receptor expression. Generally, there is a very low expression of CB_2 receptors in the central nervous system, and really, they are only found on certain brainstem nuclei and maybe in the cerebellum. There are usually more CB_2 receptors in astrocytes and microglia than CB_1s. Thus, primarily the brain's endocannabinoid signalling is expressed through CB_1 receptors on neurons, and glial cell CB_2s.

CB_2 receptors are mainly expressed on microglia. When CB_2 is activated, immune cells enjoy increased migration and adhesion, so fewer proinflammatory cytokines are released. Apoptosis – programmed cell death - is triggered in dendritic cells too, and it is suspected that it may not only be CB_2 receptors that initiate this. CB_1 may do the same, leading to the hypothesis that endocannabinoid signalling plays a pivotal role in the development of neurodegenerative diseases. Recognising that neurodegeneration and neuroinflammation contribute to aging, it's suspected that if scientists could find a way to regulate glial responses via the endocannabinoid system, they may be able to influence how fast the brain ages too.

The method of communication for a neuron is down the axon of a nerve. But the extraordinary thing is they either fire or they don't. This is called the "all or nothing" phenomenon. That is: regardless of how strong the signal comes in for a muscle to move, it either will or it won't. There is no middle ground.

So, this seems quite straightforward, doesn't it?

Yeah, right! Have you only just started reading this book? Nothing related to cannabis, in some way, is simple! We need to dig deeper, so we'll have a more detailed look at how a neuron fires.

Right, here seems as good time as any to introduce you to another new word (at least this one you can get your tongue around!).

Depolarisation
–the alteration of the electrical charge between the inside of the membrane of a nerve or muscle cell, and the outside. This happens as the permeability of the cells softens and sodium cells migrate to the interior of the cell.

You will understand this better in a moment.

Before we start, can you remember what an ion is?

It's a molecule with an electrical charge.

That will help you as we boldly enter The Matrix. Do you remember how Morpheus explained to Neo that we were nothing more than batteries in a machine?

Terrifying, but the truth is potentially stranger than fiction because he is nearly right... Although our brain is closer to being equal to a collection of around 80 billion batteries. Each neuron in the brain has the potential to accumulate a charge across its cell membrane. This results in a tiny, but nevertheless useful, voltage.

On average, a neuron contains a resting voltage of approximately -70 millivolts, or 0.07 volts. Compare this to the 1.5 volts in an AA battery (doing the maths, it is 21 neurons to a battery!).

So, let's think this through a bit...

The neuron is at rest and has a potential of -70 millivolts (I like to think of the neuron as a tranquil living room where potassium sits. I think he is reading his paper with his feet up).

The neuron is stimulated (his wife is moaning from the kitchen that it must be his turn to wash up... There is a gentle irritation).

Since the signal was fired upstream, a channel will open and sodium ions enter the cell (the door opens and in comes sodium with curlers in her hair and a pinny on!).

The sodium keeps coming and coming and soon the flood barrier is breached and so a floodgate opens. It explodes to +50 milivolts. As sodium rushes in, potassium rushes out (potassium can't take the nagging any longer, explodes to his feet with some very spicy language *"I can't get a moment's peace in this place. Fine, I'll go and do the fenugreek-ing washing up, if it'll shut you up. At least it's fenugreeking quiet in the kitchen!"*).

There is a resting period until electrical potential reaches -70 again.

During this resting potential, the neuron is unable to fire (hyper-polarisation)

(the radio goes on and the Tremolos drift out "Silence is Golden" while everything calms down).

So, this sodium/potassium exchange is what happens when a neuron fires. Then, when the signal reaches the end of the axon, there is a communication in the synapse, the gap between the first and second neuron.

Calcium Ion Channels

Glia communicate in a way that is more complex. They communicate in waves through calcium ion channels. Where **CB_1 & CB_2 receptors *open* potassium channels**, they ***inhibit* calcium channels**. The sole means of access of entry into the part of the nerve that forms a synapse with another cell - the bouton - is through a calcium ion channel. CBD restricts calcium access, thereby stilling the mind and giving the brain a few moments respite.

So, what do you know about calcium? Anything? Nothing?

Okay, let's have a quick jump in the time machine and travel back to Harvard, 1966. Researchers Kuffler and Nicholl are eager to understand how potassium changes the electrical potential of a cell (yes, it's kept me awake for many a night too...).

What they inadvertently discovered was that when they stimulated the **neuron** it depolarised (that's the sodium/potassium interchange we have come to understand), but that wasn't the only thing. The **glia** depolarised too. At the time, they surmised this was probably caused by the potassium. Now, scientists understand many factors are involved, but the main catalyst is *not* potassium, but rather calcium.

So, skipping forward to 1986 to the Open University and a guy with a name to warm any Irish grandmother's heart, Sean Murphy. Whilst experimenting with rats he noticed that when neurons released transmitters, these stimulated astrocytes in the rat's neocortex and this caused an influx of calcium. Interesting, because less than a year after Kuffler's depolarisation paper another study had elucidated that there had to be calcium at a synapse for a neuron to be able to release neurotransmitters.

Now, where my books are always oozing with the blood of tortured rats I'll admit this section is distinctly froggy looking!

Sydney Ringer (1836-1910) was a British born physician from Norwich (I love Norwich, very pretty). He had spent most of his career working for University College, and then went on to be assistant physician at Great Ormond Street Hospital. Ringer's *Handbook of Therapeutics* was a classic of its day and passed through an incredible thirteen editions between 1869 and 1897. This book had been originally commissioned as a revision of Jonathan Pereira's (1804-1853) massive *Elements of Materia Medica* (first edition from 1839), you might remember Pereira as one of the early authorities who had found that spikenard helped epilepsy. Now, Ringer wasn't really interested in the minutiae of traditional medical botany and materia medica (who would be? Strange people, them!). Instead, he produced a practical treatise where he concisely summarized the actions and indications of drugs.

Sydney Ringer had four papers published in The Journal of Physiology in the early 1880s. These are acknowledged as the starting point for the development of our modern understanding of how calcium contributes to the contraction of the heart. In them, Ringer established the relative importance of sodium, potassium, and calcium ions.

Ringer explained how he had discovered that if you put a frog heart into sodium it would stop beating. But, if you removed the blood and added a saline solution, it would still stop but it would slow gradually over a period of about 20 minutes.

Ringer and his associate had tried to restart the heart, using shocks, but to no avail. They next tried potassium chloride and then the darling of all internet cleaning recipes – bicarbonate of soda, but still, the heart would not beat (I'll bet there were no smears though!).

Then there was a fortuitous accident. He had instructed his student to place the heart in water and the student had done what I would have done. Rather than getting the distilled stuff he was supposed to have used he turned on the tap. Not only did the heart freakishly re-animate, but it continued to beat for four hours. As serendipity would have it, the amount of calcium put into London water supplies in the 1850s was almost an exact match to what we have in our bodies (Universe, which did you arrange first, the water or the frog?).

So, astrocytes communicate with one another, and with neurons and neurotransmitters through calcium waves. But what else does calcium do in our body?

Well, calcium is a cellular regulator to every bodily system. It is fundamentally important to reproduction, for example. When an egg is fertilised, a calcium wave through the ovum initiates conception. Both cellular division and development are calcium-dependant processes, and without enough calcium an embryo will not develop properly and sadly, it will die. Calcium also plays a critical role in oligodendrocyte function and survival.

So, how does it work?

Well, a cell is like a calcium TARDIS! It has internal complexes that means it can store between 10-50 times the rate of the intracellular space (that is: inside of the cell!). When the electrical signal reaches the end of the axon, calcium from the extracellular space floods the synapse. There is a mahoosive 20,000 times more extracellular calcium than there is inside of the cell. This flux encourages the internal complexes to release their own calcium and then these can be used to release neurotransmitters. It has been proven that this transmitter release from the calcium is instigated by the astrocytes.

Extracellular calcium stops a muscle from contracting, but when it drops below a certain level, muscles start to twitch uncontrollably.

Okay right – just for a second, stop reading. I want you to think about all the conditions that you can where there is some kind of uncontrolled twitching. I urge you to write these down now.

Done it?

Okay, moving on....

Most of the calcium inside of the cell attaches itself to proteins since calcium simply can't exist without interacting with *something*. It also particularly likes water molecules and nitrogen, for example.

Astrocytes communicate between themselves through calcium ion channels but it is thought that they communicate with neurons through a release of an important amino acid called glutamate, used in the synthesis of proteins.

Let's just have a recap on the functions of the astrocytes, to wrap it up in your head. They:

- Make up the BBB
- Provide nutrients to nervous tissue
- Regulate the repair and scarring processes of the brain and spinal cord after someone has sustained a traumatic brain injury
- Release gliotransmitters in a calcium dependant manner
- In contrast to neurons, which have two "processes" (axons and dendrites), glial cells just have the one
- Neurons generate action potentials…but glial cells can't do that
- Glial cells have a resting potential
- Very importantly, neurons have synapses to use neurotransmitters but glial cells don't
- There are between 10-50 times more glial cells in the brain compared to the number of neurons

So, after all that, how many of you are asking yourselves…

What has this got to do with cannabis?

And the answer is nothing.

But it has everything to do with the endo-cannabinoid system…

Because **glial cells also express *endocannabinoid* receptors.**

It is through them that the endogenous mechanism is built, that protects the brain and nervous system against inflammation and damage. All those amazing things we want to learn about cannabis, well, they are predominately done through glial cells.

Now, do you love glial cells?

I thought you would!

The Chemical Nervous System

Now, when I did my aromatherapy diploma when dinosaurs roamed the Earth in 1993, our learning only covered the electrical nervous system. In our very bones, we holistic therapists knew emotions affected disease, but nothing in physiology told us how. It wasn't until later that glia, endocannabinoids, and neurotransmitters literally filled the gaps.

The electrical system relies on chemistry to send messages to other neurons.

Some of the main neurotransmitters it uses are:

- Acetylcholine
- Dopamine
- Epinephrine/Adrenaline
- Norepinephrine
- Serotonin
- Glutamate
- GABA
- Endorphins

Serotonin

Let's start off simple.

Serotonin, you know.

It's the mood modulator, right?

Yyyyesssssss…

But also…

No.

It does *so* much more.

It's a neurotransmitter, of course, so it signals along and between nerves. About 80-90% of it is found in the gastrointestinal tract, but it is mainly found in the bowels, brain, and blood platelets.

It's especially important for constricting smooth muscles. It regulates cyclical body processes and contributes to wellbeing and happiness. With regards to mood modulation, doctors still can't decide if low levels of serotonin lead to depression or depression causes serotonin to drop. Either way, when we see low levels of serotonin, the person is rarely wearing a smile. Now, what's lovely is that CBD potentiates the GPCR $5HT_{1A}$, or the serotonin receptor.

Potentiate? Increases the power or likelihood.

Happier? Yep…

Regularly visiting the toilet? Yes. Or at least...not being punished by constipation.

This same 5HT receptor is involved in a whole host of processes, from how we perceive pain to how hungry we are, if we feel sick or anxious, and is even connected to sleep and addiction mechanisms. It is likely that CBD's interaction with this receptor is the reason for its anti-psychotic effects but also its anti-emetic, anxiolytic, and antidepressant prowess.

Interestingly, CBDA – the precursor to CBD - is only found in raw cannabis and has an even stronger affinity to this receptor, leading to possible innovations in anti-depressant and anti-nausea meds.

Dopamine

One of the rock stars of neurotransmission, I suspect we have all heard of dopamine and have at least a small understanding of what it does. In fact, the brain has several distinct dopamine pathways all affecting different aspects of movement and cognition.

The media is full of stories of how dopamine probably underpins our reward systems and may lead us to an understanding of addiction. More recent research leads to the suspicion that the mechanisms may be more complex. Undoubtedly, dopamine (DA) is released by dopaminergic neurons during times of pleasure. However, we now know it can also be released in nastier situations too. It seems it is how important or noticeable a person *expects* a situation to be that is the governing factor. What's more the signals will still fire, even if the occurrence doesn't actually come to fruition. It is the **_expectation_** that seems to fire the dopamine across the synapse.

Certainly, it plays a part in addiction, not least because drugs like cocaine and amphetamines directly release dopamine at the receptors, in a part of the brain called the mesolimbic pathway, causing this massive rush (through varying mechanisms depending on the drug of choice), as does cannabis. Dopamine is released across the synapses in times of pleasurable behaviour: during sex, on a winning streak at the roulette table and, of course, when eating cake! Consequently, dopamine is capable of persuading our mind to go and find the activity again. Mine kicks in before I have swallowed the frosting and so I reach for the next slice. However, it's not the pleasure we are feeling...it is the desire...and this party is all going on at the nucleus accumbens and the pre-frontal cortex.

Dopamine is produced by **_dopaminergic neurons_** in several brain locations: in the *substantia nigra pars compacta,* in the part of the midbrain called the *ventra tegmental* area, and in the *arcuate nucleus* of the hypothalamus. The name "substantia nigra" refers to the darkened colour of the neuromelanin filling the dopaminergic neurons and means "black substance."

It's a very temperamental thing, dopamine, and balance is absolutely vital. Too much or too little, both can send the system into melt down.

It's very, very, *very* delicate.

The main systems we know it controls now are as follows:

- Movement
- Memory
- Pleasurable reward
- Attention
- Inhibition of Prolactin production
- Sleep
- Mood
- Learning

Let's get the awkward one out of the way first…prolactin…manufactured by the pituitary when we give birth, this creates breast milk. During pregnancy, the levels sky rocket and then when baby appears we get melons that feel like bowling balls. Depending on your view point you may decide this is pleasurable or a really painful bind. Either way, potentially dopamine might be behind both your opinion and any potential pain you feel. Not to mention whether you find the experience utterly blissful or Hell on Earth, of course! Failure as a woman as I am, I fall into the latter, and I feel happier now I can potentially lay the blame neatly at dopamine's door.

Movement then.

Too little dopamine and movements become delayed and uncoordinated. If there is too much, then there are unnecessary and additional movements, like shaking or repetitive tics.

We spoke of how addiction seems to happen in the pre-frontal cortex. Well, so does memory. What's interesting is that scientists now suspect that dopamine might have some bearing on the choices our brain makes about whether it should stay in short term memory or whether it should be moved into the long-term archive. We'll look at that a lot more in depth in the PTSD clinical evidence. If you mull over the ramifications of the new hypothesis that dopamine is expectation, does that mean we make a choice on what we choose to store based on whether we think it will be important in the future? Yes, potentially it does. That's flipping clever, isn't it?

Goddess, I love neuroscience!

Balance, again, is quintessential here. Excess or deficiency...both will screw the memory.

One of the triggers for dopamine, bizarrely, is vision. What we see triggers dopamine release and that helps us to focus our attention. But...if dopamine concentration drops in the pre-frontal cortex, our attention is shot. Those who are still able to focus now might have guessed that there seems to be a link between reduced levels and attention deficit disorder.

The foreman of the dopamine factory is the frontal lobe. This seems to control how effectively information flows in from other parts of the brain. Communications commander, he keeps thinking clear. When he goes off sick, because his levels are low, we feel confused and unable to connect clear thoughts.

There are five dopamine receptors. For a change, this bit is easy. They are called D1-5!

D1 is the body's most abundant receptor, and along with D4 it controls our cognitive processing. We can expect to see low binding at D2 receptors in people suffering from social phobias and social anxiety. Evidence suggests some of the negative features associated with schizophrenia – apathy, anhedonia, and social withdrawal - must be associated with this deficient binding at this receptor.

Too much dopamine?

Bipolar behaviour.

The patient becomes hyper social or even hyper sexual and their thrill seeking goes off the scale. Mania can be blocked by using dopamine antagonists.

Psychosis too, seems to be related to abnormally inflated levels of dopamine at the neurons in the mesolimbic pathway. Remember cannabis supercharges dopamine release. This, in part, is accredited with contributing to later life psychosis and schizophrenia in patients who have been early life smokers of weed.

Very briefly, dopamine seems to be implicated in the control of vomiting and nausea.

It plays a huge part in the way the central nervous system processes pain. These are processed through the spine, thalamus, basal ganglia, insular cortex, singular cortex and the periaqueductal grey. In particular, we might think of how dopamine is responsible for how painful Parkinson's can become, mainly caused by the nerves been trapped at the base of the spine. Distress signals are sent out by the neurons, and the dopamine very kindly sends a massive ouch signal up the spine to the brain.

Lastly, returning to the idea of expectation, it seems likely that dopamine is involved in a person's decision-making process. I can see how that might play out, based on how scary an event might seem or how painful they expect it to be when they move, they become less and less likely to interact with the world and stay firmly in the chair.

Without getting too technical (because Goddess knows this book needs no help with that!), CBD modulates DA activity states in the mesolimbic pathway.

Balance, baby.

It's all about the balance.

GABA

Gamma Amino Butyric Acid is an amino acid functioning as a neurotransmitter. Its primary function is neurotransmission, calming the nerves and regulating muscle tone. It is estimated that between 20-50% of synaptic transmission is mediated by it.

It is very much associated with cognitive function such as memory, attention, and the specific learning associated with that. GABA is also implicated in psychiatric disorders such as anxiety and panic but also schizophrenia and addiction. GABA also plays a critical part in the dopamine system and these interactions have been hypothesized as contributing to bipolar disorder.

Organically, GABA is synthesized from glutamate in the brain. Many internet pages recommend to supplement with GABA, but that's probably a futile endeavour since it doesn't pass the blood brain barrier (there are some exceptions where the "net" is less dense in parts of the brain and specialised injections can permeate the barrier, but for the most part, GABA is denied entry). It acts at inhibitory synapses in the brain, binding equally to both pre- and post-synaptic receptors. When working as a ligand, activating the receptor, ion channels open. Negatively charged chloride ions flood out of the cell and positively charged potassium ions flow in, inducing hyperpolarization. Incidentally, neurons that ***produce*** GABA mainly have an inhibitory function in the system and are referred to as ***GABAergic neurons***.

GABA produces this inhibitory effect by binding to two types of receptor.

- $GABA_A$ receptors – Here the GABA works as part of a team in a complex signalling system, thereby controlling chlorine ion channels. These mediate both tonic and phasic signalling.
- $GABA_B$ receptors – Directly use G Proteins to open ion channels.

Much to my Mind-Body Spirit delight, GABAergic mechanisms also creep out of the brain and into the periphery, creating this glorious body-mind bridge. These mechanisms have been discovered in intestinal, stomachic, and pancreatic tissues, in the fallopian tubes, the ovaries and testes, in kidney tissue, and the tissues of the bladder, lungs, and liver. Recent advances also uncovered the same GABAergic mechanism seems to exist in the respiratory airways, possibly influencing asthmatic stress mechanisms.

It is very clear that cannabis has a positive effect on GABA, and that CBD is the master coordinator, but until very recently it was not understood how (just for you to see how new this research is I am typing this on April 25th '17 and the paper I am citing is dated for next month, May 2017!).

So, it has all been happening at The University of Sydney, Australia. They wanted to understand the same as we do: that CBD possesses anti-epileptic, anxiolytic, and hyper-analgesic properties, but how specifically is it making that happen?

Brace yourselves people, we have two electrovoltage clamps...

These are used to study the electrophysiology of the brain and here we are looking at comparisons between what 2-AG does to the receptor and what CBD does.

Now, theoretically over 800 receptors *could* exist in the brain, but thankfully for you and I (and particularly my increasingly exhausted typing fingers), there are only 9 unequivocally identified as being GABA receptors. Their subunits are important and interesting because they act like "*x* marks the spot on a physiological map", identifying which synapses they influence. For example, in the limbic system there are lots of GABA$_A$ receptors containing the A5 subunit, and these are involved in learning and memory.

The trial isolates two:

- A synaptic receptor - **α1-6βγ2**
- And an extra-synaptic receptor - **α4β2δ** (known to mediate tonic currents in a large range of cells)

They found that CBD and 2-AG were both positive allosteric modulators of α1-6βγ2. In other words, they steadied the G protein at the allosteric site (that's not the enzyme's usual site on the cell, but the back door). However, this effect was at low micromolar potency...so just itsy bitsy tinsy wincey amounts. The greatest effect of either the CBD or the 2-AG, was on any GABA$_A$ subunits that contained α2.

I know, I know...I haven't told you what α2 is.

That's because it is the most glorious punchline. As a holistic therapist, I feel like screaming it from the rooftops...

It's an adrenergic receptor – one that responds to adrenaline or noradrenaline.

In other words, the strongest effect of the CBD or the 2-AG was by calming receptors that were on the hunt for stress hormones.

If you watched the G Proteins video, you might remember me saying it's usually the alpha subunit that binds, but sometimes it can be the beta. Here is an example of that because the CBD also exerted a strange preferential effect, preferring to bind with B2/3 subunits over B1, if it had the choice (there are 8 different types of beta subunit in total). The anxiolytic, anti-epilepsy, and the hyper-analgesic effects of CBD may come about through interaction with the $GABA_A$ receptor.

I hope you were listening then, because I intend to test you on that later!

Gruelling, isn't it? But my goodness, what a sense of achievement to understand that.

And y'know...wow!

Since the blood brain barrier restricts access to GABA, supplementing people with Alzheimer's, ADD, anxiety, schizophrenia, or any of the other things implicated is futile and yet...CBD gets there all by itself, it leapfrogs the blood brain barrier and gets to work.

It flabbergasts me. The truth is weirder than MLM fiction.

Going back eons in history now to October 2016 when I started writing this book, this paper from the University of Barcelona was one of the first studies to make me cry (many hempen tears have been shed since then). They built on the existing data that showed that a combination of CBD and THC could reduce the symptoms of an engineered Alzheimer's - like rat illness, when it was chronically administered in the early stages of the disease. Their trial continued that work and proved that it would also help to alleviate symptoms if used later in the illness too. This was due to increased level of $GABA_A$ RA1 (receptor alpha 1 subunit), and that it reduced the activity taking place at the glutamate receptor GLR2/3.

So that's memory...but what about anxiety?

Well...

In 2015, a paper was published by The Department of Pharmacology at The University of Sao Paolo, Brazil, entitled: *"Dissociation between the panicolytic effect of cannabidiol microinjected into the substantia nigra, pars reticulata, and fear-induced antinociception elicited by bicuculline administration in deep layers of the superior colliculus: The role of CB1-cannabinoid receptor in the ventral mesencephalon."*

Snappy, isn't it? I might have it printed onto a t-shirt.

At first glance the paper is overwhelming, but if you stare at it for a couple of hours with your eyes half closed and kind of try not to focus, it is a bit like one of those 3D pictures. It starts to make sense and, actually, it's incredibly exciting.

It explains that panic seems to emanate from a GABA pathway that runs through neostriatum-nigral disinhibitory and nigro-tectal inhibitory, which are found in the basal ganglia. Now, I can't really fathom what these men in white coats did to my furry friends, but I can promise you it was not nice because they aimed to make them scared and to inflict lot of pain, which seemingly they achieved. They found that by blocking $GABA_A$ receptors in the deeper layers of the superior colliculus (in the midbrain), they could terrify our rodent heroes into fiercely defensive behaviour; poor mites. I might be able to forgive the aggressors though, because they uncovered a thoroughly exciting nugget that proved everything mums say about *"try to think about something else"* is right. As the furries panicked and tried to escape, there seemed to be a significant reduction in how much pain they were experiencing.

Then the scientists micro-injected cannabidiol into the substantia nigra (again, the basal ganglia), producing what was deemed to be a clear anti-aversive effect. They noticed the length of time they were defensively alert diminished, the frequency of them being immobile from their defensive reactions, and how long they stayed still was also reduced. The frequency and duration of explosive escape behaviour, expressed by running and jumps, were also calmed.

In short…relaxed rodents.

But as the Irish comedian Jimmy Cricket used to say:

"Come here, there's more…"

As the escape behaviour decreased you might expect they would remember they were in pain and let their minds dwell on that again…but they didn't.

The antinociceptic properties continued and their perception of their pain was diminished.

Glutamate

One of the main reasons CBD brings about such positive changes in mood and wellbeing is deemed to be because it modulates how excited the glutamate receptor gets. Just as CBD wades in to take THC's toys off it, she also acts as if she is snatching a bag of sweeties from a hyperactive glutamate. She calms the surplus secretion of glutamate, and then levels of tranquil GABA begin to rise to fill the gap. This GABA tone environment is a whole site more relaxed…no longer bouncing off the glutamate ceiling, CBD has worked its chill pill magic.

I think it is time we got a bit more acquainted with glutamate, don't you? He's no small player in the neurotransmitters arena, but he doesn't seem to have the sexiness of dopamine or the sunshine disposition of serotonin, and if I am allowed to say…I do think glutamate gets a rough deal, because everyone paints him as the bad guy. Having said that, glutamate is the body's most predominate excitatory neurotransmitter, and you might remember that astrocytes communicate to each other via its release.

Let's start with where he comes from, because he starts his biological life cycle as a different chemical…as glutamine. Glutamine has several key functions in human health, but most notably he forms the building block for the body's antioxidant complex glutathione. Glutamine is one of very few molecules able traverse the blood brain barrier to be converted from glutamine into glutamic acid, a precursor of GABA. So, GABA is then synthesized in the brain from glutamate.

Meanwhile, out in the body, glutamic acid (an amino acid) is converted into glutamine and then undergoes a reaction with sodium, which produces glutamate.

So, you will have grasped by now he's a neurotransmitter, but glutamate is also one of the twenty amino acids the body uses to assemble proteins. Its neurotransmitter action was identified in the early 1950s, but it wasn't really until the 1980s that the scientific community started excepting it as such. We primarily find it in the nervous system, but in other parts of the body too, notably in cerebro-spinal fluid.

It operates on three cell compartments:

- on the pre-synaptic neurons
- the post synaptic neurons and glia
- Together this is called the "tripartite glutamatergic synapse"

Between the three compartments, they control the release, uptake, and activation of glutamate by the different receptors. The main glutamate receptor has the enchanting name of N-methyl-D-aspartate. From now on we'll call it its more popular name of the NMDA receptor.

What does glutamate do?

Physically, when the conversion of glutamic acid and glutamine takes place, it also detoxifies the system of ammonia.

Most ammonia in the body forms from proteins broken down by bacteria in the intestines. The liver cleanses the system by removing ammonia via two pathways, through urea and through this glutamine synthesis. Likewise, skeletal muscle relies solely on glutamine synthesis to remove ammonia, as does the brain.

If we are unlucky enough to have a raised level of ammonia in our blood, then we are going to experience muscle weakness and fatigue. If we are very unlucky we might even suffer liver and kidney damage or failure. Left untreated, raised levels of ammonia in the blood can affect brain tissue, leading to confusion and delirium. Expect to see a rapid change in cognitive function.

Not much fun, and so we applaud glutamine for sorting this particular source of chaos out for us.

So, half close your eyes and maybe you'll see the most glorious rainbow bridge forming between the body and mind, because while glutamate and its predecessors clean the system, they also affect the mind.

For cells to communicate across the nervous system they need glutamate. Memory formation, learning, and general housekeeping of the nervous system all rely on its turning up to work each day. It processes information, regulates brain development, and measures information about the survival of each cell.

Glutamate forms and eliminates synapses.

So, when the doctor recommends doing your brain training as you get older, it's because glutamate assesses which thought processes haven't been used for a while, and then he declutters. Use them or lose them, is wholly glutamate modulated. Hence, glutamate must be present in the right concentrations in the right place at the right time. Too much glutamate is harmful, but so is too little. If you have too much glutamate, very much like cannabis, it turns from friend to foe.

Used in myriad different ways in a multitude of system junctures throughout the body, it's easy to see how signalling dysfunction could be implicated in so many diseases.

Glutamate Receptors

Now, I made a fundamental error when I was researching this area. I surmised there was a glutamate receptor.

There's not.

That is, there is not only one. There are more than twenty different glutamate receptors found in the mammalian central nervous system, and they are extremely complex.

They fall into two main categories:

- **ionotropic** – sensitive to changes in voltage across the cell membrane
- **metabotropic** – These bind with ligands

Then, each ionotropic or metabotropic receptor has three different sub types decided by their binding specificity, ion permeability and conductance properties, as well as other factors.

So, each type has multiple subtypes.

Let's get a bit more specific.

Ionotropic receptors act speedily. When they open they alter the flow of current into the cell. Significant changes occur, even if the differences in voltages across the membrane are minute.

So, if glutamate works as a ligand here, it binds to a metabotropic receptor then its relative channel undergoes a conformational change. Extracellular sodium and other ions rush into the cells and potassium rushes out. When depolarization is triggered in the post-synaptic cell, it's enough to transmit a signal. This will seem very intangible now, until you get to the sections on memory or epilepsy for example, when you see how startling a difference it can be when CBD says: *"No more firing, you guys, let's give her head a chance to catch up"*, or likewise it says: *"Bit more, bit more, bit more, we need to get those galloping so they catch up the firing by such and such a receptor."* CBD is all about balance and its ability to get these receptors to move in harmony that allows it to do truly impossible things, ease epilepsy, straighten out memories, even perhaps make the voices in someone's head stop.

In a 2011 paper from Sao Paulo University in Brazil *The interplay of cannabinoid and NMDA glutamate receptor systems in humans: preliminary evidence of interactive effects of cannabidiol and ketamine in healthy human subjects"*, it was suggested that interactions between glutamatergic and endocannabinoid systems might contribute to schizophrenia, dissociative states, and other psychiatric conditions. Working as a weak partial agonist to both CB_1 and CB_2, Cannabidiol (CBD) potentially plays a role in future treatment of schizophrenia through its interaction with NMDA receptor.

So, we have all these different kinds of glutamate receptors and the properties do differ somewhat, as does their distribution throughout the body, but for the most part, glutamate receptors are best known for looking after learning and memory, for modifying properties of different ion channels, for enhancing glutamate neurotransmission, and for the gene expression that ensures the perpetuation of disease/health.

Our brains are immensely capable of learning, remembering, and recovering from injuries and plasticity. Endocannabinoids tend to congregate at sites of traumatic brain injury and dictate how fast or well it will heal. CBD can often help such healing and this can be attributed to improvement of how well synapses work in relation to NMDA signalling, particularly in the hippocampus.

The basic mechanisms that support plasticity – your brain/mind growing and changing – include:

- neurogenesis – where the brain grows new neurons
- activity-dependent refinement of synaptic strength (the way we remember things as part of our experience of them but also by repetitive "doing")
- pruning of synapses – getting rid of the ones we don't need

Now, as I said, I had erroneously concluded there was just the one glutamate receptor. That one is NDMA (*N*-methyl *D*-aspartate) which is expressed on neurons. It is one of the *main* glutamate ionotropic receptors, but it works in a rather peculiar manner. It's what's known as a **coincidence detector**. In other words, it needs two specific things to happen at the same time for it to work. In this case, to get the channel to open:

- glutamate must bind to the receptor (obvious)
- but the post-synaptic cell also needs to be depolarized (i.e. it needs to have a negative charge)

And this is because magnesium blocks entry into the channels. The gateway can only open when the negative charge has kicked magnesium out of the way.

So that was **ionotrophic** glutamate receptors. How does that compare with **metabotropic** ones?

Well, metabotropic glutamate receptors act far more slowly and they exert their effects *in*directly. They make their changes in the body through gene expression and protein synthesis.

Broadly, there are three groups of glutamate metabotropic receptors. Again, distinguished by their pharmacological and signal transduction properties. In total, scientists have thus far cloned eight subtypes of metabotropic glutamate receptor. Each group is positively affected by CBD.

Group I metabotropic receptors are predominately expressed on the postsynaptic membrane of a cell, and are suspected to be implicated in learning and memory problems, addiction, and motor regulation, as well as Fragile X syndrome, one of the most inherited common causes of learning disabilities. Affecting about 1 in 4000 males and 1 in 8000 females, this Fragile X anomaly contributes to a whole host of learning difficulties, as well as language, attentional, emotional, social, and behavioural problems.

Group II metabotropic receptors are also situated on postsynaptic cells, but can be found on presynaptic cells too. Potentially, this might be an elaborate mechanism that nature created to suppress glutamate transmission. If group II metabotropic receptors are dysfunctional, expect to see anxiety, schizophrenia, or Alzheimer's disease.

Group III metabotropic receptors are also presynaptic and their function is to inhibit the amounts of neurotransmitters released. Found within the hippocampus and hypothalamus, they may be involved in Parkinson's disease and some anxiety disorders.

Okay, so we understand how the signalling works on the most minute monomolecular level! But let's have a look at what the body might look like if too little glutamate is circulating, and likewise too much.

Glutamate deficiency

I've noticed a very strange connection between glutamate and cannabis. Look at symptoms of low levels of glutamate, and it reads like a synopsis of someone who has been smoking marijuana for a long time:

- Depression and poor attention span
- Fast heart rate (tachycardia) or slowed heart rate (bradycardia)
- Decreased feeling or loss of sensation of pain
- Loss of appetite or decreased perception of taste
- Weakened emotional response: apathy, anhedonia, where a person does not show anger, joy, and sadness
- Mental fatigue
- Difficulty collecting thoughts, demotivation, passivity
- They show weird eye responses, sometimes delayed, untimely movement, or fixate on a specific object/target (that really sounds stoned, doesn't it?!)
- Profound hypotension (low blood pressure), or they are likely to go dizzy when they stand up too quickly

Now the similarities become utterly bizarre.

Glutamate deficiency gives an:

- Altered perception of time and movement (sometimes overestimation, and more commonly, underestimation of internal time)

- Impaired perception of one's surrounding environment (how tall people are, objects, form, and writing appearance/placing)

Low levels of glutamate are linked to depression, obsessive-compulsive disorder, and schizophrenia.

How freakin' strange is that?

Glutamate Excess

So, deficiency was fairly straight forward, and to be fair, it is very rare. Excess, not so much. Perhaps you've never heard of glutamate, or even its excitability, but it's a very common problem. As it spirals out of control all manner of nasties climb out of the woodwork.

Neuro-degenerative conditions featuring glutamate excitotoxicity is a growing list. Some of these include:

- ALS
- Alzheimer's
- Autism
- Brain trauma and brain injury
- Huntington's
- Multiple sclerosis
- Parkinson's
- Schizophrenia
- Seizure disorders
- Stroke and ischemia

Excitotoxicity can come from two things. Firstly, that there is far too much glutamate in the system, but also secondly, receptors become hypersensitive, needing the very tiniest of nudges to activate them. It destroys neurons. Diseases of this kind often develop after some kind of traumatic brain injury. The assault causes a rapid increase in glutamate receptors, then subsequently leads to neuronal cell death. Recent studies show altered levels of glutamate taken from the cerebrospinal fluids and serum of patients with mood disorders, often exhibiting altered levels of glutamate. This is especially so for people with bipolar disorder and major depressive disorder. Likewise, glutamate is implicated in seizure disorders. In 2012, a paper was released entitled *"Towards a glutamate hypothesis of depression"* which suggested signalling impairments might underpin that disease too. A study by Zheng *et al.,* 2016, proposed blood glutamate levels as a potential biomarker of autism spectrum disorder.

Glutamate imbalance then... Seriously bad news...

Activating CB$_1$ receptors reduces glutamate release, but CBD acts in a far more dynamic way. It harnesses and controls glutamate _modulating_ receptors, always working as a buffer to send levels of glutamate back to a point of balance.

Truly incredible when you let the ramifications of that flood over you.

Glutathione

CBD strongly affects and regulates the glutathione system.

Anyone's hand up on what glutathione is?

No? I'd have been looking sheepishly around the room, hoping the teacher didn't pick me too.

This is an exciting one peeps…

Serious healing here.

Glutathione is an antioxidant that prevents damage by ROS, free radicals, peroxides, and heavy metals. In particular, it cleanses the body of mercury accumulated through amalgam in your fillings or from seafood (since eating more fish oils is advised to reboot your endocannabinoid system, knowing that fish can poison me with mercury makes me feel like I am on a conveyor belt of doom!).

Now, mercury poisoning… Here's a strange thing.

Checkout the effects it can cause. It reads very much like a list of conditions where cannabis would be indicated.

Incidentally, I flagrantly stole this list from:

http://www.dentalwellness4u.com/layperson/symptoms.html

Digestive System
- Colitis
- Diarrhoea/constipation
- Loss of appetite
- Nausea/vomiting
- Weight loss

Head
- Dizziness
- Faintness
- Frequent headaches
- Ringing in ears

Heart

- Anaemia
- Chest pain
- Rapid or irregular heartbeat

Lungs

- Asthma/bronchitis
- Chest congestion
- Shallow respiration
- Shortness of breath

Muscles & Joints

- Cramping
- Joint aches
- Muscle aches
- Muscle weakness
- Stiffness

Neurological/Mental

- Fine tremor
- Lack of concentration
- Learning disorders
- Short and long-term memory loss
- Numbness
- Slurred speech

Nose

- Inflammation of the nose
- Sinusitis
- Excessive mucus formation
- Stuffy nose

Oral/Throat

- Bad breath (halitosis)
- Bone loss
- Burning sensation
- Chronic coughing
- Gingivitis/bleeding gums
- Inflammation of the gums
- Leucoplakia (white patches)
- Metallic taste
- Mouth inflammation
- Sore throats
- Ulcers of oral cavity
- Allergies
- Anorexia
- Excessive blushing
- Genital discharge
- Gland swelling
- Hair loss
- Hypoxia
- Frequent illnesses
- Insomnia
- Loss of sense of smell
- Perspiration excessive
- Renal failure
- Skin cold and clammy
- Skin problems
- Vision problems (tunnel vision)
- Water retention (oedema)

Emotions

- Aggressiveness
- Fits of anger
- Anxiety

- Confusion
- Depression
- Fear and nervousness
- Hallucination
- Lethargy
- Manic depression
- Mood swings
- Shyness
- Energy Levels
- Apathy

Now look at *conditions* exacerbated by mercury poisoning.

- Chronic tiredness
- Restlessness
- Acrodynia
- Alzheimer's
- Anterior lateral sclerosis (ALS)
- Asthma
- Arthritis
- Autism
- Candida
- Cardiovascular disease
- Chronic fatigue syndrome
- Crohn's disease
- Depression
- Developmental defects
- Diabetes
- Eczema
- Emphysema
- Fibromyalgia
- Hormonal dysfunction
- Intestinal dysfunction
- Immune system disorders
- Kidney disease
- Learning disorders
- Liver disorders
- Lupus
- Metabolic encephalopathy
- Multiple sclerosis (MS)

- Reproductive disorders
- Parkinson's disease
- Senile dementia
- Thyroid disease

Mercury has a cataclysmic effect on the immune system and its inherent detoxification systems. Many symptoms we see throughout this book result from chronic mercury poisoning (directly or indirectly). How many of these symptoms, and how bad you experience them, can depend on a whole cocktail of factors. We need to be considering:

- how many fillings you have had
- how long you've had them
- how often they are being rubbed by food, toothbrushes, etc.

Mercury is classified as a neurotoxin. It causes or contributes to emotional and psychological issues, such as depression, anxiety, mood swings, and memory loss. It's all looking awfully familiar, isn't it?

Mercury also indirectly harms the system, depleting essential antioxidants like glutathione and alpha lipoic acid. The body needs these to rid the body, not only of mercury, but other harmful toxins and free radicals too. Thus, it could be indirectly contributing to even more symptoms and diseases than appear on this list.

What's rather fortuitous, then, is CBD increases glutathione. Much of the wonder of the medicine is through its anti-oxidant genius.

Chemo-protective genes work tirelessly as anti-oxidants to fight free radicals.

Phase II and phase III detox genes are very good at linking to toxins like mercury (and other heavy metals) and transporting them out of the body. One lecture I listened to described them very eloquently, the tutor called them *"molecular chaperones"* or *"repair molecules"*.

Let's hit the time machine again and head for Naples. We're going back to the university mouse labs in October 2016. I will warn you though, we are heading straight into torture.

Our four-legged friends had high levels of inflammation and hyper motility induced in their intestines. In other words, they were given colitis. They were then given CBD oil inter-peritoneally and then orally. The volume of CBD was assessed in the colon, the brain, and liver after the oral treatments, and then again after the injection in their tummies. Analysis showed CBD reducing damage to the colon, attenuating injury and motility. *"These findings sustain the rationale of combining CBD with other minor cannabis constituents and support the clinical development of CBD for IBD treatment."*

Now what's weird and hideous and scary, is these diseases and neurological problems can arise when there has been an infection and the activity of the glial cells has been activated.

Infection in the brain? So how on Earth does *that* happen?

Too blinking easily for my liking!

Truly, it is like some kind of terrifying horror movie, gals.

I'm warning you: brace yourselves.

We need to think about every aromatherapist's favourite bit of the body, the blood brain barrier (BBB). Strangely enough before this research, I had never really considered what it was made of or how it did its job. So, let's start there. It's made up of epithelial tissue. Oddly, the network of cellular elements that make up the BBB are very similar in constitution to the tight junctions in the cells that line up the digestive system. That is: they have intricately tight junctions present between each part. This forms a *diffusion* barrier, like body guards, showing real prejudice about who should and should not come in. It is a successful system. By monitoring the entry of substances into the brain, it protects it well. It allows essential nutrients to cross over into the hallowed realms but bars the way to toxins and other harmful particles.

And it is great...when it's working.

So, what can affect it?

Terrifyingly, it seems like *everything*:

- stress
- infection
- changes in our gut flora
- poor diet
- food sensitivities

The link with food and stomach is a big one. All of these "challenges" loosen tight junctions in our gut and make it more permeable, thus compromising the barrier. Our gut lining becomes inflamed and leaky. Suddenly, unfriendly particles are escaping from the gut and entering the blood stream and then career headlong to parts of the body that really shouldn't have them.

Heavens a-plenty, it is like a scene from The Walking Dead!

Zombie intestinal cells on the rampage!

Bad huh?

I haven't even begun...

Research published in 2011 in the Physiological Reviews Journal terrified the pants off me. It speaks about a lovely protein called zonulin. Now, between you and me, zonulin is a door supervisor of the very highest order. As such, he works two jobs simultaneously. He regulates the function of the tight junctions in the blood brain barrier but he also looks after the intestinal barrier of the gut. Thing is, zonulin is a bit of a soft touch and he is easily persuaded to let the odd unsavoury type in.

Now in 2006, the Scandinavian Journal of Gastroenterology found that **gliadin**, (a protein found in wheat and gluten) increases levels of zonulin. So, if someone is having an adverse reaction to wheat, zonulin increases his shifts, so the soft touch is on the barrier more often letting far too many toxins in. Those previously tight junctions become more permeable. The barriers don't work properly, leading to *both* a leaky gut *and* a leaky brain...and there is no defensive wall between them.

It's a whole new dimension to "*S**t for brains*" really, isn't it?

But in this story the sky is going to turn even darker and the background music becomes tenser, because what happens now is truly sinister.

The leaky barrier brings all kind of unpleasantness into the brain, so then the body shouts *"invader, invader",* a band of astrocytes and microglia wage war on the infection. The problem is...*they're* not supposed to be in the brain either...they are Roman conquerors in an unknown land. Confused and power hungry, what would normally have been rather *pleasant* microglia turn *mean,* and start to attack the brain.

Microglia release ROS, which in this context work as neurotoxic agents. They release TNF alpha and Interleukin 1, both of which are perfectly designed to create a large inflammatory reaction designed to kill any infection. But now, the insidious truth becomes clear...

This will now continue to happen in the absence of the infection.

The body is now creating inflammatory responses in the brain that really have no place being there. When you see chronic illnesses, you can bet you will see these low levels of infection that seem to be on a continuous loop inside of the brain.

Some more delights that can activate this:

- Lyme Disease – a horrible disease caught from tics.
- HHV6 – Human herpes virus 6 (most people have this but it lies dormant in the system until it is activated). Then we see astrocytes being recruited into the brain, causing even more inflammation.

- Beta amyloid plaques - It used to be that scientists thought these caused Alzheimer's, but now it seems likely that it is the inflammation and background infections that tend to be found beneath them that cause the issues.
- Mould toxins – Here, it is not only the mould itself, but also the immune reactions that they provoke that can cause problems with the BBB.

So, we see this proinflammatory loop, but then it becomes self-propagating, activating, activating, activating.

Now, we want to add to the cocktail of doom with lipopolysaccharides (LPS). These are found in the outer membrane of Gram-negative bacteria. They elicit very strong immune responses and can often find their way into the system, either from a leaky gut or from a sinus infection. Again, these LPS activate the immune system, provoking the glia to emit proinflammatory cytokines. These damage neurons, which then squeal to the big boss "*Skipper, I'm down*" and so more immune signalling comes pouring in. At every turn, they are ramping up the inflammatory release of glia.

So, we have this wheel feedback effect, don't we? Think of it like the wind turning the sails of a mill. The wind here might be immune-based triggers, or equally it might come from some kind of neurotoxin.

Whatever happens, in this situation the toxin will always activate the **NMDA receptor,** the glutamate receptor.

Right, so if you were in The Waking Dead...what strategy or weapon would you employ to keep yourself safe? (well, I wouldn't be going into sheds that's for sure! Why do they always do that, please?). I think I would be building barricades, wouldn't you?

How about if it told you that there was a way to plug those gaps in the gut and contain the scary stuff inside? Sounds like a plan, doesn't it?

Well, it *is* possible, if you can find a spectacular thing called claudin. Claudin creates proteins that seal up the gut. The only thing is they don't set it in Tesco, or Aldi, or even in the poshest aisles of Waitrose. You need to make it yourself.

Well that's rubbish then, I hear you cry.

Oh, just a minute, I forgot to say....

Both CBD and THC affect glutathione triggering the body to manufacture claudin, seal up the gut, and tone those helpfully tight junctions.

With CBD-rich cannabis oil...ain't none of those zombie cells gettin' out.

(I feel the need for an epic soundtrack of victory here, don't you?).

Adenosine

Adenosine occurs naturally in every cell and is the creator of cellular energy by forming the "cell batteries" ADP and ATP. It's a neurotransmitter and appears to play an important role in sleep initiation. If concentration of adenosine in arousal centres of the brain increase, you stay awake longer. By contrast, partaking of a steaming cup of caffeine blocks adenosine and thus gives us the wakeful boost we need to get through the day. It's thought caffeine gives us the jitters (increased alertness or anxiety) because adenosine receptors that would normally inhibit how much glutamate is released are now being blocked so levels sporadically surge.

Adenosine's got other jobs too of course, just as these neurotransmitters always do.

It dilates coronary blood vessels and so improves circulation to the heart and increases the diameter of the blood vessels, supplying peripheral organs and giving them more flow too.

By contrast it decreases renal flow, reducing the amount of the blood flow enzyme, renin, produced in the kidneys.

In the lungs, adenosine constricts airways. In the liver, it constricts the blood vessels that break down glycogen to make glucose. It's a busy little bee and CBD ensures adenosine receptors are always engaged and healthy. It's thought that CBD's activation of these adenosine receptors contributes greatly to its anti-inflammatory power, but also make it such a spectacular anti-anxiety agent.

Adenosine receptors contribute to the release of dopamine and glutamate, indirectly affecting cognition, motor control, motivation, and reward mechanisms.

In 2010, Hospital Universitario Fundación Alcorcón, Madrid, discovered brain damage, caused by a drop in oxygen, could be helped by CBD. Here it's neuroprotective mechanism derived from a beautiful interplay between the adenosine receptors and CB_2.

Glycine

Again, an amino acid and a neurotransmitter, this binds to GlyR – the Glycine receptor. One of the most widely distributed inhibitory receptors in the Central Nervous System, the actions of GlyR are mediated via chlorine flux.

It seems to be implicated in neuropathic pain and inflammation signals transmitted through the spinal cord to the brain stem.

When glycine levels go out of whack, the patient experiences exaggerated responses to unexpected stimuli going completely, albeit temporarily, rigid. A clue to glycine problems is chronic and repeated falling, resultant from these nasty jumps.

It can play a stimulatory or depressant role in the nervous system and seems to be related to sleep and cognition. Clinical trials showed supplementation of glycine improves sleep quality and reduces fatigue. Supplementation of glycine also reduces symptoms of schizophrenia, but sadly the amount needed would be unmanageable as a prescriptive treatment.

Formidably, research shows CBD strengthening glycine channels.

Acetylcholine

One of the major neurotransmitters found in the peripheral nervous system (along with noradrenaline), acetylcholine is found at neuromuscular terminals and controls muscle function.

It usually, although not always, exerts an excitatory effect on the body, and works within the autonomic nervous system (ANS). The ANS brings the body back into homeostasis using automatic functions like heart rate, respiration, or pupils dilating. It controls how much saliva we produce, our digestion, urinary output, and sexual arousal.

Emotionally, its job is to temper some of the more severe effects of hard emotions. If we are angry, the acetylcholine weakens our heart and stiffens our arteries, protecting the body against the biological changes of fury. Problems naturally occur if you have high cholesterol, because then this stiffening easily leads to heart attacks.

Depleted levels are related to the memory loss seen in Alzheimer's. Magnesium levels preserve and protect acetylcholine, inhibiting its release. Deficient magnesium/excess of calcium also results in too much acetylcholine circulating in the system, and thus hyper-exciting the nervous system.

It binds to the nicotinic receptor, and although it's not closely implicated with CBD, Mahgoub *et al.* established CBD interacting with α7-nicotinic acetylcholine receptors in a 2013 study.

Chapter 7 Lessons from Homeopathy

Cannabis in Homeopathy

When I took my Advanced Diploma of Aromatherapy in 1994 we had to complete a module on miasm. It is a contentious issue and many homeopaths often discount it as far-fetched. To make things more difficult, it is very confusing. I must say, though, that in conditions such as psoriasis, for example, I have found it to be an illuminating and helpful tool. I think it adds a very useful dimension to understanding how cannabis might be helpfully used as an essential oil.

Miasm

The theory of miasm belongs to Samuel Hahnemann M.D (1755-1843), the founder of homeopathy. You may hear him referred to as the Father of Experimental Pharmacology because he was the first physician to prove medicines on *healthy* human beings. He did this because he wanted to understand the actions each medicine went through to their outcome of curing diseases. In other words... *How* did each medicine heal?

Prior to this, people had only really ever gone on indicators and anecdotal evidence rather than trying to obtain documented physiological evidence. It is kind of where we are at now with cannabis oil, I suppose, thanks to political restraints on testing.

His research was vast and marvellous. He discovered incredible healing abilities of inert substances such as gold, platinum, silica, vegetable charcoal, etc., as well as in plants. He processed these medicines in a dosage-related system called *potentization* and, in doing so, he managed to create substances that were soluble in alcohol or water (not normally possible for something like gold, for instance) and found these substances held medicinal forces.

He became a very well sought-after physician with a great deal of healing success. In due course, though, he became troubled by the fact that his successes seemed to be confined to acute conditions. *Chronic* conditions didn't seem to respond as well to his remedies and he undertook to understand why that might be. After many years of study, he presented his ideas about miasm in his book *The Organon of the Healing Art*, published in 1810. The sixth edition of this, published in 1921, is still a foundation work of homeopathy today.

The way I was taught miasm was that it was an inherited disposition to disease, and whilst oversimplified, this is by far the easiest way to understand and remember it. It is a complicated system and so any kind of leg up you can secure to getting your head round it is okay with me, so...**Miasm is an inherited disposition to disease!**

Hahnemann proposed three main types of miasm, these are:

- Psora
- Sycotic
- Syphylitic

He was certain all chronic disease was underpinned by at least one of these and often two, or more infrequently all three. Miasmic healing went out of fashion for a while, but recently there has been a resurgence of interest into it. Since then, several further miasms have been added to the list. For the purposes of this book, these three will suffice.

He considered most illness stemming from psora, and that sychotic and syphilitic probably made up about twenty percent of chronic disease, but also had elements of psora within them.

I will warn you that the whole of this section is pretty mucus-laden and grotesque! The word *miasm* itself means infection, dirtiness, stain, and blotch. We can deduce then, a blotch on one's constitution.

Psora

A very quick overview of psora, since it's not *really* relevant to this work but for roundedness… Hahnemann described psora as one of the oldest diseases into existence. He felt that it originated from ancestral suppression of leprosy. Psora disease had, he felt, spread throughout the world from around 600 BC up to the middle ages.

The word comes from **scabies** in Greek. He suggested the moment the scabies itch touched the skin an infection began to form. We now know he was very close to the truth. It takes about 6 to 10 days for the infection to take hold, but by the time a vesical has formed, he was right: the whole body has been infected.

The psora miasm describes "the intolerable itch". Think of skin eruptions described as dirty, dry, or itchy. Consider eczema, and how cracks appear in the hands and feet. Sufferers might also smell because they sweat so much. This perspiration is worse in sleep, so patients can often smell offensive (it's a bit different to the sweet fragrances of aromatherapy, isn't it?). It becomes a syndrome of symptoms.

When recognising expressions of miasm, we notice how the mind and body work together as a unit, and how things will also disturb it. In the psoric miasm we witness the body reacting in a specific way when exposed to environmental stimuli. We might say to one's surroundings things like light, noise, particularly fragrance. Think of how these disturb the body in conditions like a headache or nausea, for example.

Physically a person will talk about how their skin itches, their burning sensations, how they are prone to inflammation, and then in turn this might lead to congestion. The easiest example to imagine is somebody with hay fever.

Psoric Physical Traits

If you try to describe the pain of the psoric miasm, it would be with words like *sore, bruised* or perhaps *neurological*. Clinically we will see *acidity, burning,* how this congestion has led to *constipation* and *flatulence*. Of course, we can see *itchy skin,* but also *burning of the spinal-cord*.

Personality Traits of Psora

A person who is predominantly this type of person will emotionally *exhibit highs and lows*. They *struggle with the outside world* and this becomes particularly important *when they're stressed*. They're *rarely confident* people, they often talk of feeling *constantly anxious,* they're often *afraid that they cannot cope or achieve new things*. These are *insecure* people, they are *anxious about the future,* but *hopeful and incredibly clever, mentally alert people.* In summary, these people are *deep philosophers*. They can be quite *selfish*, though very *restful in their outlook*, *physically and emotionally weak,* and often *very fearful*.

Syphilitic

Syphylitic has a central theme of hidden-ness. The person experiences an innate sense of something being very wrong inside of them. Emotionally, this might be expressed as dreadful guilt or self-criticism. They will go through life afraid to show others their true self, often projecting their feelings of self-dread onto the world, being suspicious, afraid, angry, or even violent. Since the dread is hidden so deep within the psyche, the individual rarely has opportunity to recognise or name it.

These fears often translate into a fear of being attacked. So, kids become terrified of going to sleep, lest the monster under the bed might get them, and people who suffer from agoraphobia live in terror of what lies outside the door. As the world becomes ever scarier, in its worst manifestation a person suffering from syphilitic miasm might feel there is only one way to end their fear cycle: kill it or kill me.

Physically illnesses often remain shrouded until they are in a very severe state. Heart disease, for example, might remain from view until the patient has a heart attack.

Sychotic

This is the miasm we are most interested in, because along with *Thuja* and a homeopathic remedy, *Medorrhinum,* both *Cannabis sativa* and *Cannabis indica* are specifically indicated as remedies for people exhibiting symptoms of the sychotic miasm.

Hahnemann initially became intrigued by this miasm when he noticed male patients who had been allopathically treated for gonorrhoea (that is to say, the doctor had treated them) and had been cured all began to exhibit the same sets of symptoms and predispositions after the gonorrhoea had left the body. Weirder, he noticed the *wives* of these men also exhibited similar traits, even if they had met their husbands after the gonorrhoea had already been treated. In other words, they had been affected by the gonorrhoea in a way that could not be attributed to the outward symptoms alone.

Even more strange is that children of these couples also seemed to have common traits, that again were not symptoms of the gonorrhoea, but seemed to derive from it and somehow impacted on the future generations of the sufferer.

He proposes that the ***symptoms are the result of the suppression of gonorrhoea***; that by removing warts and taking away the outward healing mechanism of the disease, it forced the gonorrhoea deep into the tissues. This simply set up a whole new set of symptoms and personality traits. The future generations of the line inherit these traits. So, to be clear, just as a person might never have a scabies rash on their skin but still experience the difficulties of the psoriatic miasm, the same applies for syphilis in the syphilitic miasm and gonorrhoea here in sychotic, Remember...

Inherited predisposition to disease.

Sychotic Miasm

If we were to make a film about sychotic miasm, and we wanted to do a trailer, we could either call it "pus filled, green, and oozing", which has its own revolting appeal, or we could put in a hunk of an actor and go far more glamorous and hype it as being "a tale of excess, escape, and decadence".

Both would be correct.

The word sychotic comes from the Greek *sykon,* which means fig because delightfully, this describes the fig warts that often display around genitals with the disease.

The sychotic miasm is a collection of many facets, emotional and physical, and so here we are looking for ***patterns*** that may fit a patient, rather than focusing on the genital warts (a little less rude, Reader, avert your gaze from the figs please!).

Let's start with physical because that is usually the easiest to perceive when learning a new diagnostic tool.

Outward symptoms, according to Phyllis Speight in her 1961 Comparison of the Chronic Miasms, are as follows:

You will see your patient as being cross a lot of the time and very irritable. What is interesting, though, is his demeanour (and symptoms) become very much worse during the seasonal changes towards damper days. He exhibits very fixed thinking, and rather than just pertaining to inflexible thinking, we might see certain thoughts bordering on the obsessive and even possibly exhibiting as psychosis. They are very jealous and suspicious by nature. This probably stems from a deep dislike of their self, which can exhibit as self-condemnation and even on bad days, suicidal thoughts.

Here, I am going to point out an area of interest and confusion, mainly because it has bugged me so I suspect it may do the same to some of you:

- Sychotic – to do with the miasm
- Psychotic – disordered thoughts
- Sychosis – to do with the miasm
- Psychosis – disordered thoughts

That being said, you will see that, whilst there is most certainly an irrefutable relationship between the two, they are different things and one is not necessarily involved in the manifestation of the other.

Physical properties

Sychotic disease moves around. So, if there is a symptom that comes and then is fleetingly gone and then perhaps moves to somewhere else, you can suspect there may be a sychotic element to it. This is particularly true of things to do with fluids.

The psora miasm is to do with the Earth but our sychotic miasm is quintessentially linked to the body's requirement to keep fluids moving effectively and healthily. Specifically, it represents our relationship with water and the watery element. Given that we are made up of 60-80% water (depending on what age you are), you can see that this is a very profoundly acting miasm that permeates right into the very deepest tissues.

To clarify, a healthy relationship would mean we are not always thirsty - we do not become dehydrated, but conversely, we do not retain fluids in the case of oedema either. It is this capability to absorb fluids, to utilise them and eliminate them effectively, that is the primary physiological influence of sycosis.

If we think for a moment about the fluids we are concerned with here, we might think:

- Urine
- Bile
- Blood
- Sexual fluids
- Mucous discharges
- Perspiration

So here we would be worried or interested by fluids which have become stagnated in some way. Simple examples are swellings in the joints, like tennis elbow, or a puffy face or swollen ankles. You might also find some patients have a tendency towards puffy ankles or feet, and in the same way some people often awaken with swollen fingers or wrists. In fact, any kind of oedema at all is of interest here. We have already grasped sinus congestion and catarrh but we might also think of humid asthma and bronchitis. Worse, this miasm tends to grow kidney stones, gall stones, growths of any kind, including keloid scars and tumours. Any of these swellings, thickening of tissues, and deposits, should make us think *sychotic*. This is particularly true if it happens seemingly out of nowhere...like a big swollen knee, for instance.

Now, I like to put a cat amongst the pigeons because just when we start to think we are getting to grips with this, we realise that we only have the smallest fraction of the picture. Here, I am going to point out that we have focussed on the element that is relevant to cannabis and it is a small dimension of the picture. Consider instead for a moment, if you will, that we were thinking about Ayurveda: regular readers will understand that whilst we are born with a dominant vipaka of vata, pitta or kapha (or a combination of two or maybe three), this is not fixed. External influences such as how hot it is, what we eat, etc., will make the energy move so we become more vata and so we get drier skin, we feel the cold more, and our thought processes become vaguer. Another day, we might be more pitta, so we have sharper tempers and our skin becomes more sensitive. These are not permanent states, they are transient health stages. This is the same with the miasm. Whilst they do not necessarily appear and disappear, think of the sychotic miasm a bit like a sleeping volcano. It can be dormant, ready to erupt at any given time. The problem is that when it does detonate, it sets up symptoms far deadlier than before.

Interestingly and frustratingly, when you treat someone's miasm you might see a circle of needs. So, one week you will treat the sychotic dimension and the next week they come back and you might think their needs have changed and you seem to be faced with the syphylitic miasm now, and then the next week they suddenly seem to be presenting all the symptoms of psora. This is not unusual. In fact, it is very *usual*. I always like to think of it as peeling away the layers of an onion and somewhere on the journey you might be lucky enough to see exactly what is wrong with the person as an absolute truth, but if usual is anything to go by...probably you won't. You just need to let the medicine take the lead and see where it takes you.

So, if we are looking for areas where cannabis medicine would be indicated, then it is useful to group the presenting symptoms of the sychotic miasm as benchmarks.

Have your medicine poised if you see any of the following...

Face

The complexion is either very congested or has a bluish pallor. Potentially they will look drawn and their complexion puffy. There are warty eruptions (remember this. The warts will be important and interesting later).

Skin

Warts, moles, wine-coloured patches on the skin. The nails are ridged and overly thick and heavy and can often become deformed. In days gone by, *barber's itch* would have been a sign, but seeing ringworm passed via unsterilized shaving equipment is probably a thing of the past, I would imagine. Maybe not. I hope so!

Overall you can expect to see an over growth, a thickening of the tissues. As well as warts, think cysts, growths, adhesions, keloids, and also profuse yellow green discharge, particularly, but not exclusively, in catarrh.

Nose

The sychotic nose is red and bulbous, and has loads of capillaries studding it. Often this miasm can lead to the loss of smell. In sychotic children you will likely see persistent snuffles. Catarrh is yellowish-green and often these people cannot breathe well though their nose because it is blocked by the mucus.

Mouth

The mouth tastes musty and fishy.

Chest

Palpitations - often there will be a description of a violent hammering of the heart. Also, they may exhibit a rheumatic pain that goes from the shoulder to the heart region.

Stomach

There is discomfort which is decidedly worse after having eaten. The patient feels much better, though, if they lie on their tummy, and in fact any abdominal pain seems to improve by being palpated, by pressure being put on it, or if they bend double. You might see colic, appendicitis, or peritonitis, for example.

Despite their delicate digestion, you will see a smile come to their face when they imagine the prospect of beer, rich foods, fatty meat, and rich seasonings.

Gynaecology

Signs to look out for are ovarian inflammation, any kind of uterine disorder, cysts, and painful periods.

Look for catarrhal changes as an indicator that the miasm may beginning to rise.

Excretory

Excretion is painful, with forceful diarrhoea often preceded by colic. You might also note that the person has a strange bodily odour, a more honey-based stench. What's more, the person is probably hyperaware of their smell.

Extremities

Probably the clearest outward sign we might see of suppressed gonorrhoea is muscular debility. We will see rheumatic conditions really ravaging the joints. The pain is often far worse when the person sits down for a while and is exacerbated by the cold damp weather. It will be better in the morning than the evening, and will be improved by stretching. Their symptoms may virtually disappear in the drier weather.

Headaches

Specifically, headaches will be felt at the vertex (on the top of the head) or at the front. Bizarrely, these headaches seem to be better after midnight and will improve if the person is moving about, particularly in the car.

Now, I was fascinated to see this because as I have been watching the anecdotal evidence of the CBD oil, there are quite a few people saying that the oil helps varying conditions that they have, but it gives them a headache. Most people seem to have remedied this by simply taking a smaller dose. It makes me think of Murphy's directive that too much marijuana makes sychotic symptoms worse. It seems likely that these larger amounts have been exacerbating the sychotic miasm.

Generalities

The sychotic patient is often anaemic. The blood cells are destroyed because of the impaired oxidation of the nutrients of their food.

Holistically, the sychotic miasm attacks the sexual organs, the pelvic organs, the circulatory system, and the bones.

By now, we should understand the differences between acute illness and chronic, that the latter lingers and does not heal over time. But the illnesses we find in this group do not go away, but neither do they really progress; they are in a fixed state of discomfort.

The patient is further exhausted by his/her efforts to try to hide or compensate for them because they tend to centre around the rather embarrassing areas of the genito-urinary systems. That being said, we might also see asthma, tumours, eczema and/or genital herpes.

Psychological

Hmm…

Secrecy.

If we compare the difference of the psychological burden of psora, which manifests in a huge sense of responsibility and duty, which then translates into guilt, we can see that sychotic disease is almost always cloaked in shame.

It makes me think of Valerie Ann Worwood's work on ancestral memory and how that passes through the generations. It seems to be that shame permeates the visceral layers too.

Often you will see the sychotic person living some clandestine existence. They wear a masked persona to the world and there is a sense that you never quite see the true personality.

You see, the sychotic person feels soiled in some way. They perceive themselves as unclean and blemished (interesting that the outward manifestation is exactly that…blemishes). They often feel a very profound sense of self-loathing. We saw this in the Helichrysum book, and particularly how this self-condemnation can manifest into autoimmune diseases. Auto-immune disease is quintessentially sychotic.

Let's just take a break from the theory and think about what we have learned. Now bear in mind I am not a homeopath. Their dried-out medicines do not speak to me at all. My learning is prosaic and is only useful as far as it helps me use my smelly oils better. Ipso facto when I say, *"We use a hair of the dog that bit you"* to treat people, that is as ideologically correct as the plastic coal scuttle I was given for Christmas. In theory it works, but a lot more thinking needs to take place.

However, the fact that we are using a herb that brings about similar conditions to the inherent ones in the body and psyche of a sychotic person is fascinating to me. It reminds me of a lecture I heard at the 2016 NAHA conference by a rather dashing doctor by the name of Dr. Pejman Katiraei, about using essential oils and tinctures on troubled children.

He proposed that as aromatherapists we may be doing a very similar thing to conventional medicine in that we are moving more and more towards *suppressing* symptoms when **actually we should be supporting the system**. That when a child is acting aggressively, it could often be seen that their hormonal levels have gone askew and we would be better served in using oils that support their endocrine function rather than reaching for the valerian or camomile to suppress the volatility. Potentially, that aggression may have a very real function for being there. It is not simply a bad temper, it is likely to be an indicator that something is hormonally awry. It is the body's way of trying to re-assert equilibrium.

Is that what cannabis oil insists we do, I wonder? It seems to be, in homeopathic. That we use it to support the sychotic system. That we use a hair of the dog that bit you!

Let's carry on, because the psychological aspect is about to get even stranger. I am going to call our guy "he" but of course it could equally be a washed out girlie with painful periods, as we have seen.

Now the sychotic (in an extreme state) is egotistical and selfish. He is very insecure. He is jealous. He struggles to be happy at anyone else's success because he is green with envy (or is that snot?!). He puts everybody under suspicion of some perceived ill motive and is bitterly resentful of his lot. When the sychotic miasm rises like a tidal wave it casts a shadow of darkness and these ill thoughts begin to manifest in truly vindictive behaviour. Spiteful, cruel, and heartless, all of his relationships will bear the brunt of the sychosis. The only redeeming excuse we can really give him is, well, he is ill. Potentially he may be coughing his guts up, and likely every bone in his body is screaming in agony. To cap it all, it is bloody snowing again! (*Remember, he gets worse with the cold weather*).

So, the differences in psychological directive are marked between the psora personality and the sychotic one. Psora guy sees the whole world as chaotic and very much out of control and that terrifies him. The sychotic person sees this as a different challenge that he is very happy to rise to. He compensates this chaos by imposing very rigid order. You might see it manifest as perfectionism driving every aspect of their lives. Indeed, for some, this imposition of control becomes their mask. It is what they hide behind. Taken to the extreme we can see obsessive compulsive traits.

So, we need to be careful. By nature, the sychotics are manipulative and deceitful, deliciously seductive and über-charming…just as long as it suits them. Often, they are riddled with guilt and an inferiority complex would not be unusual to see. We can see how these people can easily move into crime…probably to fuel their addictions by now.

As I write this section, we are just four days away from the US election, so it gave me huge amusement to read that these people also move very easily into politics. My initial thought was to say "He" about obvious psychological parallels. But then I remembered "She" famously stumbled because she was suffering from pneumonia (yellow green mucus), and there had also been rumours of a neurological/autoimmune disease. Not that I believe much of anything I have read in the papers about this election, but it is interesting, isn't it?

Did excesses of a sychotic mind (no *P*, you note, lawyers and lynch mobs) eventually take on a physical manifestation?

Leaving politics behind then, let's think of the other *P* we have all been avoiding: the P in psychosis, and remember, here we are talking about sychotic miasm, not cannabis (but there is evidence that cannabis can ramp [p]sychosis up in certain individuals).

Often, there is an unconscious sychotic survival strategy to split, to disassociate, or to float. This splitting is fascinating because if you look at the gonorrhoea bacterium under the microscope it is dual (incidentally this splitting phenomenon is often seen in sexual abuse victims too).

Sychotic Challenges

Puberty. Nature's joke, right? And with puberty we start to gain these irresistible urges. Now for the psora teenager, the challenge is to do with the protection of the self and it would not be that shocking to see him carrying a gun, or worse, a knife. But the sychotic teenager, well he is interested in the perpetuation of the species and here we see a real shag-nasty. Don't forget, too, he has the charm to pull it off, and his pallor probably makes him look like something out of Twilight! This lad is onto a winner.

The problem being for Casanova, is that he carries all this sychotic shame of all the cultural overlays our society has about sex. We have countless religious connotations bringing up feelings of guilt, if not internally then probably mum is urging him to have a little more respect. Social and cultural taboos are piling up, shame is bickering at his shoulder, so what goes out of the window…?

Visits to the sexual health clinic. And what predator is lying in wait? Potentially a little bacterium called *Neisseria gonorrhoea* I would imagine. And when the bacteria takes hold, the condition is back, and what do we do…? We seek to suppress it again.

Mental

The sychotic miasm has a peculiar relationship with time. Often the specific remedies are used for strange memory traits, but in essence, they are time-related, or perhaps more specifically, our relationship to time. Sychosis distorts our time sense.

There was a sign in one of the shops that really made me giggle last week. It said *"Sometimes I amaze myself by my brilliance. Other times I put my keys in the fridge."* Completely astute. Could have been written by me. What the actual writer probably had no perception of, is her statement is a complete giveaway to sychotic miasm. There is concentration but in very short bursts of time. It evaporates before actions have been completed. In actual fact, homeopathy has a specific remedy for this exact kind of forgetfulness. They use Nux vomica.

Medorrhinum is used for people who lose the thread of conversations all the time and struggle to find the correct word. Often a person may sense the word sitting right on the tip of their tongue but their memory cannot stay strong long enough to help them to utter it. For this they use thuja, a plant whose essential oil dwells on many hazardous oils lists because of its high levels of thujone. It's not really poor memory, is it? More poor attention span or absent mindedness. In themselves they are an irritation, nothing more, but in the scope of sychosis, they bear the markers of a far darker malaise, a veritable syndrome, no less.

In reality, all of these are actually manifestations of our perception of time being distorted. Sychosis is forcing our minds to rush, but likewise it can affect our time sense in the opposite way. The leading sychotic remedy for this is *Cannabis indica*. Taking the homeopathic remedy and smoking the drug can make a minute seem like hours. Time passes inordinately slowly and feels as if the person has all the time in the world. Very irritating for everyone around them, but blissfully relaxing for them. Interestingly, this distorted experience of time is common in every type of hallucinogen.

In his book *Homeopathic Miasms - A Modern View* Ian Watson describes how the psora person, preoccupied with survival, becomes focused on the changes of the seasons as a means to ensure he has "enough". His perception of time comes from an external factor - from the planet. But the sychotic person's perception comes from internal factors. It is his own private perception and the sychosis and sychotic remedies have the power to change and control this. Time then, can seem to expand and contract. This can be a gift, of feeling like we have all the time in the world, but of course, conversely it can feel panicky, like time is running out.

It is important to state here that there has always been a relationship between marijuana and sychosis. On one hand, they (*Cannabis indica* and *Cannabis sativa*) are both cited as leading sychotic remedies, but also when the sychotic miasm begins to take dominance you are likely to find a history of marijuana or other hallucinogenic abuse.

Mind Body Perception

It never ceases to amaze me how the energies of plants change and how they present themselves to the world in different ways. In the Helichrysum book, I pondered on how the oil had remained hidden, for the most part, until the 1980s and then come to the fore just as the planet, which was to rule the Mind Body Spirit movement, also made itself known.

There seems to be a similar correlation here with cannabis. Somehow, the sychotic miasm seems to be concerned with the energetic body as a whole. We think of the fluid permeating every cell, even at the deepest level, but also in the brain, and we might also think of the more obvious mind body connection. Just as the world is starting to recognise the quintessential link between the two, but also man has been able to breed strains of the drug that can treat the body and leave the mind, for the most part alone. In recognising the link, he has been able to stabilise the plant to become a medicine that is simpler to use.

Cosmic Ordering

On the surface, it seems like sychotic miasm speaks to reproduction. Actually, what it speaks to is attraction. Where psora is concerned with keeping itself safe and secure, sychosis says:

"Now what would I like? What brings me pleasure?"

We see it in the negative aspects of the glutton, who has bellyache, but he isn't going to give up his fatty meats; and the sociopath, who just sees something they want and takes it with no regard for the consequences. But there is a far more positive aspect to this.

This is the mastery of cosmic ordering.

In my very first aromatherapy workshop we were given an experiment to do. I'm not kidding you, it made me feel like some kind of Jedi! You should do this because it really awakens your mind to new possibilities.

Work in a two with a partner. One stands in front of the other person about five feet apart with their back to the second person. The person in front closes their eyes and stands still. The person behind reaches out their hand, as far as they can in front, but does not touch their partner. Instead, she imagines pushing the energy surrounding her partner forward, then pulling it back. Focussing hard on the energy, pushing and pulling it, like a rope, within seconds the front person starts unconsciously rocking in exactly the same rhythm as their partner is pushing. It is clear they are being moved energetically.

This is the same phenomenon as stepping up a step on an escalator. The person in front automatically steps forward without openly being aware that you are there. You have stepped into their personal space, into their aura.

For those of you interested in this, there is an English Biologist who has done a great deal of research on what he calls *morphic resonance*. Rupert Sheldrake shows how people can perceive that someone is watching them even if they cannot see them (pretty scary if you are psora, I should think!).

But this idea of being able to feel someone else's presence without their fingers touching you, without being able to hear them, or indeed see them, is a vital element of healing. But it's more than that, isn't it? It is a new understanding of connectedness. That just because our physical skin does not touch or is not even close to another, does not mean we cannot feel a connection, so something bigger and wider must be at play. Once one begins to perceive the etheric bodies and energetic connection, then there is a real step forward in ego development. It takes our understanding of the human experience into a whole new multi-layered place. In some ways, there is no turning back from that. One learns from an entirely different viewpoint from that moment on.

Once we understand that we are all ultimately connected, so therefore we can never be separate, then empathy is the only possible outcome.

Spiritually, sychosis speaks to boundaries between us and the universe. For people like you and I this is a particular life lesson, isn't it? How do we remain open enough to fully absorb experience and enjoy the bounty of love, but also have effective boundaries around us so we don't let too much in? Now on a physical level, I am going to say like nurses learn not to absorb germs and bugs. But on a spiritual level, I think we need to acknowledge whole realms of malefic presences that we don't really want to think about.

Just as sychotic miasm is to do with boundaries, these bleed and become more fluid and so bringing thoughts into manifestation is very much easier for these people. There is a birthing of capacity to feel energy as vibration in our bodies, and this is not only the cosmic awakening, for as every gal knows, the bigger the vibration the more the pleasure! Since the sychotic is all about *"I'll have a bit more of that please..."* this idea of attraction has positive and negative aspects to it. The positive will all be obvious and not need elucidating but it is worth thinking of the greed that cannot be satisfied, the sexual appetite that cannot be sated, and the need to want more, more, more. For the guy who is loving this expansion of consciousness, who feels that he has the secrets of the universe at his fingertips – and maybe he does - but it is beyond him to make himself a sandwich. He is so far off with the cosmos that the most basic things become neglected. Likewise, the gentle creature who becomes so sensitive to others, so empathic that she walks around with everyone else's negativity drowning her into chaos. Conversely of course, since she has not protective shell – no boundary formed - then the chances are she will become bitter and cruel too.

These are fertile breeding grounds for addiction.

The Rise of Sychosis

Modern homeopaths say Hahnemann's statement that psora is the largest miasm underpinning the largest number of chronic diseases is outdated. They assert that balance has now changed and that about eighty percent of men are carrying the traits of sychotic miasm.

How can this be? One assertion is that we are more promiscuous than we were a hundred years ago, but this seems unlikely. Common thought follows a theory, originally expounded by Dr. J Compton Burnett, that it may be down to disturbances in the system caused by small pox vaccinations.

It is thought that sychosis very rarely results after that first vaccination because a pus-filled pustule usually follows it. The theory is the problem becomes more dangerous if the patient has a repetitive dose, because the first vaccination did not take. Impossible to know for sure really, isn't it?

Energetically, if you were to look at the chakra functions of a person drowned by sychosis, then potentially you are likely to see the sacral chakra (pertaining to the gonads) and problems with the third eye.

The following is taken from *Principles and Practice of Homeopathy*. The therapeutic and Healing Process – (Box 17.4)

Indicators of sychotic Miasm:

- Escapism
- Autism, refusal to incarnate fully
- Duality - False front, closed, secretive, control, perfectionism, fastidiousness, OCD
- Fixed ideas
- Hedonism; high sexual energy
- Sexual perversions, creatures of the night, self-abuse, alcohol, recreational drugs, excess, extremism, fanaticism, passionate, intense
- Addiction, habitualism
- Jealousy, possessive, suspicious, vindictive hate
- Deceitful, manipulative, exploitative
- Over-growth of tissue, infiltration, thickening, adhesions, tumours
- **The mental state is relieved by the appearance of warts, growths and abnormal discharges and is aggravated by its suppression**
- Sychotic discharges are green to greenish yellow and are fish brine in odour
- Herpetiform eruptions
- Streptococcal infections

Sychosis attacks tissue of:

- mesodermal origin
- mononuclear phagocyte system
- connective tissue

Blimey, it is a list, isn't it? Where to start? Well, at the end I think, because these are physiologies that are pretty much unknown to most of us and yet, in this context, are really very fascinating.

Mesoderm

For this we need to think about germ cells which are, *not* as you might expect, carriers of bacteria. Rather, they are sexual reproduction cells.

The mesoderm is the middle layer of germ cells appearing in the third week of embryonic development. Later as the foetus grows, mesodermal tissue goes on to form muscular tissue (smooth, cardiac and skeletal) such as tongue muscles and the pharyngeal arches that enable us to chew and give us facial expression. It creates connective tissue, the dermis and the subcutaneous layer of the skin, and bones, as well as cartilage. The dura mater, the membrane that envelops the brain and spinal cord, is also formed from mesoderm. The endothelium of the blood vessels, as well as both red and white blood cells, are also all formed from it. It constitutes the basis of kidneys, adrenal cortex, and the excretory units of the genito-urinary system.

Homeopathy uses cannabis medicine to treat sychosis.

Sychosis attacks tissue of mesodermal origin.

Blimey...that's just a few applications then!

More, sychosis attacks:

The Mononuclear phagocyte system

Remember, microglia? Those tiny glial cells functioning as macrophage scavengers in the central nervous system, protecting us from infection? And the Kupfer cells that form the lining of the sinusoids of the liver? You know, the cells that clean up the body's internal streets, gobbling up dead or dying cells, bacteria, or any invading foreign invaders?

Both microglia and Kupfer cells are derived from mesoderm.

Connective tissue

A reprieve at last. An easy bit...

Sychosis attacks tendons, ligaments, and cartilage.

The ramifications are endless, aren't they? Sychosis forms in the most primitive of our cells from our earliest moments of development, then shapes our personality, physical health, and emotions through its manifestations. Cannabis has the power to free us from its grasp.

Chapter 8 Clinical Evidence

Many glimpses of biological secrets unfold herein. There will be moments of belief that you hold the very secrets of the universe in your hands. I know that, because too many have slipped through my fingers like grains of sand these past few months, as I have researched, felt the elation, then given myself a reality check.

If curing cancer or Alzheimer's were as easy as putting a bit of cannabis into a test tube then we would all be millionaires, and very healthy ones at that. Not every finding leads to healing, or is even of that much relevance when making drugs. For us, as aromatherapists, this is a distinct advantage. Sometimes it is enough not to understand every mechanism taking place, simply the situations where we can *expect* cannabis to work. In phytotherapy, where the onus is on empirical evidence, there is a requirement to go further. Traditional use does not necessarily constitute valid evidence for recommendations in modern medicinal practice.

The effects of cannabis, and indeed THC, CBD, or any one of the constituents found in any plant medicine are, for the most part, pleiotropic; that is, they are capable of creating more than one effect. You'll find that a lot through the evidence and it's terribly exciting, but also scary too, because it does make you [me] feel like you [I] might have missed something that could be adverse. There is no getting around that. It's just a biological truth. What's more, understanding contraindications is part of what makes a good therapist and protects you from becoming complacent.

On reviewing the evidence, it is important to remember that most of these experiments are performed in test tubes, under microscopes, or even on mice and rats. Rodents are chosen because they are evolutionarily similar to Homo sapiens, but they are still different. Often, when drug experiments move along to human trials, very different reactions might take place. The slow progress can't be entirely blamed on cannabis's legal restraints (although that plays a massive part), it is also very sensibly legislated to reflect and protect.

A horrific tragedy in 2016 might give us pause, when we hear how an FAAH drugs trial took a horrible turn.

Remember FAAH? It's the serine hydrolase that breaks down endocannabinoids. Inhibiting FAAH is anticipated to be a successful target in the war on chronic pain, so it makes very good sense to imagine that this might be a novel drug design.

Think it through…

FAAH breaks down the bliss molecule, anandamide.

Anandamide's the ligand that binds to the CB_1 receptor.

The CB1 receptor controls pain.

So, if we can prevent this breakdown and maintain levels of anandamide, perhaps pain can be brought into abeyance.

It makes sense.

It should work.

Agreed?

In January 2016, Rennes Hospital Centre, France, reported a dreadful misfortune had befallen a tiny clinical trial run for the drugs company, Bial-Portela & Ca.

All six patients in their trial had been hospitalised, one had been left brain dead. The drug, BIA 10-2474, had been designed to inhibit the breakdown of anandamide, working on the same pretext as we just did, that if they could slow down its degradation then it might help reduce pain.

Trial information sheets promise hopeful treatment interventions for motor problems found in Parkinson's disease, multiple sclerosis, cancer, hypertension, and obesity. Again, from what we understand of the CB_1 receptor, we would concur with that hope.

The *Agence Nationale de Securité du Medicament et des Produits de Santé, in* their final report, concluded that some unknown secondary reaction must have unexpectedly taken place. Perhaps the drug had also inhibited other, more protective, servine hydrolases, or maybe it had harmfully affected the imidazole pyradine "Leaving Group" which might, otherwise, have stabilised the reaction. In truth, it was impossible to say.

The horror had taken place alarmingly quickly. One patient suddenly started showing symptoms several days into the trial after previously exhibiting absolutely no adverse effects at all. The trouble seemed to take place when dosage was quickly ramped up. When symptoms did begin to appear, they seemed entirely unrelated to the condition being treated and so were deemed to be unrelated to the drug. Ignorant of the horror taking place, scientists gave other participants a further dose of the meds. Their symptoms very quickly followed suit. A post mortem MRI, taken from the unlucky braindead participant, showed they had suffered deep cerebral haemorrhage and necrosis.

Translating plant medicine to pharmaceuticals is not as easy as it looks and there is a very good reason that the FDA and Medicine's Control boards insist on clinical trials for drugs to be licensed. Please be mindful as you read, that just because a rat's memory gets better doesn't necessarily mean ours will. On the other hand, every condition here has plenty of **anecdotal** evidence that our herbal medicine gives people a great deal of help.

Bioavailability

Another challenge placed comes from CBD itself and its bioavailability - how it transfers from the site of administration into the blood stream. In other words, how well it absorbs. In fact, CBD has very *poor* bioavailability. A lot gets lost in transit as it travels through the digestive system and liver before it can be absorbed into the blood. We will look at the ramifications of that in the actual aromatherapy section, but here it is enough to understand that injecting it inter peritoneally means that 100% of the CBD gets into the blood. Taking it orally, which is the most common application, is far less efficient. Only about 6% of the dose finally makes it into the circulatory system. In canines, it is much higher, 13-19% per cent, so a) watch how much give to the dog, and b) understand that the species bioavailability mechanisms can be very different.

So that's quite a fall, isn't it? 100% down to 6%.

Where does it go?

Well, for the most part it changes into other metabolites as part of a process called **First Pass Metabolism**. This, very much, reminds me of a question I had on one of my O Level papers at school: "**Describe the journey of a ham sandwich.**"

Looking back, I am pretty sure I missed the entire point of the question and wrote about its adventures when it reached the sewers! What I should have mentioned was how it was met by enzymes in the gastrointestinal lumen, how the gut wall enzymes then got involved and then finally the liver enzymes blasted it...because these also happen to the CBD. Interaction with one particular enzyme (CYP450 mixed function oxidase) transforms it into over 100 *different* metabolites.

In other words, the reaction you get from taking the oral version of CBD, or using it topically, or even inhaling it, may not be the same outcome as we see in the trials.

Further, CBD exerts such low binding affinity with CB_1 and CB_2 receptors that amounts used in test tube experiments, designed to investigate the mechanisms, are vastly larger than would need to be used to affect the human body. Although, one would suspect that if they could find a potentially effective healing avenue through the eCS then potentially they could nano-encapsulate it to increase its potency, but that remains to be seen. The amounts that get through to the body are infinitesimal in comparison to those used in a petri dish.

What's more, scientists and aromatherapists are in agreement that the majesty of cannabis comes from the **_entourage effect_** of the plant, and that whilst CBD does its job, other terpenes, cannabinoids, and the rest of the army are also affecting and potentially modifying that solitary studied event.

But...

You work with what you've got, and we are thankful for the research done so far, although as I write this, I wish they would book themselves a ticket for two weeks in the Bahama's just so I have a chance of keeping up. The very day after this is published I promise you it will be out of date. Research is that fast. Whether the obsession for it stays with me, remains to be seen. Will I return and update? Since it has been so consuming, I can't promise that, no.

Perhaps.

Maybe.

Probably.

We'll see!

So, let's get to it. None of this is in any specific order, but I found it easier to do the mind, then the brain, then the body, so that's what you get too.

Psychological

Stress

The mechanisms of stress are well elucidated in my book *The Professional Stress Solution*, in particular, commentary of the way the hypothalamus, pituitary, and amygdala kick into gear – the HPA axis. Glucocorticoids are released during times of tension and act as anti-inflammatory and benign helpers against resulting endocrine and behavioural changes. In short, they are friends. But in periods of long term stress, the axis seems to turn and inflammatory markers are despatched, weakening the body.

Endocannabinoids are produced by cells found in almost every brain region. Recent evidence seems to show that when glucocorticoids are produced in the stress response, they trigger production of endocannabinoids which then diffuse retrospectively across the synaptic cleft to bind to CB_1 receptors.

As the receptors are then activated, it calms how much of the second messengers, CAMP and adenylate cyclase, are made at the GABA and glutamate terminals.

This in turn inhibits the release of neurotransmitters and depolarisation then either excites or inhibits the receptor.

As your mind follows the journey you might erroneously perceive this as a solitary chemical reaction taking place in isolation, but that's not so. It happens at every point of the axis, at the hypothalamus, amygdala, hippocampus, and the pre-frontal cortex. Little by little, endocannabinoids switch down each part in turn. As they activate each CB_1 receptor, the voltage sensitive Ca2+ channels (calcium channels) are suppressed and subsequently the volume is then turned down on how much adenylate cyclase is produced. Meanwhile, it also enhances conductibility of inwardly flowing potassium. Sound confusing? Yep! Really you only need to understand the outcome of each cells' interchange, which is fewer neurotransmitters and thus a calmer demeanour.

Fascinatingly, the nature of the stress you experience affects functions differently. The negative effects of long term chronic stress may come from reduced numbers of CB_1 receptors. But acute *repetitive* stress alters that, gradually sensitising the receptor and dampening the stress response.

Stress, of course, elicits a myriad of delightful effects on the body and cannabis treats this with ease - so let's have a look at how its medicine might be able to rectify some of those problems.

We'll begin with the mind.

Depression

This is a very interesting healing mechanism because there is a very clear correlation between cannabis and depression. In a poll of young people, 69% of them said they used cannabis because it made them feel better, but there seems also to be a strong indication that long term use of marijuana will eventually *lead* to depression, potentially through decreased regulation of the CB_1 receptor.

It seems a deficiency in eCS signalling is enough to bring about a "depressive-like" phenotype, eliciting changes in the reward mechanisms as well as cognitive and emotional behaviours. Outside of the mental faculties, physical traits echo this with the HPA axis kicking in more quickly, thereby causing more stress responses. This reduced stress adaption is coupled with reduced neurogenesis, so the brain cannot heal. Since the person is now very unhappy, as you would imagine, we also see altered serotonin feedback.

CBD, however, elicits both anti-depressant and anxiolytic effects, independent of the eCS. It's been deduced it probably does so by propping up the serotonin receptor.

Anxiety

The relationship between the endocannabinoid system and anxiety is more complex than it is with depression. Certainly, a deficiency of anandamide is a certain predictor of stress-induced anxiety, but other evidence shows that so can too much in some people. Regardless, evidence proves CBD reduces anxiety.

The Department of Neuroscience at The University of Sao Paolo did a lovely experiment in 2011 where they placed twenty-four students with Social Anxiety Disorder (SAD) in a simulation of a public speaking exercise. The participants, none of whom had been treated before, were given either CBD or a placebo an hour and a half before the presentation.

Then they were assessed against psychological questionnaires and biofeedback of their blood pressure, heart rate, and skin conductance (incredibly, the skin is a better conductor of electricity if it's under the influence of internal or external stimulation from arousal!). Feedback scores were taken six times throughout the test.

CBD reduced their anxiety and cognitive impairment. It calmed their speech, taking away the shrillness of stressful anticipation. Altogether, the CBD team were all more comfortable during their performance.

When assessed in 2011, at least some of the success of CBD in this area was unveiled as being the way it modulates uptake of endocannabinoids in the brain. Interestingly, it reduced uptake in the left para-hippocampal gyrus, in the inferior temporal gyrus, and in the hippocampus itself, but then it decreased how many endocannabinoids were taken up by the right cingulate gyrus. Another trial, the same year, watched the changes on blood flow through the brain after a person had taken CBD. They saw drastic effects on the limbic and paralimbic systems, with altered blood flow in the left amygdaloid nucleus, extending down into the hypothalamus and then up to the left posterior cingulate gurus. In 2014, The Vanderbilt Medical centre demonstrated that anxiety relates to endocannabinoid imbalance in the amygdaloid complex, the bed nucleus of the stria terminalis, the medial prefrontal cortex, the periaqueductal grey, and the hippocampus (how any of us are *ever* calm, looking at that list, is beyond me!). Fundamentally though, reduction of anxiety requires neurogenesis in the hippocampal regions…again, anxiolytic prowess of CBD.

By far the strongest effects though seem to come from the actions on serotonin and CBD's actions on receptors in the bed nucleus of the striatum accumbens, which we will meet more in depth in a moment.

PTSD

Cast your mind back to when we were talking about glutamate and calcium. We talked very briefly about memory and how the doctor tells us to exercise our brain power with sudoku puzzles, because if we don't use it, we will lose it. glutamate and . We talked very briefly about memory and how the doctor tells us to exercise our brain power with sudoku puzzles, because if we don't use it, we will lose it. glutamate and . We talked very briefly about memory and how the doctor tells us to exercise our brain power with sudoku puzzles, because if we don't use it, we will lose it. glutamate and . We talked very briefly about memory and how the doctor tells us to exercise our brain power with sudoku puzzles, because if we don't use it, we will lose it.

Potentially some of this research would be better placed in that section, but I feared our heads might explode at that point. So, I separated it. But you will probably find it useful to read that section again, if PTSD is an area of interest to you. I would also recommend having a look back at the Professional Stress Solution and read up on the HPA axis and how the hypothalamus and pituitary, and adrenal glands process stress.

Research in this area is vast, thank Goddess, but it does mean that you and I have a lot of fetching and carrying of great scientific tomes to do, if we want to catch up. There is a ton of A & P that is completely off the usual aromatherapy certification map. So, make sure you have your sneakers on, because high heels and library steps simply will not do. The one blessing is the experiments are all fairly recent, so there is not too much dust to choke us as we sift and compare.

Where to start...?

I think... With LTD and LTP.

Not a limited company (Ltd.), but instead **Long-Term Depression** (not to be confused with chronic depression – a completely different thing) and **Long-Term Potentiation.** (Memorise them. I'll be abbreviating them from now on).

This is how the strength of a synapse changes.

In this section, it pertains to memories and how the brain sifts them, but the process works similarly wherever a synapse has taken place. We touched on how NDMAR - the glutamate receptor - was vital to that. Now we are going to take that deeper.

It's jolly interesting stuff...but complicated. Grab yourself a cuppa and check you have your comfy knickers on. We may be sitting here a while!

I'll cut to the chase this time...this involves CB_1 receptors on a very large scale.

So, imagine you are learning to do something and it takes a while. I can see my dad ruefully grinning in my mind's eye about how long it took him to teach me to ride a bike and to skip, so we'll use those as an example.

The first time I got on the bike, I was apparently on it for 20 minutes before I took my foot off the floor. In that time, I kept trying, but the bike wobbled and the foot went down again. Within seconds of getting my confidence, I fell off.

Then I fell off again, then I'm crying, dad's trying to stay patient, but we decide to call it a day.

The next day he says: *"Get on the bike"*. But I don't want to. Why the hell would I? I have grazed knees and knocked-up palms, and yesterday I could see mum was none too happy about the fact I'd put holes in my new dungarees. Thus, I pretend to have a million more important things to do, until finally I am persuaded to get back on the bike…and I can't get my foot off the floor again.

Three weeks later, after him patiently trying to get me to do it every day, I managed to ride down the road. Three weeks. Skipping was just as bad, took weeks and never even got close to Double Dutch! As for juggling…I've nearly made it to one ball, but don't hold your breath!

Now imagine how, as I learned, the thought processes went through my mind. The neurons are firing, the synapses are overloading, telling my foot to get up, trying to listen to dad, there is another voice in my head saying: *"who's he trying to kid? That's never going to work, get that foot DOWN!"* My hands want to know if it is a good idea to pull the brake or not…there are a million things going on.

And every synapse leaves a kind of footprint, so the brain gets untidy, until something called synaptic deletion takes place…they are washed away. Consider if they didn't…they would pile up into a massive junk mountain so there is no room for more learning or for new synapses to be squashed in. So at night as we sleep, a cleaning crew comes in and tidies up.

So, we need this synaptic deletion, but what is important is that the brain recognises the synapses we need and those we don't. It's a bit like clearing out the kitchen drawer full of "stuff". I *know* you have one. That place full of homeless creatures! The key to success is to be ruthless and ask yourself honestly *"when was the last time I used that?"* then to start throwing away. The brain does the same thing.

Or it should…

But sometimes it gets screwed.

Sometimes it makes us forget everything and just as cruelly it refuses to wipe memories away.

Now, functioning correctly, LTD and LTP control how long a synapse will keep working after the neuron fired. Effectively, these are the janitors in charge of the cleaning schedule. LTD diminishes the synapse, and LTP controls plasticity, in other words it creates new ones for the neurons to use.

In Liz's merry little kingdom: LTD cleans the table after dinner, LTP lays it again for morning.

Together, they control how long the synapse will last after it has been stimulated for a period. Found throughout the entire central nervous system, these processes are perhaps best understood in the hippocampus and the cerebellum.

Cerebellar LTD is believed to assist our motor learning (*so pedal faster Liz, head up, pedal, pedal, pedal...*) and the hippocampus is involved in the decay of memory (*remember what I said, that's it, keep that foot up, keep pedalling...*) and also spatial memory (*look where you're going...don't forget to turn, Liz...turn, pedal, turn... Oh, never mind, let's have a look, does it hurt?* ☺).

Conversely, where LTD **wipes out** the synapse, LDP **potentiates** it...it strengthens it...keeps it going... The hippocampus gradually says, let's keep the ones where it is working, and clean out the mishaps. Then we'll see how we go from there.

Ideally, that means I should be able to get on a bike and ride it after all these years; that my brain can find where it stored the successful synapse that holds the secret to getting the foot up and pedalling fast. Likewise, one day it might be able to manufacture a two-ball juggling synapse...ya' never know. It would not only be a miracle if it did, it would also be LTP.

Now, let's the leave the traumatic bike incident and go to something more pleasurable, like conjugating French possessive adjectives... (I know. It takes all sorts...).

I can hear myself now, walking to school chuntering so no-one could hear my weird little obsession...

Mon, ma, mes

Ton, ta, tes,

Son, sa, ses

Notre, notre, nos

Votre, votre, vos

Leur, leur, leurs

(*my, your, his or her book etc*).

I could sing this waltz-like chant in my sleep, and alone in my room I would wing my arms around to it in *port de bras* so I could practice for my ballet exams at the same time! Consequently, I can still do it now, and that is because high frequency firing of a synapse drives LTP. Do it loads, then it sticks!

This long-lasting plasticity depends on endocannabinoids. CB_1 receptors regulate the pathways and act as retrograde messengers reporting backwards about which tables need clearing and whether Liz has actually left the stage of putting her foot down, or whether she still needs that particular synapse leaving on the table, because she hasn't finished - she has just popped for a loo break!

You can picture endocannabinoids in their high viz jackets on their walkie-talkies saying, *"I think you can safely clear away the soup bowls. She seems to have grasped the foot thing now, but I wouldn't make any plans for this evening, it's gonna be a good while until she gets the hang of pedalling and looking forward, and we can actually get on and wash up the dinner stuff!"*

Now, one thing that affects the strength of a synapse and thus whether it is strong enough to be kept or discarded, is called Spike Timing Dependant Plasticity (STDP). Again, this is controlled by several factors, including endocannabinoids.

STDP adjusts how strong synapses are between neurons, based on the timing that passes between the first neuron firing and the second. When the neurons on either side of the synapse (input and output) trigger at about the same time (in other words, that they are somehow correlated), the synapse between them becomes stronger. Essentially, when the firing of the input neuron frequently leads to the firing of the output neuron, the synapse gets stronger and stronger. Clearly the strongest outcome will be when the pre- and post-synaptic neurons are able to fire simultaneously. *"Those that fire together, wire together."* When we get this precise timing of both neurons firing synchronously, LTP kicks in.

It's like learning to time step in your first tap lesson.

Shuffle...

Ball

Change

It's slow and awkward but then it gets easier...

Shuffle

Ball Change

Shuffle ball change

ShuffleballchangeShuffleballchangeShuffleballchange.

Yay...she's got it, fast, fluid, and automatic. The synapses are firing closer together until they are in synchronicity.

Then it's time for the eCBs and their walkie-talkies to update the waitresses.

"Yep, yep, yep, I think the penny's dropped. Yep, she's got it. Get clearing LTD, then send in the LTP. Great work LTD, you can go home now. Thanks for your efforts. It's been a long night." Since the job of the cannabinoid receptors on the pre-synaptic neuron is to regulate *how many* synapses are released (excitatory or inhibitory), they can now dim their lights, inhibit release, and rest until they are needed again.

(Actually, darn it! Maybe I should have used a different metaphor. All I can see now is Jacques, the shrimp from Finding Nemo, running all over someone's brain shouting "Clean!". Oh well. Hopefully you get the picture).

For transparency, eCBs are not the only stars of the show, you may have guessed from what we learned earlier about glutamate that LTD depends on fully functional metabotropic glutamate receptors in the hippocampal and cortical regions of the brain, the serotonin levels need to be booming in the pre-frontal cortex, and the circulating dopamine, in the striatum, must also be willing to join the dance. Also, vital for the interchange are calcium levels. If the cell is strongly depolarised, this will lead to LTP, thus weaker depolarization keeps LTD working. Low calcium levels mean no plasticity - no new synapses - because LTD prevents LTP from kicking in. It's likely that CBD's powerful action upon calcium homeostasis probably explains its powerful neuroprotective properties.

Okay. So, from here you should be able to see that if the endocannabinoid system goes out of whack, then memory becomes an issue. Let's work out from there.

In 2013 in France, it was determined that stress sends this system haywire. This data was ascertained by studying some mice to take a good look at the band of fibres that runs across the surface of the thalamus called the *bed nucleus of the stria terminalis* (BNST). These fibres serve as the exit for messages travelling from the amygdala to the hypothalamus. Its function is very clear, it **monitors threats** and **modulates our anxiety responses** thereof. The BNST controls levels of stress by modulating the HPA axis, by sending either inhibiting or exciting messages to the organs.

Interestingly though, it works like a relay switch controlled by a kind of timing mechanism that will only kick the HPA axis into action if it comes under fire from stressful situations lasting for more than ten minutes. So if, for example, someone plays a trick and makes you jump, that *won't* trigger the mechanism, nor "take years off you" which is what we always say here in England.

But, if a stressful situation endures for more than 10 minutes, then the lever is pulled and something rather strange happens.

LTD changes to LTP.

Suddenly, this chronic stress wipes LTD from the receptors around the synapses and LTP holds memories hostage, refusing to let them go (I wonder if that's why dad felt the bike riding trauma so acutely!).

Going back to the French experiment... The mice endured a restraint test for an hour. Then results collected from the rodents elucidated that this switch out, to which we refer - the LTP change - happened independent of the usual cortisol stress response we would expect to see. The CB_1 receptors controlled it. Glucocorticoid hormones then piggy-backed off this eCB signalling to ensure a memory was either consolidated or driven to extinction.

In other words, it was never the cortisol, he was just the hanger-on henchman, it's the CB_1 receptor calling the shots.

This is a huge breakthrough for many different drug therapies, but particularly for PTSD research, since existing treatments are often little more than happy co-incidences as people get a bit better from taking meds for something else. Sadly, however, doctors enjoy little success prescribing traditional SSRI anti-depressants for complex PTSD where the sufferer has been kept captive in a long-term situation they couldn't escape, for example, sufferers of early life trauma or veterans. Perhaps this holds the key.

Animal studies reveal the CB_1 receptor is one of the key controlling factors in fear. When activated in animal experiments, creatures take on exaggerated characteristics of anxiety and depression. Endocannabinoid signalling controls the stress response by either activating or terminating the HPA axis in the stress sensitive nuclei of cells in the hypothalamus and in other stress-y structures like the amygdala. Further, this happens regardless of whether the patient endured acute stress (where there is one overwhelmingly terrifying event) or prolonged and repeated terror.

But is this what causes PTSD?

We could safely say, *partially*, I think.

Experts suggest the PTSD phenotype may be created by a four-pronged curse scattered across the brain.

1. Certainly, PTSD seems to be characterised by heightened activity in the amygdala. It's here we acquire fear associations, but it is also where we begin to express responses to those fears. Hence, both become exaggerated.
2. Deficits in the prefrontal cortex make it harder to distract attention away from worries. Complex memories linger, with triggers shooting attention right back to them.
3. LTD is no longer active, cluttering the hippocampus with conflicting synapses. The chaos makes it impossible to assess which contexts are safe and those that are not. Sensibly, it remains on high alert.
4. Anomalies in the function at the basal ganglia then cause difficulties in moderating *responses* to triggers. *They* become exaggerated. Over time, reactions and motor habits are being conditioned and then re-enforced.
5. CB_1 signalling is disrupted, meaning that the normal fear extinction mechanism no longer functions effectively.

In short...

It's all bad.

Now, any or all of these, alone or in tandem, might serve as avenues for treating PTSD. For obvious reasons, we will pick up the CB_1 trail and see where that takes us.

We'll visit 2013 first. A good year for eCB research.

Scientists at the NYU Langone Medical Centre presented a fascinating study at the Annual Meeting of the Society of Biological Psychiatry in San Francisco, reporting discoveries of a connection between PTSD and the number of cannabinoid receptors in the brain.

Sixty study participants were divided into three groups:

- Participants with PTSD
- Participants who had experienced trauma but not developed PTSD
- Those who had no history of trauma or PTSD

A radioactive tracer was given to all three groups illuminating CB_1 receptors when viewed with a pet scan. Those with PTSD, especially the women, had a **surplus of CB_1 receptors** in the brain, as well as significantly **reduced** levels of anandamide. Ever brilliant, the body seemed to generate extra receptors in a bid to try to increase the available surface area to catch the anandamide. Hence, in PTSD patients, we see these high levels of receptors but very little anandamide to lock to them.

Scientists still have very little understanding of what anandamide does in *humans*, but, in rats, we know it impairs memory.

Also in 2013, eCB research took us to Ground Zero and the aftermath of the World Trade Centre coming crashing down to Earth. More specifically, it takes us to a lab at the Hotchkiss Brain Institute from the University of Calgary, and looking at the blood serum belonging to forty-six willing volunteers who had all been in physical proximity of the WTC at the time of the 9/11 attack.

What had the trauma done to them in those twelve years after that horrific day?

Amazingly, twenty-two had avoided PTSD, but sadly, twenty-four of the group had lifetime diagnoses. Their blood results were fascinating. The PTSD group had significantly reduced levels of 2-AG circulating in their serum. The report reads: *"The effect of the 2-AG content in PTSD remained significant after controlling for the stress of exposure to the WTC collapse, gender, depression, and alcohol abuse"* I'm not sure how one vets for the stress factor, but it sounds very clever to me!

Now, no significant differences were observed in the circulating levels of anandamide or in the cortisol levels, but there did seem to be a clear correlation between patients who had very intrusive symptoms and low levels of 2-AG. Further, the study concluded that PTSD is most certainly associated with this reduction of circulating levels of 2-AG.

Y'know, when I come back in my next life I am going to come back as a malevolent, masochistic, mercenary mouse to take revenge on every lab tech who has exploited my beady eyes and those of my rodent compadres. I realise it is in the name of science, but I feel torturing empathy with my mouse-mates living in a cage in Sao Paolo University in November 2012. For a whole hour, a cat stalked their cage in a bid to induce terror. An hour later they were stabbed with needles, and some of them endured repeated shots. The syringes contained CBD.

Seven days later, the mice were given a further treat of being put out into an elevated maze. Those who had been given repeated doses of CBD showed no fear, scampering out into the open arms.

Now just as a reminder, treating CB_1 problematic conditions is going to be more effective with marijuana. There, THC mimics anandamide, giving them more opportunity to lock with CB_1 receptors. As anandamide becomes more available, then more receptors are produced. In an ideal world, you would hopefully see PTSD symptoms receding.

Marijuana obviously has its own pitfalls and concerns, though. And in any case our medicine is high CBD hemp oil. Now if you are like me, you'll be asking yourself, can CBD help these people if it doesn't bind with the CB_1 receptor?

Doesn't it?

It's more complicated than that, isn't it?

Although it's the tiniest amount THC *is* present in our oil. It needs to be to get the entourage effect with CBD. But CBD modulates it, just as it curbs the psycho-activity of a joint.

And CBD *does* bind to the CB_1 receptor, just not *directly*.

It interacts allosterically, (remember the two places on the cell?).

It is a **negative allosteric modulator**, meaning it changes the shape of the receptor, thus inhibiting the strength of signal that the receptor puts out.

But, if CBD is helping these people, (and it does) it's probably *not* through the CB_1 receptors, is it? Because its binding action is simply too weak. Something else must be going on.

Exactly so, and these scientists weren't so interested in what the CB_1 receptors were doing, but instead how the <u>serotonin</u> was working. So, they used an agonist to block the CB_1 and CB_2 receptors to prevent them from kicking in at all.

They wanted to measure two things:

- 5HT1a receptor MRNA (need a recap? It is the messenger RNA that is building new serotonin receptors)
- BDNF protein (used for building brain function. Poor levels are linked to brain aging, Alzheimer's, neurotransmitter function...all that jazz...)

Sensible thinking, since a functional relationship has been established between serotonin neurotransmission and BDNF expression in mood disorders.

They measured levels in the hippocampus, frontal cortex, amygdaloid complex, and dorsal periaqueductal grey.

Amazingly, seven days after their feline frightener, the mice that had had repeated doses of CBD were still singing that Pharrell Williams song. Serotonin levels were still high, they were *happy* and feeling like a "room without a roof!" The CBD had modulated the serotonin gene expression, guarding against it faltering and then keeping levels of the neurotransmitter high enough in the frontal cortex and the hippocampus to prevent anxiety from taking hold after that dreadfully scary event.

The important thing...<u>repeated doses</u>.

Mind, it had only taken seven days to attenuate mousey melancholy, so *repeated* need not necessarily mean prolonged.

I suspect I may have found out why "repeated" was important in a trial that went onto the internet just last week!

May 2017, our friends in Sao Paolo analysed how the CBD influenced memory to try to ascertain how it worked on the mind's conditioning.

Acquisition of fear memories comes from a concerted effort between the Pre-Frontal Cortex, the amygdala, and the hypothalamus. But where originally it was presumed the affects were linear, it is now understood that memory associations seem to be recruited at specific time windows after the event has taken place, through interactions with the serotonin and dopamine receptors.

If CBD was given immediately after the event, no change was seen. But given five hours after the terror, CBD interfered with processes in the prefrontal cortex and to impair the conditioning process. By tampering with the gene expression in the limbic circuitry, it was able to say, *"no thanks we don't need to keep that one"*, refusing to let LTP win the race. The conditioned memory was released into the wind and allowed to drift off into the past where it belonged.

The University of Ontario, November 2016, and there is another trembling cage of rodents; this time, rats. Here, the team of scientists acknowledged that CBD is an effective treatment for fear and anxiety, but wanted to better understand why. Was it the cannabinoid receptors, serotonin, or dopamine receptors that were doing the dance with CBD? This time they focussed in on *freeze behaviour*, by using a combination of fear conditioning and then recording electrophysiological feedback.

Freeze behaviour is common to all prey animals. It is the body's survival strategy. For example, when caught by an owl, a mouse might possibly still be able to get free by pretending to be dead or by fighting. Changes in blood pressure and heart rate respond to the situation, shortness of breath and even adopting a crouching position all get the mouse ready to spring, should he gain the opportunity. If he does get away. however, it's usual he will be left with heightened expectancy and anticipation of another event. Many of those effects are difficult to measure and so most experiments will zoom in on watching the crouching position that the subject takes.

Now, CBD is proven to stop mice adopting this crouching position and, in turn, to protect against conditioning that something else bad is going to happen. So, scientists blocked all avenues that might be doing the deed. They blocked the cannabinoid dopamine, and serotonin receptors, and one by one, removed the agonist to see which one let the CBD through to do its job.

Serotonin again, guys.

CBD prevents the freeze behaviour conditioning (in rats) symptomatic in PTSD through interaction with the 5-HT1A receptors.

One last study before we leave, again from Sao Paolo. I'll paraphrase because it was easier to untangle the delight of four Slinkies mashed up together by Dex last week than it was to unravel this study! It's mice, being given to all manner of stressful situations for a fortnight, then given CBD inter-peritoneally two hours after the terror, to see which part of their bodies responded to it. *"Repeated administration of CBD (30 mg/kg i.p., 2 h after each daily stressor) increased hippocampal progenitor proliferation and neurogenesis in wild-type mice."*

Remember the progenitors? They are the stem cells. So the CBD encouraged more cell growth in the hippocampus and sprouted more neurons. Then, when they watched what was happening in a test tube, the scientists saw the CBD was mimicking and activating the CB_1 and 2 receptors bringing about an anxiolytic response as if it were preventing FAAH from degrading endocannabinoids.

Fear and anxiety are, of course, defining features of many serious psychiatric illnesses. Inappropriate fear responses are symptomatic of PTSD, but also panic and phobia disorders, as well as myriad other conditions. Usually, these illnesses might be treated with traditional extinction therapy, where the subject is exposed to their stressor over and over again and then when their terrifying outcome does not come to fruition, the extinction changes expectation, hopefully alleviating fear. It might be that in these cases, cannabis extracts could gain a better traction dealing with the physiology at source.

Sleep Disorders

A little story from the saddest of sad places, about a ten-year-old girl treated in January 2015 for PTSD by Professor Shannon, an Assistant Clinical Professor of Psychiatry from the University of Colorado School of Medicine, and Ms Opila-Lehman, Naturopathic Physician from the Wholeness Center in Fort Collins. The child had been sexually abused and had very little parental supervision as a young girl under the age of five. The doctor's medications had given some relief, but she suffered terrible side effects and any beneficial effects soon wore off.

She suffered dreadfully from anxiety and insomnia. School was problematic, and she had very low self-esteem. She had become very prone to outbursts and was displaying sexually inappropriate behaviour. She was aggressive, disobedient, and impulsive. Worse, she had begun to imagine ways to end her life.

Her sleep was restless and interrupted, totalling about two to three hours a night. She was unable to sleep without her younger brother.

Her mother had suffered from bipolar disorder and depression. Having a methadone addiction, as well as being an alcoholic, she had smoked marijuana throughout her entire pregnancy with the child.

Both parents were emotionally absent. Then, when she was three, the girl had been molested by an 11-year-old boy. In 2011, trauma hit again when her father was killed in motor accident. Subsequently, the girl's maternal grandparents took over her permanent guardianship.

Initially, her treatments had begun with Clonidine, a drug traditionally used to treat anxiety, drug withdrawal, and high blood pressure. In addition, a recommendation was made for her to receive some Eye Movement Desensitization and Reprocessing therapy. Sadly, the wee thing began to suffer hallucinations from the drug, so she ceased taking it. Her medication was altered and she began a series of counselling where, although she was anxious and traumatised, her behaviour and mood did seem to improve.

But when she was reassessed three years later – after receiving psychotherapy twice a week for the entire duration - her behaviour and mental state had deteriorated horribly. She had ceased taking her medication 18 months prior. And subsequently begun to self-harm, cutting her leg.

At this point she was prescribed with Melatonin, 5 mg; St John's wort, 450 mg twice daily; magnesium, 300 mg; and diphenhydramine, 25 mg per night.

When appraised three weeks later, she was still difficult to manage and having outbursts at school. Magnesium and St John's wort were stopped. Treatment was then continued with EPA fish oil, 750 mg per day and diphenhydramine at night (this is Benadryl, the stuff you would normally take for hay fever, presumably, because it makes you drowsy). A conversation was had at this point with the grandmother about the possibility of CBD. Understandably, given the child's history with pharmaceuticals, her grandmother had reservations so it was decided to see observations for the next two months to see how the other medications faired.

Since no improvement was seen in that time, in March 2015 it was recommended that our little friend begin CBD, as well as starting animal assisted therapy. Granny gave consent. So, to gauge the improvement, child and grandmother completed two separate questionnaires:

A *Sleep Disturbance Scale,* where a score of over 50 is considered indicative of a sleep disorder, and a SCARED test (*Screen for Child Anxiety Related Emotional Disorders*). Here, a score of over 25 indicates a high probability of a childhood anxiety disorder.

Watch what happens...

Date of visit	Sleep scale score	SCARED score
March 16, 2015	59	34
May 25, 2015	42	24
July 22, 2015	41	19
August 24, 2015	37	16
September 22, 2015	38	18

A quick review of treatment shows us:

March: Started a regimen of CBD oil, 25 mg (1 capsule) a day to be taken at 6 pm, an addition to EPA fish oil, 750 mg per day; and diphenhydramine, 25 mg per night.

April: The scores showed she was sleeping better with CBD treatment. She was experiencing some stomach aches but her mood was more at ease. CBD, fish oil, and Benadryl all continued.

May: Patient complained of "ghosts" waking her at night. Benadryl ended. Treatment of fish oil & CBD oil continued the same.

July: Sleeping better; able to sleep in own room 3–4 nights a week. EPA fish oil, 750 mg per day remained the same. CBD capsule was changed to 12 mg (in 4 sublingual sprays) per night; a further 12 mg more (in 4 sublingual sprays) during the day as required for anxiety, typically 3 or 4 times a week.

And now for the happy ending. The report ends in August.

Sleeping well. Handling school well.

Final recommendations:

CBD oil, 25 mg (1 capsule) a night; CBD liquid, 6–12 mg (in 2–4 sublingual sprays) as needed for anxiety, typically 2 or 3 times a week. EPA fish oil, 750 mg daily.

Addiction

Shannon and Opila-Lehman also describe how another of their patients, with a long-standing diagnosis of bipolar disorder, had become profoundly addicted to marijuana. Making no changes to his medication except to add gradually decreasing dosages of CBD (24 to 18 µg) they were able to prize him off his joints. Their patient described feeling less anxious and began to maintain more regular patterns of sleep. He also reported using no marijuana since using CBD oil and was able to maintain non-usage of marijuana at the dose of 18 µg.

Now, to me, after everything we have learned about the entourage effects of cannabis constituents, that doesn't really surprise me, but what does is it seems to also apply for heroin, cocaine, amphetamines, nicotine, and alcohol too. Looking at the mechanisms it affects, I can't see why it would not work for gambling, sex, or shopping too...I'd certainly be tempted to give it a try on any addictive behaviour.

Now here's a scary stat: between 162-324 million people took some kind of illicit substance between 2012-2015 worldwide. Not everyone would have become hooked, some would have had lucky escapes, but 183,000 deaths in those years were drug related.

It's well understood that the dopaminergic and glutaminergic signalling play an important role in re-enforcing substance seeking behaviour. Likewise, endocannabinoid signalling is implicated in whether we will acquire or maintain the seeking behaviour too. It seems odd to think of addiction in the same way as we think of cardiovascular disease, diabetes, or arthritis, but all of them are chronic diseases, addiction by virtue of the fact it is a chronically relapsing disorder.

The most important dimension to getting clean is neuroplasticity, just as addiction is learned behaviour, re-enforced by repeated behaviour so it must be unlearned. To do that, the brain needs to be able to re-enforce new synapses, which as we know from PTSD, CBD is well-equipped to do.

I'm sure it will surprise few people to discover that addiction seems to be closely related to dysfunction in the CB_1 receptor, which again CBD allosterically influences weakly. Neuro-physical symptoms should be well-recognised now as anandamide binds to TRPV1, stimulated by CBD. Meanwhile, it inhibits FAAH , alters hydrolysis of anandamide and maintaining heightened levels of endocannabinoids.

Stress responses and compulsive behaviours are very much co-ordinated by the serotonin receptor, and as agonist to 5HTA1, it calms and soothes the psyche.

Now...are you ready for this? Because we are about to step into freaky land because which other receptors do you think our beloved molecule influences?

Only the bloody opioid receptors!

I know, right?! Is there nothing this chemical cannot do?

For the swots amongst us...it allosterically affects μ and σ opioid receptors, which would normally react to enkephalins and morphine. In just the same way as she waded in and took the toys off them for their own good, she's found another game to spoil too.

In March 2017, a joint study by Universities of Birmingham and Loughborough, UK, with Universities of Sao Paolo and St Caterina, Brazil, found cannabidiol acutely reduced how drug memories were expressed and disrupted their consolidation. Scientists at the Mount Sinai Centre in New York had come a little closer to understanding the drive mechanisms in 2012 when they discovered CBD steadied brain signalling known to lead to people seeking out heroin. It normalised a well-recognised anomaly in glutamate signalling at AMPA GluR1 and CB_1 receptors in the nucleus accumbens, thus confounding the usual conditioned stimulus cue (I'm going to try this out to see if I can get rid of the sugar craving that overwhelms me the second Dex goes to bed and I settle into the chair at 9pm!).

Cocaine, however, seems to have a different effect. When scientists in Mallorca looked closely at the brains of addicts, they could see the CB_1 receptors worked differently in heroin users, or indeed those who used cocaine or heroin together. They had 44% deficit of the protein that creates CB_1 receptors in the prefrontal cortex. The membranes of their receptors were increased but they had much less cytosol in them. There were fewer receptors and kinase, suggesting the receptors had become desensitised over time. Scientists believe this could lead to neuroplasticity (and we're back to the beginning again) and to neurotoxicity.

Now, we haven't talked about magl yet, have we? Remember the serine hydrolase that sounded like an investment banker? Well here's the thing...it seems it might be her fault people get addicted to fags! Since CBD affects her levels, perhaps it might be able to help people to give up the REALLY evil weed, tobacco. A 2012 study from the University College in London suggests it stands a good chance. Twenty-four smokers were given either an inhaler of CBD or a placebo and were told to use them every time they felt the urge to smoke.

So, twelve smokers puffing away, what percentage less cigarettes do you think they smoked?

Forty percent!

Holy smoke, Batman! Just imagine the effects CBD and hypnotherapy, or CBD and acupressure could have!

Now, though this area of addiction is now being well researched, it is still very sparsely populated. One interesting take away though is that CBD can't seem to do the job on its own. It needs THC to potentiate the action (just as a reminder, yes, it's in the oil) and also Cannabinol, each of which do their own important part in reducing addiction.

Schizophrenia and Psychosis

Potentially, the most controversial debate regarding cannabis must surely surround schizophrenia. It forms the most passionate arguments both for and against the plant. In one camp, you have people screeching that smoking causes psychosis, and in the other, that weed is completely innocuous and has no effect.

Now, I have to admit that I would probably have been teetering on the first camp, or even had one foot fully in perhaps, but research has shown me to be wrong. Neither of the extremist views is rooted in science.

It is true that when healthy volunteers were given high doses of THC they experienced psychotic-like symptoms, but unlike schizophrenia, the effects were transient; they quickly went away. In addition to that, historical studies show that smoking weed was virtually non-existent in the West until the 1950s, but then skyrocketed as so many people toked up in the sixties and seventies. The diagnosis figures for schizophrenia stayed the same.

Likewise, there is a clear correlation between sufferers of schizophrenia and smoking weed. A far higher percentage of schizophrenics enjoy a smoke than the number in healthy population. So, then we ask ourselves, are they perhaps self-medicating? But surveys largely say that the cannabis use predates their onset of symptoms.

But the least controversial viewpoint seems to be that cannabis can provoke psychotic symptoms in individuals that already have a predisposition to the disease. So why?

Who knows?!

Several theories abound.

The first pertains to the pre-frontal cortex as it enjoys huge surges of growth during the period of adolescence. Laden with CB_1 receptors, perhaps the THC affects how it functions and matures.

Similarly, observations show that people with schizophrenia, and those with a first-degree relative with the illness, have a strange disruption on the dopamine signalling. During adolescence, the dopamine signalling shifts in the PFC, altering how it communicates with the surrounding neuronal populations. In provoking dopamine release, perhaps cannabis skews this? It's not clear.

We do know that CB_1 signalling changes through our lives. It ascends its power through childhood, peaks during adolescence, and then falls throughout the rest of life. Perhaps having so much stimulation from THC during that ripened time is simply much too much.

The jury is still out.

What is agreed is that CBD seems to cancel out the effects of the THC and has the power to reverse psychosis.

It's so well agreed now that GW Pharmaceuticals completed a Phase II placebo control trial of using their liquid CBD, GWP42003, with standard antipsychotics in 2015. The trial consisted of 88 volunteers who had not been responding to their prescribed meds. Adding CBD was deemed to bring significant improvements to outcomes. The results were so good that they then took out a patent protecting the use of CBD and other cannabinoids, in combination with existing antipsychotic meds for the prevention and treatment of psychosis and psychotic disorders. That patent is in place until 2029.

At every point in the trial, CBD proved superior to the placebo, causing fewer headaches and less drowsiness than its counterpart. There did seem to be more diarrhoea and a much higher incidence of nausea (7% opposed to none from the placebo). Two people did withdraw from the trial because of side effects but one was taking CBD and the other was taking the placebo.

The fascination for creating drugs for schizophrenia is clear. Existing ones just don't work very well. Ones that do have horrible side effects, ranging from a dry mouth to tremor and muscle spasm. Often the patient can feel so out of it the psychosis seems preferable to the fog they're living in. Consequently, they won't take their meds. It's that horrible dilemma. They'll only take meds from people they trust. As they become more ill, they trust fewer people's opinions about taking their meds, thinking they are being misled, but in reality they need their meds more. It becomes an impossible spiral and the question becomes where does personality end and neurological damage begin? Dreadfully and frighteningly sad.

Diagnosis of schizophrenia is dreadfully complicated, with psychosis only being a part of the disease. These delusions, or hallucinations, can just as likely stem from a brain tumour. Even long-term depression can result in psychosis.

It's almost like a syndrome of symptoms, classed as positive and negative. Positive symptoms that seem to have been added or driven to excess above the norm, hallucinations and delusions yes, but also racing thoughts. It's imagined these might derive from an increase in the signalling in the subcortical parts of the brain. When you consider these as controlling movement, emotions, sleep, and attention, you can start to imagine the mania they feel.

Likewise, the negative symptoms seem to take away from life. These, thought to come from decreases in the PFC, tend to lead to a loss of social interaction, difficulty organising and planning, changes in personality, and poor judgement and decision-making.

The side effects people experience are because the antipsychotics alter the signalling of the DA2 receptor, thus you no longer have visions and paranoia, but it does create excess movement and shaking. Hence, finding a way to treat the psychosis outside of the dopamine receptors is pretty much the Holy Grail.

The discovery that CBD alleviates psychosis dates right back to 1982, when two cannabinoids, THC and CBD, were used to measure psychosis. It was noted that CBD produced less anxiety and psychotomimetic symptoms. Evidence grew and grew, but even though it is clear people's psychosis recedes when they use CBD, it's still not really clear *why*. Antagonising the CB_1 with CBD seems to inhibit the metabolism and uptake of anandamide. So, then it makes the endocannabinoid system stronger. But how does that help? Anandamide affects the GABA receptors in several parts of the brain. In fact, medium spiny GABARergic neurons make up 95% of the neuronal population of the nucleus accumbens, so that's a lot! Animal studies suggest the dopaminergic receptors in this area might be super sensitive. Perhaps they inhibit the GABA neurons that then release less GABA at the ventral palladium. It's all very complex!

Perhaps easier for us to understand is the theory that since anxiety also recedes with the psychosis, perhaps CBD is exerting its power through the serotonin receptors. Not only through 5HTA-1, but also 5HTA-2.

Interestingly, CBD affects CB_1 receptors and the TRPV channels in a contrary manner, indirectly activating it where it has switched CB_1 down. Its hypothesised that this activation facilitates glutamate release and then, in response, GABA release is slowed.

CBD calms the glia, preventing them from releasing inflammatory messengers. It might be that THC causes psychosis because it lacks this powerful anti-inflammatory effect. CBD draws the activity away from the CB_1 receptor over to CB_2, and in so doing also stabilises the glutamate receptor. Effects in the CB_2 receptor seem to block psychosis.

Whatever the mechanism, CBD ameliorates both positive and negative symptoms of the schizophrenia. Their thinking become clearer but they seem more able to function on a day-to-day level, dressing and cleaning themselves better, anxiety falling, and better able to interact with the world.

When tested in a clinical trial next to the traditional treatment of clozapine, it performed equally as well, but it was found that it also interacted with the glutamate receptors that the clozapine hadn't. This meant that the locomotor behaviour - wringing hands, biting of nails, etc. - also calmed.

One of the biological markers for schizophrenia is believed to be a disruption in PPI signalling (no, that's not the insurance on your banking that everyone is trying to sell you!). **Pre Pulse Inhibition** is related to our startle response and how it responds to weak stimuli. It's thought it might reflect the massive amount of sensory information that is being handled at one time and involves a complex interaction between dopaminergic and glutamatergic receptors.

Now, if ever there was an occasion that makes us stop and think through the science, it's this.

CBD reverses the signalling disruption, for instance it puts it right in mice experiments. But in rat studies, it doesn't. No-one can really say why that is. It's easy to shrug it off as differences in species, but then of course, homo sapiens are a different species still.

A couple of interesting adjuncts.

Morgan and Curran, in 2008, assessed psychosis of marijuana users smoking in a natural setting. These who had levels of a combination of CBD and THC in their hair samples experienced less psychosis than those who had THC alone.

Then, in 2010, Morgan *et al.* assessed how well 132 very stoned users could recall pieces of prose. The smokers had all chosen their particular favourite brand of weed. Those with CBD THC had no problems with recall, but those with only THC remembered far less.

All that debate aside, the science is in agreement. Once a patient has onset symptoms of schizophrenia, it's important they get off the THC. Using cannabis is clearly adverse and is also related to them discontinuing their meds, and thus a poor prognosis. It is vital you get them off the joint and onto CBD.

Bipolar

Throughout the experiments I reviewed for schizophrenia, one name came up over and over again. Zuardi, again from the University of Sao Paolo. A great deal of the movement forward with schizophrenia research has progressed because of him, so when I see a trial where he said CBD might not work, I feel inclined to believe him.

The aim of the report was to focus on efficacy and safety of CBD on Bipolar Affective Disorder - BAD. This was the first time this had been done and the team selected two female patients in their thirties who were suffering from manic episodes but were free from co-morbid conditions. Both women were given a placebo for the first five days. Then, from the 6th to 30th day, they were given CBD.

Then the treatments were separated. The first patient also received an oral dose of olanzapine on days 6-20. On day 31, CBD was taken away and for five days a placebo replaced it.

The first lady seemed to improve while on olanzapine and CBD cocktail, but didn't get any better with the CBD alone. The second woman didn't improve on any dose of CBD during the trial. That said, there were no side effects either.

I'm surmising that CBD could help other aspects of bipolar, but I cannot find data either way.

OCD

Very early days, but CBD seems to inhibit OCD behaviour in rats.

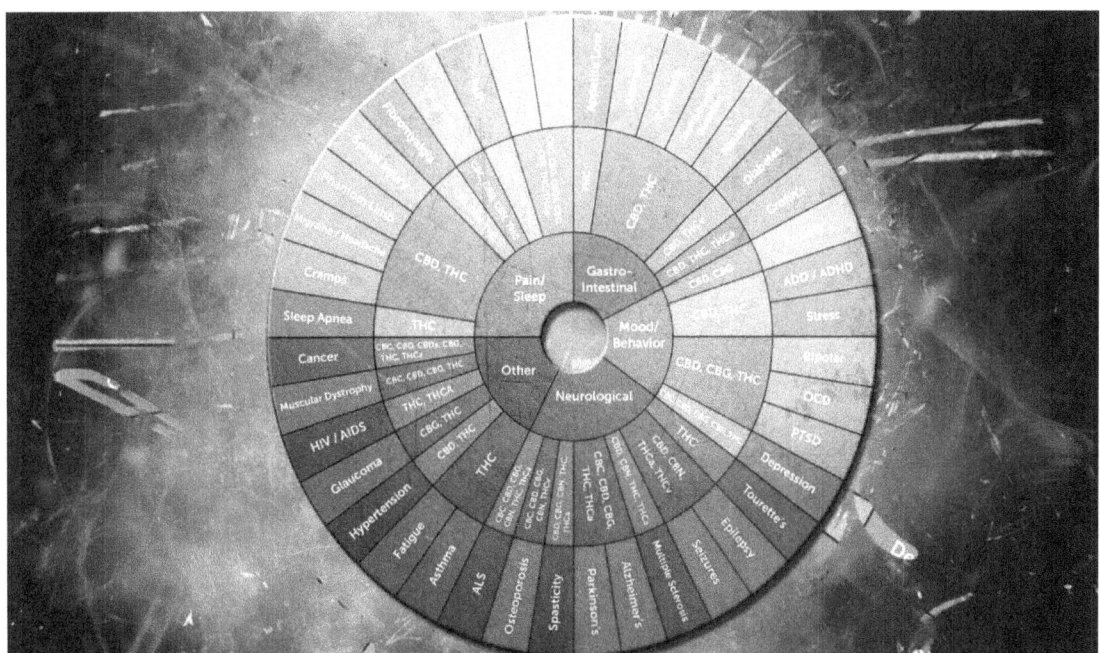

This image is available to download in A4 should you want to file it or

put it on the wall:

https://buildyourownreality.lpages.co/cbd-actions-wheel/

Neurological

Epilepsy

I opened the book with the story of lovely little Charlotte Figi, the tiny dot having seizures in her nappy. It doesn't bear thinking about how hard it must be to watch your child suffer with Dravet's Syndrome or any kind of epilepsy. Charlotte, a fraternal twin, was enduring twenty, thirty, sometimes sixty seizures a day. She had injured her head several times and even had broken teeth. By the age of two, Dravet's babies start losing the power of speech and development slows as they become ever more neurologically challenged by their faulty synapses. By the Winter of 2011, Paige and Michael Figi had signed a DNR for their daughter, feeling she was no longer human, failing in their arms. They had navigated their way around twelve different medications, none of which had helped. They were at a loss of what to do, until one day, Michael, working abroad, called home with details of the possible effects of cannabis on epilepsy.

They lived in a compassionate state.

Anything was worth a try.

When she started taking the CBD, benchmarks were small but very significant; Charlotte forming some words, perhaps eating, drinking, or even managing to stand and take some steps. Big achievements for any toddler, massive leaps for a little girl with a disease of this magnitude.

Six years on, Charlotte's episodes have fallen from 1200 seizures a month to just three.

How?

In truth, science has still not satisfactorily yielded that answer, but research does reveal compelling clues.

Epilepsy is characterised by frequent seizures, neurodevelopmental delays and, over time, a reduced quality of life. It develops through a process called epileptogenesis, causing neurons to occasionally slip out of kilter and fire in a hyper-synchronous manner (to peasants like you and I, hyper-synchronous means "out of synch" or "a lot"). Hyper-synchronous firing of neurons is recognised as a seizure.

Both CB_1 and CB_2 receptors are highly expressed in the hippocampus and within other parts of the central nervous system. CB_1 receptors calm how many synapses are being released at calcium and potassium channel gates. But CBD's not a CB_1 dude. That's not where he is doing his job. So where?

Many of these CB_1 receptors are expressed on glutamatergic synapses and it is suspected that these probably modulate where a person's threshold for a seizure lies. We know CBD seemingly inhibits how much glutamate is released at these synapses. Perhaps it's this action that is the secret.

Also, while CBD has does have a very low binding affinity for CB_1 receptors, it also powerfully decreases the activity of G proteins. In other words, perhaps it's not the receptors CBD interacts with. Maybe it's the ligands.

In addition, it's likely that CBD probably helps epilepsy by affecting the orphan receptor GPR55, as well as modulating TPRV1 signalling. There is evidence supporting effects on the 5HTA1 receptor, as well as the alpha 3 and alpha 1 glycine receptors.

It seems that the entourage medicine of cannabis (CBD, with cannabadivarin (CBDV) and THC (and possibly other constituents) controls **epileptogenesis,** thereby affecting the seizure threshold. CB_1 receptors act differently during epileptogenesis and after recurrent seizures. Again, CBD is able to modulate this by controlling glutamate release. Finally, Cannabidiol also prevents the spread of seizure activity through the brain via its influences on GABA.

I say finally, but I doubt it stops there. There will be more, perhaps, that I have missed or they have yet to find. Either way, that's probably still an incomplete assessment. I can feel it in my waters!

Many of the most beautiful research papers about cannabis come from Israel. This especially applies in epilepsy. We'll begin right back in 1980, in one of the first experiments done by Mechoulam, the father of cannabis medicine.

He created a two-phase study where, in the first phase, healthy volunteers were either given CBD or a glucose placebo. Then in the second phase, 15 volunteers with temporal-focused epilepsy were either given 200-300mg of CBD, or a placebo, over a period of up to four and a half months. Every participant continued to take anti-convulsant meds, even though the group had been screened as medication no longer helping their symptoms.

No toxicity or side effects were seen in either group.

At the end of the trial eight out of the fifteen were almost free of the seizures. Three had seen partial improvements and CBD had proved ineffective in one patient (I can't identify where the other three participants went I'm afraid!).

Good first results.

Over time, many different trials have taken place, first to isolate what kinds of epilepsy CBD seems to help, and secondly to try to elucidate the mechanisms that create the epilepsy phenotype.

A retrospective study from February 2016 by paediatric neurology units from seven different hospitals in Tel Aviv described how five paediatric epileptic clinics were using a regime of medical cannabis oil to treat children and adolescents. All participants were described as having intractable epilepsy, which means the condition refuses to come under control with conventional treatment. Their epilepsy was resistant to any one of seven antiepileptic drugs. 66% of them had also been tried on a ketogenic diet, and had had a vagal nerve stimulator plantation, but their conditions still refused to respond.

The study included 74 patients in total, with a wide range of ages from 1 to 18 years. They'd all started being treated with the cannabis oil in 2014, between the months of February to November.

Every participant stayed on the treatment for at least three months but most had continued treatment for an average of nine months. The selected formula contained CBD but also tetrahydrocannabinol at a ratio of 20 to 1 (this has higher levels of THC than we work with in the hemp oil). The blend had been dissolved into olive oil.

The CBD dose varied, ranging from 1 to 20 mg per kilogram of body weight per day. The parents then reported on how frequently their children had experienced seizures.

The effect of the cannabis treatment was remarkable.

89% of the children experienced a reduction in seizure frequency.

13 of 74 even reported a 75-100% reduction.

Twenty-five children experienced a reduction of between 50 to 75%.

Nine had had their seizures reduced by between 25 to 50%.

Only 26% of the group reported a reduction of less than 25%.

Sadly, **five patients reported seizures worsening with the CBD** so had been taken off the oil. Presumably these are the ones that only completed three months of treatment.

These effects on the seizures would have been wonderful in their own right, but there was more. Behaviour had improved, so had their alertness. Language and communication was enhanced. They were sleeping better and they were finding motor skills easier too.

Some adverse reactions were noted, again leading to cannabis being taken away from five patients. These included sleepwalking, general fatigue, disturbances in their gastrointestinal movements, and general irritability.

The report labels the results as *highly promising* and warranting more clinical trials to further investigate the effects of CBD on intractable epilepsy.

In December 2013, The University of Stamford Department of Neurology appealed on Facebook to a dedicated group of parents of epileptic children who were using a page to pool their experiences of using CBD to help their children. The university wanted to glean data about their outcomes.

Of the respondents, nineteen had children who matched the criteria of the survey.

Thirteen had Dravet's.

Four had Doose Syndrome.

One had Lennox-Gastaut Syndrome.

One had idiopathic epilepsy.

I won't go into the differences, suffice it to say they are all nasty strains of different types of epilepsy that refuse to submit to the will of medications. In fact, on average, these parents, like the Figi family, had all gone through twelve different treatments (none of which had worked) before they had started treating their children with CBD.

The results of the survey were published:

84% said they had seen a reduction in the frequency of the seizures.

11% of these – 2 people - said there had been no more seizures at all.

42% - 8 people – said their kids had benefited from a greater than 80% reduction in seizures.

32% - 6 parents – said the reduction of their children's seizures was somewhere between 25-60%.

The overall opinion was that the children were more alert, had better moods, and were sleeping better too. Although it was also reported that the treatment made some of the kids feel drowsy and fatigued.

I will point out that this is a slightly biased survey since it is taken from already converted people, but it certainly tells a story, doesn't it? However, a 2015 paper by Katona *Cannabis and Endocannabinoid signalling in Epilepsy* expresses a concern that not every patient will respond well to cannabis. Katona writes:

"*However, emerging data show that patient responsiveness varies substantially, and that **cannabis administration may sometimes even exacerbate seizures**. Qualitative and quantitative chemical variability in cannabis products and personal differences in the etiology of seizures, or in the pathological reorganization of epileptic networks, can all contribute to divergent patient responses. Thus, the consensus view in the neurologist community is that drugs modifying the activity of the endocannabinoid system should first be tested in clinical trials to establish efficacy, safety, dosing, and proper indication in specific forms of epilepsies.*"

Right through the traditional medicine and in the homeopathic process, we are advised the amount of cannabis we should be using is small. Modern recommendation is the same, to start off on very low doses to monitor effects before building up. Be observant and document well. At all points, aim to ensure that you are not being led by what you *want* to see happening rather than what actually is.

Neurodegeneration

A report undertaken by Reading University, UK, in connection with G W Pharmaceuticals, gives us a sobering glimpse into the current status of research into CBD for degenerative neurological conditions. It gathered together all available research papers in an effort to prioritise the next steps for exploration.

It explained the challenges the vast array of data now presents.

Their data collection identified over 65 separate mechanisms that CBD uses to protect the brain.

- 15% were through ion channels
- 15% were through receptors
- 20% were exerted through actions on transport proteins
- 49% of CBD's effects were due to how it related to enzymes in the body

(Hmmm, we mislaid one percent somewhere. I'll attribute it to rounding, but you'd like to attribute it to magic, that works for me too!).

More than enough to go on, but then many avenues could be ruled out. Most required concentrations of CBD that were far too large to be adaptable. Sometimes experiments had elucidated how reactions had been triggered, but the studies had then not adequately proved this reaction as the actual catalyst of the disease. Other targets uncovered were entirely irrelevant to neurodegeneration. Occasionally, an active molecule *had* revealed itself as a potential target, but other experiments had already proved that molecule would be unhelpful further down the line. Lastly, studies had shown that it might modulate a certain enzyme but it had already been found that messing with that might have a bad outcome (ironically, this was written just months before the FAAH tragedy we spoke of earlier).

The recommendations were that from this point onwards research should now focus on GCPR55, voltage anion channel 1, and calcium sulphite in the body, all of which are associated with intracellular calcium. Although it has not yet been proved that calcium is causal to neurodegeneration, focusing research is expected to bring them closer to the truth.

Autism

So, what about our miracle of the mute boy made to speak? How did that happen, and can it be replicated again?

There seems no reason why not. All the evidence stacks up.

Neuroligins are proteins on the surface of cells and their job is to connect the network of cell signalling. Connecting pre- and postsynaptic signalling, they shape the network of messages that pass through the brain and body.

Deficits in the genes that code neuroligins seem to be implicated in autism and other cognitive disorders.

The body needs Neuroligin 3 (NL3) for tonic endocannabinoid signalling to work properly. Scientists suspect problems here might underline autism. To assess whether their theories hold water, they are focusing on Fragile X Syndrome known to be one of the most common causes of autism. It happens because the body lacks a protein (FMR) that is supposed to regulate signal transduction. Without it there is nothing to stabilise neuronal excitability, and so you will see issues like hyperactivity, deficits in attention, and seizures.

The endocannabinoid system is vital to modulating key parts of this. It underpins synaptic plasticity, how well our cognition works, levels of anxiety, levels of pain via nociception, and again, seizures.

Strange anomalies seem to exist in both CB_1 and CB_2 receptors. Firstly, there is a huge upregulation of CB_2 receptors in autism, possibly in response to inflammatory nature of the disease. Potentially, the inflammation might be blamed on the fact there is a huge surplus of cytokines. This may be because of the problems with NL3.

We also know that anandamide seems to be inhibited at their CB_2 receptors.

CB_1 is interesting because it is linked to basic emotions and helps you to distinguish a happy face from a sad one. Where there is a deficit, and there is in autism, it's much harder to recognise facial expressions. This might explain the atypical stare people on the spectrum can have, and their reluctance to make eye contact. Potentially, they don't get the same reward feedback from a smile as we do; these standard societal rules seem rather odd.

Tonic signalling modulates the genitourinary system and, most notably, metabolism. Again, issues with NL3 skewing the signalling has deleterious effects on key processes, like digestion.

Since the stress response is encoded via our sunshine 5HT receptor, we can see how CBD might be able to help from a different angle. That said, experiments show that activating PPAR α, PPARy, or the GPR55 with cannabinoids all reduce autistic symptoms in rats.

ADD/ADHD

I couldn't find loads on this area, which disappointed me, but here goes.

There is a distinct correlation between people with ADD/ADHD and marijuana use. Somehow, they are self-medicating, it seems. There also seems to be a relationship between a child who has ADD/ADHD and becoming an adult who is at higher risk of cannabis disorders. They suffer more cravings and more "use-related conditions" – I've taken that to mean psychosis and paranoia, but I concede that I am not sure.

I could only really find one trial that helped us, but it was a good one from Melbourne in 2012. Hyperactivity and social withdrawal were inhibited by a cocktail of cannabidiol and clozapine. What's more, the social withdrawal wasn't just normalised to benchmark levels, it was better than the control subjects in the trial (which were rats).

It's enough, I think, don't you?

Multiple Sclerosis (MS)

Sativex, also known under the INN as Nabiximols, is a 1:1 THC:CBD drug designed to treat spasticity on MS patients. Trials also show it reducing neuropathic pain, muscle spasms, and sleep disturbance, however, it remains a controversial treatment here in the UK. It is recommended for treatment within the NHS under the NICE guidelines (National Institute for Health and Care Excellence) as it has still not received a full technology review, however, the organisation feels it may not become part of standard treatment plans as it is not a cost-effective treatment. Those who are able to get it (must be under NHS Wales) are subject to close observation and must prove a significant reduction in spasticity within the first four weeks of prescription, or treatment is stopped.

Around 10% of patients experience adverse effects from the drug such as sleepiness, dizziness, fatigue, or feeling like they are drunk, and it tends to create a nasty taste in the mouth. So, the quest continues and naturally, scientists are interested to understand CBD's part in the treatment, and whether that can be exploited further.

Inflammation in the CNS happens because leukocytes travel across the blood brain barrier and then activate resident immune cells. In 2013, Madrid published their results of their voyage of understanding of why CBD had such strong immunosuppressant properties.

Clearly, as the leukocytes find their way to the brain, they need to find a way to anchor themselves on vascular cells as a means of feeding and replicating. They do this via adhesion molecules, such as VCAM1. The team found that CBD calmed the cell migration by downregulating VCAM1, the chemokines CCL2 and CL5, as well as the pro-inflammatory marker IL-1β. This in turn calmed down how microglia were despatched to the site. This action seemed to derive from one of the adenosine receptors $A(2)A$.

In January 2017, a new pathway was elucidated that might offer help for MS and other conditions with cannabidiol. The P13/Akt/mTOR pathway regulates the natural cycle of a cell, particularly proliferation. As you might imagine, this is an important treatment pathway for research into cancer too. It is believed the pathway also contributes to the long-term potentiation of synapses we talked about in PTSD.

Italian scientists created an experimental Autoimmune Encephalomyelitis model in mice and treated them with CBD. After 14 days of observations they euthanised the mice (their word, not mine, and I've never seen it used in trials before so I dread to think what rodent symptoms they were seeing), and analysed spinal tissues.

The assault had caused a stark downregulation of the P13/Akt/mTOR pathway which CBD restored. It had reduced production of proinflammatory cytokines such as INFy and IL-17 by switching up activity in the channel, PPARy. Then, by inhibiting kinases such as JNK and P38 that are triggered by heat shocks, cytokine activity, or UV radiation, it had stopped their influence T cell differentiation and apoptosis. The CBD restored the function of P13/Akt/mTOR signalling.

Magical, magical stuff.

The stuff of science fiction, no less, but true!

Cannabis, people, one spectacular plant. What a flippin' amazing healer.

Parkinson's Disease

Anecdotal evidence shows CBD producing beneficial effects in Alzheimer's and Parkinson's disease, and MS, but so far scientists don't feel that for Parkinson's they have enough evidence yet to create a cannabinoid drug. Animal evidence certainly seems to indicate good opportunities, but in the few cases where humans have been assessed, sample sizes are still too small to be confident that effects can be generalised. It is frustrating, but so far, inspiring.

Sometimes that inspiration concerns me. I worry that I get so excited by what I see in a paper that I fail to see the patient and what the disease is doing to them. Mostly I love my job, but sometimes looking this deeply into an illness feels suffocating. It was like that with the correlations between Alzheimer's and hot flashes in the clary sage book and now it feels that way here, again, with Parkinson's disease. I always aim to remain human in these books and likewise to try to understand the holistic nature these afflictions bring to someone's life. Nevertheless, there is something about neurodegeneration that completely rips my heart out. I find these sections terrifying to write.

There can be a danger of washing over the seriousness of illness, and whilst that would be true of every condition in the book, I wanted to use Parkinson's disease (PD) as a demonstration model of how illness ravages every area of a person's life. How the emotional impact of the physical condition becomes just as much of the horror as the presenting symptoms. A good tool for this is to use condition benchmark questionnaires.

When study groups want to monitor changes in condition they will use scales to gauge the changes in disease. The two main ones in Parkinson's are the UPDRS (Unified Parkinson's Disease Rating Scale), and the PDQ-39 (Parkinson's Disease Questionnaire). The UPDRS gauges the stage of the illness with regards to speech, depression, and how bad hallucinations are getting, whether they are benign hallucinations where the patient retains insight, or the condition has deteriorated into florid psychosis.

Can the person still turn over in bed okay? How are they managing to swallow? Are they dribbling a lot now and how often are their movements freezing?

The PDQ39 is more focused on understanding their quality of life at any time. Are they having trouble cooking or carrying shopping bags? Are they managing to leave the house, do they need to be accompanied and how far can they walk? Are they now having difficulties dressing or tying their laces? How well can they manage to write now or cut up their food? Are they managing to drink without spilling? Then, also, how often do they feel isolated and lonely? Are they feeling bitter or angry about their condition? Are they becoming weepy and tearful?

It all tells a particularly distressing story.

But, CBD does seem to help, although as ever mechanisms are still very hazy.

Do you remember the substantia nigra, where the blackened dopamine neurons live? Parkinson's is characterised by the death of these neurons in this area.

Cell death seems to take place after times of oxidative stress or energy crisis, but rather than killing them instantly the body gently, and cruelly, kicks apoptosis into gear. They die gentle and natural deaths as part of the brain's natural growth pattern. The problem is of course, they are not supposed to be dead.

When you look at a post mortem brain of a person who had Parkinson's you will find anomalies in the number of CB_2 receptors in the glial elements of the brain and in some sub-populations of neurons. Downregulation of CB_2 receptors is common to Parkinson's patients, in response the receptors then dramatically **upregulate** as the body tries to battle the damage of the failing neurons. It seems likely that CB_2 receptors in the brain form a dynamic internal defence against oxidation. What is certain, is activating CB_2 receptors slows the progression of neurodegeneration.

The United Arab Emirates University proved in 2016 that they could manipulate the brain's neuroprotective capacity by using beta caryophyllene to upregulate the CB_2 receptor.

The beta caryophyllene rescued the dopaminergic neurons and their fibres by reducing how many glial cells had been activated by a chemical attack. This is a significant breakthrough for Parkinson's research, but also for you and I as aromatherapists, because this is one of our most simple tools, inherent not only in CBD, but also **hemp essential oil**, black pepper, and so on. It showed significant neuroprotection via its anti-inflammatory and anti-oxidant abilities, which are executed through the CB_2 receptor.

Now, before you get carried away…

Remember, these trials were not on people, they were on ratties. And there is more.

In 2006, the University of Madrid had already proved that if you were able to treat the patient with CBD **immediately** after a lesion had formed, it could help restrict the depletion of dopamine, but the same would not be true if it were administered a week later. The treatment must be immediate, and since we still don't really understand what causes Parkinsonian lesions – a whole cocktail of age, environmental, genetics – it's almost impossible to supplement with CBD on demand…unless you are taking it habitually, of course.

Symptomatically then, what possibilities does CBD hold?

Well, when I read a study from Sao Paulo in 2014 (they are busy there, aren't they?) it lifted my heart.

A trial of 21 patients split into three groups of seven. One group was given a placebo, the second was treated with cannabidiol (75 mg per day) and the third with CBD (300 mg per day) (just in case that has confused anyone and you think *"They're the same thing!"* In essence you are correct, but here scientists wanted to see how the single cannabinoid would compare against the entourage effect of the high CBD cannabis oil). The participants had been screened to ensure there were no incidences of dementia or comorbid psychiatric conditions.

Now, I might be being thick here, but I am fairly certain they don't say how long the trial was. Certainly, it was more than two weeks because they assess patients during the last week of the trial and prior to the first. On assessment of the scores at the end of the trial there were no differences in the UPDRS, but in both the placebo and CBD groups there were significant improvements in the PDQ39 scores. It seemed the CBD had affected their general wellbeing and quality of life, but since there was a placebo improvement, so had the *expectation* that it might. Hope is a powerful thing.

Strangely, the Sao Paolo team had seen the opposite outcome on the UPDRS score in 2009 when they had focused on assessing CBD's effects on Parkinson's patients who were now in the grip of psychosis. It was a tiny study of four men and two women who had been suffering from psychosis for more than three months. They were given a flexible dose, starting at 150mg per day for four weeks. At the end, all four of them were much better. Their motor skills had not worsened and this time, they *did* see an improvement in the UPDRS scores. Likewise, when they were assessed against the Brief Psychiatric Scale and the Parkinson Psychosis Questionnaire, there has been a significant decrease in their psychotic symptoms.

One last study, before we leave this topic, is the 2014 Sao Paolo evidence that CBD also helps a sleep disorder, specific to Parkinson's, called RBD. This is a strange phenomenon occurring in the REM stage of sleep that results in night terrors, sleep walking, and other dangerous incidents.

The write up in the paper is short and sweet:

"Four patients treated with CBD had prompt and substantial reduction in the frequency of RBD-related events without side effects."

Alzheimer's Disease

Alzheimer's affects 3.3 million people worldwide and this number is expected to triple in the next forty years. Consequently, huge numbers of research hours are taking place in this arena. Cannabis remains subject to legal restraints and the studies that *have* taken place give us hints but not much more. Again, anecdotal evidence of symptoms improving is everywhere, but it is still not clearly understood why.

Studying what cannabis does to the brain has illuminated grey areas about a disease in which we previously had very little comprehension. Evidence carries the same burdens: small sample sizes, lack of placebo controls, and studies that are simply too short. Consequently, we are at the same frustrating crossroads as with pretty much every other condition.

In post mortem analysis, Alzheimer's-afflicted brains demonstrate anomalies in CB_1 and CB_2 receptors. The expression of CB_1 receptors has been reduced, but CB_2 has been enhanced, and there seems to be a correlation between the number of CB_2 receptors and a protein that makes plaques on the brain, $A\beta42$.

A correlation also seems to be evident between cortical CB_1 levels and cognitive test scores taken in the final year before a patient's death. CB_1 in the patient's brains had remained intact in those scoring higher, suggesting that these may have protected and preserved their cognitive function.

When frontal and temporal cortices of the brain are analysed (post mortem), levels of anandamide and its precursor, NArPE, are found to be reduced. This also seems to correlate with a person's speed of information processing and their language abilities. No changes in 2-AG are observed.

In brain locations exhibiting plaque pathology, there seem to be raised levels of FAAH. A recent popular hypothesis is that FAAH degrades anandamide, and in so doing releases arachidonic acid. This results in proinflammatory eicosanoids being despatched, leading to even more inflammation.

On another tack, since MAGL degrades 2-AG, it's been suggested genetic deletion of MAGL might be beneficial. Since this, too, is a precursor to the harmful eicosanoids, slamming the brakes on here reduces activation of glia, curbs associated neuro inflammation and, finally, reduces amyloid plaques.

Or that's the theory anyway!

Despite so little evidence, what we do have about CBD is compelling and has been filtering through since the turn of the Millennium. In Naples in 2004, scientists proved that if you treated cells with CBD just before injuring them (with a chemical Aβ peptide), you could significantly raise the cells' chances of survival. CBD decreases ROS, reduces lipid peroxidation, fragmentation of DNA, and stabilises intracellular calcium levels. It was also proven to reduce levels of caspase 3, a programmed mediator of cell death.

Subsequent studies have also demonstrated CBD's ability to protect the adrenal cells, PC12, and microglial cells, N13, as well as other primary microglial cells from the rigours of Aβ toxicity.

So, CBD protects the brain magnificently through diverse several mechanisms. Neuroprotective, anti-oxidant and anti-apoptotic, CBD-rich hemp oil marches like a well-trained army to wage war against Aβ toxins.

In August 2007, the University of Roma further announced their discovery that CBD also blunted the gene expression of *Glial Fibrillary Acidic Protein,* a long chain protein that brings rigidity to structures such as keratin and collagen. Apart from one of the precursors to amyloid plaques, GFAP may also be a precursor to tumours.

Impeding the mechanism, it also impaired the release of the pro-inflammatory marker IL-1 beta protein and its related nitric oxide.

When scientists experimented using Sativex in test tubes, they also found that the 1:1 ratio of THC:CBD blunted microglial reactivity of a protein called tau, abundantly found in the CNS and in oligodendrocytes. Mesmerised by the outcomes, they were surprised to find that despite all that they had learned about Alzheimer's and the CB_1 and 2 receptors, this mechanism seemed to be completely independent of either. Rather than CB_1 or CB_2, the magical effects came from the PPAR pathways. Subsequently, other mechanisms have been discovered exerting their influences through PPARα, PPARγ, and TPRV1.

Recommendations about treatment seem to be to blockade the CB1 receptor and then try to enhance the CB_2 receptor's action. Whilst we do not yet have an aromatic way to manipulate CB_1, outside of CBD's ability to curb the action of THC there, we have a brilliant tool in beta caryophyllene as a mechanism to curb the inflammation. Blend CBD-rich hemp oil with hemp essential oil for a real leap ahead of the drug companies right now.

Huntington's Disease

A central nervous system disorder, Huntington's is an inherited disease. Symptoms usually develop in adulthood somewhere between the ages of 35 and 55 and derives from damage to nerve cells in the brain. Symptoms are distressingly intrusive and tend to get progressively worse until the patient dies, usually from some infection that the body can no longer fight off.

It affects movement and behaviours. It impairs cognition, distorts perception, and influences a person's awareness, thinking, and judgement. Their personality changes radically, no longer taking family members' feelings into consideration. They become extremely agitated or excited, but they also have long periods of being plunged into the darkest depression. Moods swing from extreme highs to very deep lows.

Over time, they find communication ever more difficult. Understanding what is said to them, they struggle to respond as it becomes harder to translate their thoughts into words. Consequently, they become less responsive and more withdrawn.

The disease used to be called Huntington's chorea, as a description of its characteristic movement traits. Chorea, the Greek word for dancing, describes how the patient seems to be dancing a jerky jig. Thank goodness we have moved further away from that delightful term! Initially, one might notice a loved one developing a tic, especially in facial movements. Then the tic develops to twitching and these seem to travel around the body, often causing them to lurch or fall. This dystonia, as it is known, gets progressively worse over time, until finally, the body becomes entirely rigid.

Huntington's sufferers tend to lose a great deal of weight even though they have good appetites. Eating is awkward, their dystonia making it difficult to feed themselves and the muscles in the mouth and throat begin to further dysfunction. Swallowing is difficult, especially of thin liquids like water, and choking is a very real hazard.

Often Huntington's suffers might seem as if they lack motivation, no longer being mindful of personal hygiene or social cues. This is not a personality trait, it is a result of the disease changing their perception. Sexual drive often plummets, but less often can also mean the patient starts making inappropriate sexual demands. In rare occasions, patients will also present with OCD or schizophrenia too.

It's very easy to see why depression can descend, and it is hard to pinpoint whether the aggression, irritability, and anger come as an emotional response to the situation or whether it is a physiological fact. Either way, suicidal tendencies are high.

As the throat becomes more vulnerable, so does the entirety of the respiratory system. Chest infections also become rifer. Eventually, it is usually pneumonia that claims the life.

Perhaps even more tragically is there is also a juvenile version of the disease, affecting children under the age of twenty.

To date, no suitable treatment has been found for Huntington's disease.

It needs all the help it can get. So, it warms my heart to see the same names on the Huntington's research reappearing over and over again.

Research cannabis long enough and just like aromatherapy has rock stars, Tisserand, Pappas, Shepheard Hyam, Price and Price, Shutes (you'll have your own list); people whose work you thirst for because you know they really know and love what they are talking about. Those cannabis megastars ignite the same sort of excitement in me as does hearing U2's new song these days. You probably clocked I feel like that about Ethan Russo, when we were reading the history (even though he is a vitally important neuroscientist). Pretty much every paper in Huntington's research is written and researched by one of these megastars, Mechoulam, Ramos, Fernandez-Ruis, Pertwee…and many more who don their white coats day after day in a bid to try to make sense of why cannabis helps this disease and in so doing, learn more about why the body attacks itself in this way. It is incredibly reassuring.

Despite this, and they would still be the first to tell you that the same restrictions apply. The studies are too few and still do not provide enough evidence for cannabinoids to be created into treatments for Huntington's. But treatment options for this horrible disease are so limited the battle is on to make sense of the understanding that the CB_1 and CB_2 receptor seem to be intrinsically linked to the neurological decline.

Here, as you might expect, a Sativex-like blend of 1:1 THC:CBD holds the promise of helping the spasticity it is so helpful for in MS, and this features highly in the research, but for a change we'll begin with some data about a different cannabinoid, also found in high CBD Hemp Oil: cannabigerol or **CBG.**

The Universidad Complutense, Madrid, seems particularly motivated in this field, and in 2012 they injured the brains of some mice using a toxin – 3-

Nitropropionate or 3NP (I'll remember that well, because 3NP is also Dexter's class at school!). Here, they found that the CBG improved motor deficits that the 3-NP caused by preserving neurons in the striatum. The 3-NP triggered a defensive microglial response, as the body tried hard to battle the invasion, and just as in Huntington's, the microglia did not know when to stop, going into overdrive and upregulating proinflammatory markers. CBG prevented this response, again, protecting the brain.

Next, they compared data they had gleaned from R6/2 mice, created to mimic the effects of Huntington's disease. Here, they were able to assess what genes might be involved. Seven genes (symplklin, Sin3a, Rcor1, histone deacetylase 2, Huntingtin-associated protein1, the σ subunit of the GABA-A receptor, and hippocalcium), were all altered in the R6/2 mice and were partially normalised by the CBG.

Neurotrophins... We like these guys.

Fighting for the survival and development of neurons, this is a family of proteins that signal to cells commanding them to survive, differentiate, or grow. Their action is described as neurotrophic.

CBG also induced an improvement, albeit modest, in the gene expression of BDNF (Brain Derived Neurotrophic factor).

It was also noticed that PPARy was altered in the R6/2 mice, as was the insulin-like growth factor. The CBG also brought about a small, but described as "significant", reduction in how the mutant huntingtin protein collected in the striatum.

Based on the results here, they wondered if CBG, alone or in tandem with other cannabinoids, might be able to offer some treatment effects for HD.

The same year, Universidad Complutense again, and this time the rats were treated using an enzyme inhibitor called Malonate that damages striatal neurons. It usually does this through apoptosis and by activating microglia. The team wanted to measure the extent of the damage and if it might be possible to somehow preserve the neurons in the striatal parenchyma.

They assessed the state of the brain using Nuclear Magnetic Resonance, the most familiar type of which is MRI scanning.

Four effects were noted:

1. Malonate increased swelling (oedema) in the brain. The cannabinoid blend reduced it.
2. Nissl is a granular substance that lives in the ribosome of the cell and enables protein synthesis. It is found on the dendrite and soma but not on

the hillock of the nerve cell. Interestingly, it can be stained blue so you can observe its changes. Clearly, less protein synthesis, less new nerve cells created. Malonate reduced the number of nissl-stained cells and enhanced the number of degenerating cells. The Sativex-like blend reversed this.

3. Malonate triggered a harsh microglial response. The THC:CBD mix reduced this.
4. Malonate increased expression of nitric oxide synase and the neurotrophin IGF. Both were reduced and modulated by the cannabis extracts.

Next, blocking the pathways of the CB_1 and CB_2 receptors, they found these improvements no longer took place, again validating the assumption that they play a vital part in controlling this disease.

March 2017, Madrid again, and our team of heroes have decided to investigate what effects the Sativex-like blend might have on the R6/2 mice.

Treatment began just four weeks after their birth. By six weeks the R6/2, our rodent friends, had started to show symptoms, and then they continued to worsen until ten weeks of age. Their behaviour mimicked the dystonia of Huntington's and the characteristic lack of coordination. This was demonstrated by mice being exposed to a rotarod experiment and also displaying clasping behaviour, their gait becoming awkward.

While the Sativex-like mix did not help the rotarod co-ordination, their clasping behaviour was markedly improved. In other words, the dystonia receded but they were still very lacking in co-ordination.

At ten weeks, it showed metabolic activity at the basal ganglia was reduced and this had been attenuated by the Sativex mix. At twelve weeks, prognostic markers such as energy failure, mitochondrial function, and excitotoxicity was gauged. The R6/2 mice looked very similar to what would be expected in this point of deterioration in Huntington's, but those treated with the cannabinoids were nowhere near as poorly.

It showed the cannabis extracts had protected several amino acid interchanges: taurine/creatine, taurine/N-acetylaspartate, and N-acetylaspartate/choline.

These interchanges, usually seen in HD decline, had been completely reversed.

A very old trial, from back in 1991, when dinosaurs roamed the world of cannabinoid research, formed the basis of our understanding of bioavailability.

15 patients were vetted to ensure they had no psychotic symptoms and then were either give an oral dosage of cannabinoids at 10mg/kg of body weight per day for six weeks, or the same dosage of sesame oil (isn't it interesting that the placebo chosen is also the alternative Sanskrit translation of the word hemp? I wonder if that is coincidence or someone's romantic nature?).

They assessed the amount of CBD in blood plasma levels weekly using cas spectrometry.

The mean range found was between 5.9-11.2ng/ml.

That's small, and it is what forms the basis of our understanding of bioavailability today…but there is more.

The levels remained constant, meaning the cannabinoids worked in a different way to essential oils. E/O usage is cumulative, it grows stronger the more you use them. That's not what we see here. The levels seem to remain fairly static, irrespective of how long they are used (not what you would expect to see given that people build marijuana tolerance over time).

Interestingly, ***no significantly or clinically important differences*** were found in the groups, so potentially sesame does the same, but that is research for another day.

Prion/Mad Cow Disease

There was some interest shown in 2007 to a study done in Valbonne, France, that showed CBD prevented the accumulation of the affective protein Prion that causes this neurodegenerative disease. Further, when they infected mice with the sheep version, scrapie, the CBD inhibited the neurotoxic effects and calmed the microglial release in a concentration dependant manner. The trail seems to have gone cold here. Perhaps the concentrations were too large or perhaps they found a more promising neurological outcome to chase, I suppose. Dunno.

ALS

Amyotrophic Lateral Sclerosis (ALS) is a rare group of neurological diseases mainly involving the neurons that control voluntary muscle movement. Voluntary muscles help us to chew, walk, breath, and talk. A progressive disease, there is currently no cure for ALS and no effective treatment has been found to halt, or reverse, the progression of the disease.

Belonging to a wider group of disorders known as motor neuron disease, a gradual deterioration and death of the motor neurons cause it. Motor neurons are the nerve cells that run from the brain to the spinal cord and then on to the muscles throughout the body. They initiate and provide the vital communication links between the brain and the voluntary muscles.

Early symptoms of ALS will often include muscle weakness or stiffness. Gradually all muscles, under voluntary control, are taken hostage. Sufferers weaken, eventually losing the ability to speak, eat, move, or even breathe. Most ALS deaths result from respiratory failure within three to five years from when the first symptoms occur. About ten percent of ALS patients survive for over ten years

Because of patients exhibiting such anecdotal success with cannabis, the Muscular Dystrophy and ALS Centre in Seattle called for further research to be focused onto ALS.

The author of the article, G.T Cater, explained that the ideal drug combination for potential treatment would have the following attributes in a bid to slow down the progression of the disease and perhaps prolong life:

- Glutamate antagonist
- Anti-oxidant
- Anti-inflammatory, working from central to the organism
- Would enhance the activity of one or more neurotrophic growth factors

I concur. That certainly looks like cannabis.

Likewise, cannabinoids work as:

- Analgesics
- Muscle relaxants
- Help with bronchodilation
- Reduce saliva
- Stimulate appetite
- Induce sleep

All of which would be blissful relief from the burdens of facing this cruel disease when you wake up each day.

Mind Body Interface

Inflammation

Every immune response is triggered and navigated by chemical messengers called cytokines. Released by immunologically responsive cells, they exert control over any cell possessing a cytokine receptor. Working as the foreman of the system they encourage or inhibit replication of different cell types. This is the fundamental basis of both immune and allergic responses. There are many different types of cytokines that can be divided into two groups: proinflammatory ones and ones that are essentially anti-inflammatory, but that will also promote an allergic reaction.

T-lymphocytes, produced by the thymus, are one of the major sources of cytokines. These cells have specific receptors on the cell surface, enabling them to recognise foreign invaders. However, in a person suffering an autoimmune disorder, cytokines also mistake normal tissues as bad guys and attack it. If the proinflammatory response becomes too excessive, it leads to tissue damage, spiralling out of control.

Most of the cytokines circulating the body are understood to be produced by a subset of T-lymphocytes known as **Helper T cells.** We can divide this subset again into Th1 and Th2, thus any cytokines produced can then be recognised as Th1-type cytokines and Th2-type cytokines (TH delineating T helper).

Bored?

Yep and me...

But, now, wake up.

Because this is kind of a turn-around point.

These cytokine profiles correspond to different types of *disease* profile.

TH1 disease corresponds to chronic inflammation and we see high levels of interleukins 1, 2, 12, 18, and **<u>interferon gamma</u>** (INF). I'm underlining that because I want you to remember it. Essentially, these are all pro-inflammatory cytokines but interferon gamma is the TH1 big guy. He's the main man.

The very shortened version of TH2 - allergic and atopic reactions - we'll return to in a bit.

So, why are these cytokines activated in the first place? What sets them off?

Brace yourselves guys...we are into the dark space of teensy little nasties again...

You need a microscope and very strong nerves.

Welcome to the microbiota. Scary little intracellular blighters including L-form, biofilm, and other bacterial forms. Sounds complicated? Well yes, it can be, but basically it is communities of otherwise healthy bacteria. So, remember the yoghurt ads that are always telling us to look after our gut flora? Gut flora are just one type of microbiota.

These intracellular parasites creep in and the body says: *"Nuh-uh, not happening, you're not welcome, I'm afraid,"* (incidentally, *my* body's that polite but I can't speak for yours, of course!).

Courteously, physiology instructs an army of Th1-type cytokines to eradicate the interlopers. The microbiota, a tad incensed by the audacity of it all, fight back, and it's this ongoing battle that is often behind proinflammatory responses. Subsequently, over time, it perpetuates an autoimmune response. So here we're thinking vastly inflamed conditions like fibromyalgia, but also Hashimoto's, Thyroiditis, pernicious anaemia, and even lupus.

Naturally then, the ideal scenario is that the body has a well-balanced Th1 and Th2 response. Out of kilter though, Th2 responds, which will counteract TH1's otherwise beneficial microbicidal action, and as we have seen TH1 going wrong, this doesn't look very good either.

What might *wrong* look like?

A couple of examples.

In 2015, after decades of tolerating labels such as malingerers, shirkers, or skivers, sufferers of Chronic Fatigue Syndrome (CFS) or Myalgic Encephalomyelitis (ME) were offered hope when scientists discovered that people who had had the condition for three years or less had significantly raised levels of cytokines and particularly high amounts of interferon gamma (INF).

INF is linked to the dreadful feelings of fatigue you feel when you have influenza (but that's not why I told you to hold on to it, so don't let go yet...). Researchers posit these as triggered by a virus of some kind that the immune system never quite works out how to switch off.

To be honest, the immune system does quite well really, perpetually working in over drive, but at three years it seems to fail and the levels of INF drop through the floor.

This is vitally important because it offers the very first marker for CFS/ME. In other words, a provable way to see the disease present in the physical body.

A study in the Journal of Experimental Biology and Medicine (2008), *"High plasma levels of MCP-1 and eotaxin provide evidence for an immunological basis of fibromyalgia"* showed cytokines MCP-1 and eotaxin were elevated in the blood of people with fibromyalgia, and if you added elevated levels of tumour necrosis factor alpha and interferon gamma into blood testing, then there is 70-80% likelihood that the person being tested is suffering symptoms of fibromyalgia.

One strategy being applied in a bid to prevent the onset of disease is a rigorous study of pregnancy and early postnatal life. Both states are generally recognised as Th2 phenomena triggered to minimise risks of miscarriage. The body needs this strong Th2 response, the Th1 response in utero. The foetus is capable of triggering an immune response in the first trimester, and since pregnancy is essentially a Th2 event, many babies are born with immune responses. It's proposed kids with aggressive allergies come into the world with a much weaker Th1 response, so the balance is tipped in favour of TH2. That said, more recent findings show that some children with allergies also exhibit both weakened TH1 and TH2 profiles.

Okay, so what if I told you that THC inhibits both TH1 response and promotes TH2?

I'll give you the primary school version first, where things are easily cut and dried...

TH1 illnesses include:

Allergies, alopecia areata (spot baldness), Alzheimer's and dementia, ankylosing spondylitis (inflammation of the spine), anorexia, anxiety, arthritis, asthma, bipolar disease, cancer, cardiac disease, cardiovascular disease, coeliac disease, CFS, COPD, depression, type 1 diabetes, type 2 diabetes, fibromyalgia, Guillain-Barré syndrome, hypertension, IBS, Lupus, multiple chemical sensitivity, MS, myasthenia gravis (neuromuscular disease leading to muscle weakness), obesity, OCD, osteoporosis, Parkinson's, periodontal diseases, pernicious anaemia (inability to make B12), psoriasis, rheumatoid arthritis, sarcoidosis (red and hardened lumps in the skin and lungs), schizophrenia, scleroderma (hardening of the connective tissues), Sjögrens syndrome, thyroiditis, uveitis (inflammation of the middle of the eye), and vitiligo (white patches on the skin).

Cannabinoids move the inflammatory markers and ask the body to strengthen immunity.

Now, this original research derives from around 1986, so in the scheme of things it is quite old and so it has moved on a bit from my toddler's lesson, but before I elucidate further, I was fascinated to find The Marshall Protocol, designed by Professor Trevor Marshall and his research foundation into autoimmunity. Google it. I promise you, you won't be sorry. Amongst other fascinating analysis and legwork, the team had trawled millions of epidemical studies of TH1-derived diseases and discovered massive overlaps where the same illnesses kept coming up co-morbid with other conditions. They have this spectacular diagram of what they refer to as TH1 Spectrum Disorder on their website, similar to the pin and string art so popular in the seventies. Take a look for yourself and I'd save it as a favourite in your browser, if I were you; but after hours of work, I've translated their exhaustive findings to give you a shortcut.

Allergies – Co-morbid with vitiligo and asthma

Alopecia areata– Co-morbid with depression, psoriasis, thyroiditis, vitiligo, anxiety

Alzheimer's and dementia– Co-morbid with depression and obesity

Ankylosing spondylitis – Co-morbid with uveitis, sarcoidosis, cardiovascular disease, both types of diabetes, IBS

Anorexia – Co-morbid with anxiety and vitiligo

Anxiety – Co-morbid with depression, sarcoidosis, vitiligo

Arthritis – Co-morbid with IBS, lupus, psoriasis

Asthma – Co-morbid with both types of diabetes, depression, cardiac and cardiovascular diseases, anxiety, allergies, rheumatoid arthritis, osteoporosis, obesity, IBS

Bipolar disease – Co-morbid with depression, sarcoidosis, obesity, anxiety, vitiligo

Cancer – Co-morbid with depression, asthma, IBS

Cardiac disease – Co-morbid with diabetes, depression, COPD, Parkinson's, periodontal disease, psoriasis, schizophrenia

Cardiovascular – Co-morbid with depression, cardiovascular, asthma, ankylosing spondylitis

Coeliac disease – Co-morbid with thyroiditis, pernicious anaemia, IBS, type 1 diabetes

CFS – Co-morbid with fibromyalgia and IBS

COPD – Co-morbid with both types of diabetes, hypertension, osteoporosis

Depression – Co-morbid with IBS, multiple chemical sensitivity, obesity, psoriasis, sarcoidosis, cardiovascular disease, cardiac disease, asthma, anxiety, alopecia, vitiligo

Diabetes type 1 – Co-morbid with vitiligo, thyroid diseases, coeliac disease

Diabetes type 2 – Co-morbid with periodontal disease

Fibromyalgia – Co-morbid with CFS and IBS

Guillain-Barré syndrome – Co-morbid with scleroderma, myasthenia gravis, MS, lupus

Hypertension – Co-morbid with rheumatoid arthritis, psoriasis, both types of diabetes, COPD

IBS – Co-morbid with MS, osteoarthritis, psoriasis, Sjögrens, uveitis, ankylosing spondylosis, anxiety, asthma, cancer, coeliac disease, CFS, depression, fibromyalgia

Lupus – Co-morbid with Guillain-Barré syndrome, osteoporosis, vitiligo

Multiple chemical sensitivity – Co-morbid with depression

MS – Co-morbid with vitiligo, Sjögrens, thyroiditis, IBS, Myasthenia gravis

Myasthenia gravis – Co-morbid with rheumatoid arthritis, vitiligo, MS

Obesity – Co-morbid with diabetes, depression, bipolar disorder, asthma, vitiligo

OCD – Co-morbid with schizophrenia, anxiety, bipolar disorder, anorexia

Osteoporosis – Co-morbid with lupus, IBS, COPD, asthma

Parkinson's – Co-morbid with anxiety, depression, cardiac disease

Periodontal diseases – Co-morbid with cardiac disease and diabetes type 2

Pernicious anaemia – Co-morbid with thyroiditis, vitiligo, coeliac disease, lupus

Psoriasis – Co-morbid with scleroderma, obesity, IBS, hypertension, depression

Rheumatoid arthritis – Co-morbid with psoriasis, vitiligo, cardiovascular disease, IBS

Sarcoidosis – Co-morbid with ankylosing spondylosis and depression

Schizophrenia – Co-morbid with cardiac disease and vitiligo

Scleroderma – Co-morbid with vitiligo and psoriasis

Sjögrens syndrome – Co-morbid with thyroiditis, IBS, MS

Thyroiditis – Co-morbid with pernicious anaemia, lupus, both types of diabetes, coeliac disease, alopecia, allergies, vitiligo

Uveitis – Co-morbid with IBS and ankylosing spondylitis

Vitiligo – Co-morbid with pernicious anaemia, alopecia, type 1 diabetes

TH2 then...

Its driving cytokines include interleukins 4, 5, and 13, which encourage the body to produce eosinophils (white blood cells), anti-inflammatory interleukin-10, and a substance called interglobulin E prevalent in atopic reactions.

Atopic reactions are covered extensively in my eczema book, so I'll steal a bit from there...

Atopy

Earlier I mentioned atopic dermatitis. The word atopy is from the Greek word which means special, unusual, or out of place. It pertains to hypersensitivity with allergens. An atopic disorder will only flare if someone comes into contact with a certain allergen...there must be a catalyst.

But a catalyst will not cause a reaction on its own. In the case of eczema, an allergic reaction happens because of a high level of antibodies in the system called IgE antibodies. Immunoglobulin E binds allergens to mast cells and causes inflammation by releasing histamine into the blood stream. Everyone has these antibodies in small numbers, but for some people they work particularly aggressively.

Where TH2 is running riot you're likely to see: allergic dermatitis, atopic eczema, sinusitis, inflammatory bowel disease, ulcerative colitis, systemic autoimmune diseases, urticaria, and viruses.

But I did I'd say admit to a first-grade explanation, because the truth is more complicated (of course it is. It's in this flamin' book!). Everybody is different. It's possible to have both TH1 and TH2 raised or diseases can have elements of both. Clearly there are many, many different illnesses not on my list, but you get the idea at least.

Now...the point.

Finally!

CBD and THC move responses over from TH1 to TH2. In other words, it calms the hyper response of diseases such as:

Allergies, alopecia areata, Alzheimer's and dementia, ankylosing spondylitis (inflammation of the spine), anorexia, anxiety, arthritis, asthma, bipolar disease, cancer, cardiac disease, cardiovascular disease, coeliac disease, CFS, COPD, depression, type 1 diabetes, type 2 diabetes, fibromyalgia, Guillain-Barré syndrome, hypertension, IBS, lupus, multiple chemical sensitivity, MS, myasthenia gravis, obesity, OCD, osteoporosis, Parkinson's, periodontal diseases, pernicious anaemia, psoriasis, rheumatoid arthritis, sarcoidosis (red and hardened lumps in the skin and lungs), schizophrenia, scleroderma, Sjögrens syndrome, thyroiditis, uveitis, and vitiligo.

Pretty f***ing amazing, huh?

There's more...

INF? Told you to remember it. Do you? Interferon gamma...

It's this little sodbag that modulates neuropathic pain through its effects on the CB_2 receptor. More than that, it's one of the main modulators of CB_2. So, if INF goes out of whack, CB_2 just doesn't work properly. One of the main ways CBD calms pain is by inhibiting interferon gamma. Hence, not only does CBD relax pain but it also modulates immunity too.

Mind blowing, isn't it?

Just as an aside...

At the beginning of the book, I found it very hard to get my head around the idea that THC is in the oil but in such small amounts. Initially, my brain kept saying, no THC, but of course there is. So, it will activate CB_1 receptors but to a very small degree. It will do other things too, but again, to a small degree. Add to that the fact that CB_2 receptors are the main ones for dealing with inflammation, my head struggled to visualise what CBD oil would look like helping pain. How great an effect could that tiny smidge have?

I asked Middle-Child-Maths-Genius to help me get some context.

I found an NIH report identifying THC as having twenty times the anti-inflammatory potency of aspirin and twice that of hydrocortisone.

THC exists in concentrations of 0.3%.

Andy explained that the THC content in just one gram of CBD oil matches the anti-inflammatory prowess of six grams of aspirin. What a massive support mechanism to the star of the show, CBD.

CEDS - Chronic Endocannabinoid Deficiency Syndrome

In 2008, neuroscientist and cannabis researcher Ethan Russo asked: *"Can this concept explain therapeutic benefits of cannabis in migraines, fibromyalgia, irritable bowel syndrome, and other treatment resistant conditions?"*

So, clinical endocannabinoids deficiency (CEDS or CECD) is the umbrella term for a group of illnesses such as fibromyalgia, migraine, irritable bowel syndrome, and other similar illnesses. The growing number of scientists feel that the endocannabinoid system may be at the root of these kinds of somatic illnesses.

Russo had reviewed available literature and verified that cannabinoids have demonstrated the ability to block spinal, peripheral, gastro, and intestinal mechanisms that cause pain and headaches in fibromyalgia and irritable bowel syndrome, as well as other similar disorders.

He describes how a migraine has several interconnections to endocannabinoid's function. For example, anandamide has an interesting relationship with serotonin. It encourages serotonin as well as inhibiting the receptors, so there are more good lock ins and matches making you feel much happier. Cannabinoids also block dopamine and have anti-inflammatory effects.

Anandamide controls receptors, migraines, and influences the periaqueductal grey, the part of the brain known as "the migraine generator."

THC modulates the neurotransmission of glutamate via NMDA receptors in fibromyalgia is now understood as a central sensitisation stage with secondary hyperalgesia. So, what exactly is hyperalgesia? Well, to you and I, it is this somatic illness we have spoken about over and over in the book, where the patient is clearly experiencing huge amounts of pain, but no tests reveal any kind of tissue damage that could be causing it. The patient runs out of patience and the doctor becomes sad, frustrated, and probably says *"sorry Mrs X, it is stress."*

Hyperalgesia is pain completely out of perspective with presenting signals. It now seems highly likely that we were right that there was a iddy-biddy connection and that this is modulated by a deficiency in the endocannabinoid system.

So, what manifestations might we see if the eCS goes out of kilter?

In a normal functioning ECS, someone would have normal mental state, be pain-free, and their digestive system would work well. Conversely, if someone is morbidly obese, then it is likely you will see metabolic syndrome rearing its vile head, inflammation levels will be raised, insulin resistance will occur, and even diabetes. The ECS has been observed to be hyperactive in such states. Similarly, an excess of CB_1 activity can be associated with hepatic (liver) fibrosis.

Chronic Pain

In his 2015 paper, Andrew Kowal explained that opioids are very well proven to treat **acute** pain, and indeed they are relatively safe. What they are not proven to do, however, is be either effective or safe for chronic pain. He recommends cannabis as a better option.

Arthritis & Rheumatism

Approximately 350 million people worldwide suffer from some sort of arthritis. In total around a hundred different strains of the disease exist, with the most common being osteoarthritis, where the joints become eroded as cartilage breaks down through wear and tear, and rheumatoid arthritis, an autoimmune condition caused by the body's innate defences going into overdrive and targeting the lining of the joints.

The common feature of the disease is inflammation, which of course should be helped by balancing the CB_2 receptors.

Several different trials point to this being a productive way to move forward, however it has also been shown that CBD may also be able to help through its activation of GPR55. Which also seems to contribute to nociceptive pain. Trials show that CBD's extremely powerful analgesic effect on arthritic conditions come from a combination of anti-inflammatory benefits, but also a limiting of immune reactions, and thus curbing the despatch of the further inflammatory markers to the site of damage.

In rheumatoid arthritis in particular, the CBD had extremely protective effects on the synovial cavity around the joint. The cavity is split into two compartments: the inner *intima*, and the outer part known as the *subintima*. The intima is predominately comprised of two types of molecules, macrophages, and Fibroblast-Like Synoviocytes (FLS). Together, these create homeostasis, but increase levels of FLS is a typical marker of RA.

When these levels rise, it triggers over-activity of immune cells and platelets that despatch even more inflammatory markers that damage the tissues and ones further.

Trials are currently underway to examine how the effects of balancing CB_2 in cases of RA. It's suspected that activating the receptor should restrict how many antibodies are produced, as well as pro-inflammatory cytokines and the matrix metalloproteinases implicated in the natural of growth/decay turnover of tissues, thereby slowing the erosion of the bones. It's hoped that calming the T Cells' immune response will also restrict the proliferation of FFLs.

Presented with an arthritic patient now, I will be especially tempted to supplement CBD with hemp *essential* oil, or even a bit of black pepper to further exploit beta caryophyllene's effects on the receptor.

Cancer and Tumours

So, here we are.

Don't tell me this section wasn't why you bought the book!

Cancer, everyone's worst enemy, the beast has stolen loved ones from almost everybody I know.

But can CBD oil help?

The medical fraternity strongly suspects that cannabinoids and their associated chemistry probably holds the key to beating cancer. THC, as you know, is already prescribed to combat chemotherapeutic nausea, and it seems likely that not only does it stop the patient feeling sick, it potentises the effects of the chemotherapy too. But our research here focuses on cannabidiol, its transport proteins, and any hopes there may be from inhibition of degradation factors.

Sun Tsu tells us in *The Art of War*:

"One may know how to conquer without being able to do it."

There are a lot of internet forums like that I have found. They are rife with vehement declarations that drug companies are conspiratorially hiding the truth, terrified their profits will crash. But few people have actually got very much of substance to say.

But that doesn't mean there is not much to be said.

Quite the opposite, I have found. And further, I had suspected it would all be THC, because in 1998, Christina Sanchez from Computense, the University of Madrid, announced that every time she added THC to a dish of brain cancer cells, the cells died, explaining that THC induces apoptosis in C6 Glioma. So in a way, THC is old news...but it's not the full story!

There are oodles more to talk about...and it is so exciting!

I'm going to skip anecdotal evidence here, because most of us are familiar. If you're not, plug "Cannabis – Cancer" into YouTube and you'll be kept busy for hours.

Many different gene mutations contribute to cancer, so every tumour acts differently. Some aspects are genetic, others environmental, or even influenced by lifestyle choices. It's a hideous cauldron of tumorous possibilities. These parasitic organisms have such a variety of personalities and agendas, it's incredibly difficult for scientists to get ahead of the game. But 2001 saw the release of a seminal paper that defined six characteristic hallmarks of a cancer. *This* was a game changer.

Understanding these hallmarks gives context to some of the actions we witness with CBD. It also fills you with awe for the strategic genius of the disease and it certainly filled me with respect. Cells seemingly operate as a supremely skilled terrorist army, gradually turning the screw, deftly acquiring new skills, feeding the strength of the battalion, and weakening its corporeal host.

Cancer cells:

1. Stimulate their own cells, self-sufficiently triggering growth signals.
2. Resist inhibitory signals that might otherwise impede growth
3. Resist programmed cell death
4. Multiply indefinitely, thereby enjoying limitless replicative potential
5. Stimulate manufacture of blood cells to supply the tumour with nutrients
6. Invade cell tissue spreading to new sites

Then in 2011, this list was deepened with four more observed hallmarks.

Cancer cells:

7. Have abnormal metabolic pathways
8. Invade the immune system
9. Owe their success to genome instability
10. Cause inflammation

By far the biggest challenge a cancer patient faces, is that tumours signal for cells to proliferate - multiply and spread - indefinitely. It's like a chronic tick, tick, tick, the metronome marking another set, and another set and another set...

On and on it goes.

What's more, healthy body cells are programmed to regulate growth hormones to maintain homeostasis. Healthy proliferation should be a balance of new cell growth and then cell death, thereby maintaining status quo. It should be a merry-go-round of life as the body maintains a steady pace and remains in equilibrium.

At some point though, one of the baddies...a cancer cell, dressed in black with a balaclava, snuck in and pulled one of the energy plugs. He successfully *downregulates* that signal. Now...rather than saying *"enough growth for a moment people, separate bedrooms and go to sleep,"* all the cells hear is an orgiastic chant of *"shag, shag, shag..."* they're like rabbits...proliferating toxic offspring in every corner. And that's fantastic for the tumour because don't forget the bad cells have already established some fantastic hiding place, circumventing the tumour suppressant gene and his special force of cell killers. The tumorous army increases in number and strength. The authors of *"Hallmarks of Cancer"* ominously describe the cells as now becoming "Masters of their Own Destiny."

But clearly this growth can't go continue for ever, otherwise we'd explode, so after a while the cancer signalling does something even cleverer. It switches the signal from proliferation to an aging process called senescence; the cells will die, eventually, but it is a slow and gradual process that the body is poorly equipped to deal with.

Apoptosis – programmed cell death — is designed with a clean-up mechanism built in. When the cell dies, neighbouring cells come in and absorb it. It's gone and the street is left clean. But senescence is nowhere near as ordered. As they age, necrosis sets in. Necrotic cells bloat and swell until finally they explode, catapulting proinflammatory signals to all the surrounding cells. Healthy tissue is now under attack.

Tumour cells overpower and invade healthy tissue sites, increasing the magnitude of their stronghold. Then, as the tumour grows in strength and capability, it spawns pioneer cells, despatches them from the original clump of mutants, and orders them to form new colonies elsewhere. For once, this is a term, sadly, all too many of us are familiar with. These new colonies?

Metastases.

Now obviously these new offshoots don't have the power and dominion of the original tumour, they are little start-up companies in effect, so their focus then must be strengthening their own little space in the world. They are going to trigger that exact same process of proliferation to create new cells, and then it is going to emulate another growth mechanism that the tumour also uses called angiogenesis...it is going to nourish those new cells with blood, fortifying them with stronger cell walls and feeding them loads and loads of protein. Sun Tze says *"Treat your men as you would your own beloved sons and they will follow you into the deepest valley."* Sorry, folks, the cancer cells have read it. They carefully tend their offspring, making chances of successful dominion ever more likely.

But take heart, dear friend, because we have two things on our side.

The first is mindfulness of Sun Tzu's advice to: *"Begin by seizing something which your opponent holds dear; then he will be amenable to your will."*

The second is the tool we are going to use to do that.

Your weapon is CBD. And the target? We're going to attack its means of growth.

In 2012 a team from the University of Insubria, Italy, explained that they could now confirm that CBD attacks cancer cells both in vitro and in vivo - so in a petri dish and also in some kinds of mammal. So now, their challenge is to understand how and why that might be, so they can capitalise on the data to defeat cancers feeding on humans.

Their experiment used HUVEC cells collected from umbilical cords. Filled with haematopoietic stem cells, this specialised blood manufactures every type of platelet, red, or white blood cell. These maintain our blood production right through our lives and donated sources are a potential gift of life to sufferers of blood cancers like leukaemia. There are even suggestions that, in the future, these unique immature blood cells might have the capacity to grow new nerve cells too, although that magic is potentially light years away.

Generating new blood, HUVEC cells are a brilliant assessment tool for potential cancer treatments. In this experiment, focus was on understanding the migration of new cells in the blood and then how the CBD affects proliferation and viability of cancerous cells in a tumour known as glioma.

In vivo and in vitro, CBD downregulated glioma signals for angiogenesis, disrupting the supply of blood cells to the tumour. It subdued the sprouting mechanism, halted migration, and prevented the cells' invasions into healthy cells. In our terrorist analogy...it hijacked new recruits headed for camp. CBD starved the militant cells of reinforcements, weakening them into submission.

With so many different types of cancer, all with their own particular strains and foibles, finding a derivative cause seems next to impossible. However, a breakthrough in 2007 identified a gene that should be fast asleep had awoken from slumber and turned anarchist.

ID1 gene is responsible for gene transcription. It's active when we are at embryonic stage in the womb. By the time we take our first gasp of oxygen, the gene has already switched off. It's done its job and its function is complete. However, studies show that, in very aggressive cancers like breast cancer and glioma, ID1 has been somehow resurrected and this zombie invader now rebels, turning benign tumours malignant.

So, where is the lever to stop its destruction?

We don't know.

But, *cannabis* does!

CBD switches the gene back off again, swiftly silencing the organic coup.

Now, I could write an entire book about cancer research and CBD, but frankly...

No, thank you!

So, to make this easy, I won't describe many of the experiments in detail, just the result. But...

Since I am slacking off, that means your brains need to work that little bit harder. Don't let your imagination leap over to human cancers, unless I say it is safe to. Take it for granted each time that we are talking about a test tube (in vitro) or rats, mice, rabbits, and other poor unsuspecting fluffies (in vivo).

Or nude mice...it could be them too.

I'm not sure why they have to be naked...but for some reason, it seems they do!

*Any*hooo...

Brain

In 2012, universities across Israel came together to compare the effects of THC and CBD working together on one of the most common solid cancers in children, **neuroblastoma**. This was human cells (cell ref: SK-N-SH) but in a test tube.

Both cannabinoids reduced cell viability and invasiveness. They disturbed the cancer cell cycle and triggered apoptosis. Somehow, the cannabinoids traced the terrorist lair and induced a mass suicide. Interestingly, both CBD and THC were effective...but CBD was the stronger!

I didn't expect that. Did you?

2013, Spain, and tumours were grafted onto mice and a microparticle mix of CBD and THC mix was given subcutaneously. The blend impeded the growth of the graft, it reduced viability and invasiveness of tumour cells, and induced apoptosis.

See what I mean...apoptosis yada yada ya.

If I'm not careful, the fact that cancer cells are dying is going to get lost! Maybe if I rap, or dance or something? No, that's not gonna do it. Let's just stick to a list.

2010, California, Pacific Medical Centre Research Centre. CBD with THC worked synergistically to inhibit cell proliferation in glioblastoma. They modulated the cycle of the cell, induced ROS, and brought about apoptosis.

Changes didn't happen with either cannabinoid independently, so it might be that there is another pathway, as yet unidentified, that requires them to work together, proving that even if you are puffing on a joint, adding more CBD might potentially help the THC work harder.

2005, CBD prevented the migration of U87 glioma cells. The action was independent of CB_1 or CB_2 receptors, so again the pathway remained elusive.

A 2013 finding by the Californian Pacific Medical Centre Research Institute showed that the evasiveness of glioma cells is directly proportional to levels of that anarchistic gene that is supposed to switch off when we are born, ID1.

In 2013, CBD modulated the evasiveness of glioblastoma cells by switching *off* ID1.

January 2017, University of Washington School of Medicine, Seattle. CBD reduced the proliferation and viability of ALL cells. Different to THC that focuses on cancer cells but leaves normal cells intact. Tested alone and with DNA-damaging agents, results showed that CBD might improve the effects of cancer drugs.

To cut the very longest story short, CBD is showing promise in many different cancers. These include skin, prostate, lung, colon, breast, and bladder cancers, some endocrine tumours, and in leukaemia.

I would suggest if this applies to you, that you visit an updated list of research on the wonderful site Project CBD.

Before we leave, we should just ruminate on a word of caution issued by the Uniwersytet Jagiellonski Collegium Medicum, Poland, in December 2016. The paper reminds us that the main way cannabinoids exert their effects is though apoptosis. They continue *"In the cellular context and dosage dependence, cannabinoids may enhance proliferation of tumour cells by suppressing the immune system and activating mitogenic factors."* (Pokrywka *et al.*, 2016).

Another good reason to proceed with care.

Appetite and Metabolism

Anorexia

In 2011, the suspicion that anorexia, obesity, and bulimia may have underlying issues with the endocannabinoid system were confirmed. Anandamide and 2-AG stimulate appetite (remember the breast milk and receptor's in babies' mouths?), so when signalling is stunted, appetite naturally drops. This action is executed through the CB_1 receptor.

In 2006, Rimonabant was released into the market, an anti-obesity/anti-anorexic drug, it worked as a reverse agonist at the CB_1 Receptor. Prescribed for patients to use alongside diet and exercise, it seemed to work very well. But after release, post-marketing data showed a disturbing story...

Based on your knowledge of the CB_1 receptor now, can you guess what that might be?

Statistics showed the drug was creating adverse side effects with the central nervous system. About 10% of the people taking the prescribed drug were exhibiting signs of depression, with 1% of the population even showing suicidal tendencies. It was taken out of circulation in 2008.

Despite this setback, scientists persevere. The benefits of medical marijuana offer so much promise in this area, the experiments continue.

It's very hard to guess molecule by molecule what the mechanism of healing might be. Cannabinoids seem to affect orexigenic signalling that controls desire for food. It is such a complex disease, with so many underlying factors. The 'hunger hormone' ghrelin stimulates our appetite, increases how much food we eat, and then encourages the body to store the fat. Neuropeptide Y acting as a neurotransmitter sending messages about food intake again, and about obesity, perpetuating anxiety about body shape and affecting mood, as well as dependency on the controlling behaviour. Dopamine triggers the reward systems from starving or binging, and serotonin wiping the sunshine out of life. And there in the background, the endocannabinoids in their high viz jackets and walkie-talkies seem to be on a fag break or are checking out dopamine in her far too short skirt...whatever they are doing, their eyes are not on the job, and day by day these poor girls (and lads of course) are getting sicker and sicker.

So, what in heaven's name can we do?

It's a shame we can't find a way to emulate Rimonabant without the side effects really, isn't it? We'd have to find a CB_1 reverse agonist again, but it would need to be backed up by a whole army of reinforcements to modulate any effects exerted through the receptor, wouldn't it? And, if we were going to do something truly spectacular, we'd need a pleotropic effect where dopamine was stabilized to calm their anxiety or even more so, serotonin to make them feel a bit happier about their place in the world.

How great would that be?

Mother Nature already constructed it guys, that's exactly what the entourage effect does to back the effects of CBD and THC.

What's more, because of the adverse effects of Ribonamant, R W Gorter from the University of Budapest proposed that closer attention should not be placed on cannabidiol as a means to curb hyperphagia, one of the main causes of atherosclerosis caused by metabolic syndrome.

Oh, you don't know what hyperphagia is?

No, I didn't either, but I am considering replacing my *"I'm not fat, I am undertall"* t-shirt with a less grubby and more impressive sounding *"Don't judge me…I'm hyperphagic!"* with a picture of me eating an éclair.

It means *"possessing an abnormally great desire for food; excessive eating."*

Atherosclerosis, Diabetes, and Metabolic Syndrome

So, here's a weird thing…people who smoke marijuana are thinner…well, they have a smaller waist circumferences anyway. Also, they have lower incidences of obesity and diabetes too. So, interested in a plausible connection between cannabinoids and metabolism, researchers from the school of epidemiology at Harvard set about seeing if they could prove that link.

They collected together a massive 4,657 people and surveyed the effects of a nine hour fast on their blood. The study took five years and in that time each person completed a self-study questionnaire about cannabis usage throughout their life and then, after a nine hour fast had blood samples taken. 579 of them were current users, 1,975 had used marijuana in the past.

You might want to sit down for this…

Users and past users had readings of fasting insulin that were 16% lower than non- users.

When tested against a Homeostasis Model of Insulin Resistance (HOMA-IR) their insulin resistance was demonstrated to be 17% better too.

Now listen here Teresa May… If the figures that you spend 14 billion pounds a year on diabetes medication (purported to be £25,000 every minute!) are correct…what would you say if I told you I could potentially slash £224 million off this year's healthcare bill?

Just through diabetes alone! No? Not tempted to reconsider legalising cannabis in the UK yet?

Glib, granted, but you get my drift!

So why?

Why is Toking Tina so tiny and trim? (I hate her, don't you?!)

Interesting question. I'm glad you asked.

About five years ago, ideas about the CB_1 receptor changed and this was mainly down to a paper by the guy responsible for the quote at the beginning of the Endocannabinoid System chapter: *"relax, eat, sleep, forget, and protect."*

Di Marzo took the understanding deeper when he and his team at the Endocannabinoid Research Group at the Institute of Biomolecular Chemistry in

Pozzuoli, Italy, recognised that it wasn't just about the desire for food and getting hungry that came into play in endocannabinoid interaction. The CB_1 receptor was also in charge of promoting how well adipose tissue stored energy and conversely how it rationed energy expenditure by modulating metabolism of glucose and lipid (sugar and fat). So, if CB_1 goes out of whack it can lead to obesity, type 2 diabetes, and dyslipidaemia (excess lipid in the blood). They found that cannabidiol could also protect against damage done to beta cells in type 1 diabetes. Beta cells? Not sure why these aren't a more popular term; they are what make insulin.

One of the main concerns in metabolic syndrome is the effect it has on ischemia and the heart. It was proven that THC could block the progression of the disease through its mechanism on the CB_2 receptors. CBD has been found to have an immunomodulatory effect on the body, lessening the effect elevated levels of glucose have on atherosclerosis. At this point though, because of the effects the P450 enzyme has on CBD (changing it into many other metabolites and thereby decreasing bioavailability further), the recommendation has been to look at ways to develop it as an adjunct therapy...as part of a bigger suite of therapies...diet and exercise one would presume, as well as other potential drug interventions.

A trial by The University of Reading in Berkshire made an interesting discovery, that THC was not the only cannabinoid to make you hungry. Cannabinol also increased feeding. The same trial also elucidated that cannabidiol reduced food intake.

One last exciting development before we leave, my fellow big bottom gals. Here, sweeties, have a syringe-full of CBD before I go.

Why?

Well let me ask you this...

Have you ever seen a new born baby shiver?

No? It occurred to me that neither had I when I read that new born babies and mammals have very high levels of brown fat to keep them warm. As they get older the brown fat turns to white fat, and not only does that accumulate around the waist, it also means we now begin to shiver! Very odd!

But here's the thing...

Scientists have recently discovered that white fat and brown fat work differently. White fat, as we know, comes from storing excess calories, but brown fat actually generates heat by burning. So why is that important? Well a study from Universite de Sherbrooke, Canada, found that not only did people with more brown fat take longer to begin to shiver, they also burned an extra 250 calories (1.8 times the usual rate) than those with mainly white fat. It is suspected that brown fat might contribute to keeping us lean, but it has also become the darling of the anti-obesity labs as everyone is racing to find a way to turn white fat into brown.

Well, I am sure you have guessed that something Toking Tina is doing must be helping that tiny 'tastic waist...

You are right. Last year, scientists in Korea found that CBD increased gene expression of brown staining markers through the activation of PPARy, leading them to excitement that they may have found a way to combat obesity.

Well guys, I don't know about you, but all this talk about fat is giving me the munchies.

Brownie, anyone? Just a small slice, eh? With all the CBD, we might feel stuffed pretty quick.

Lordamercy...sure sounds like happy cake to me!

Diabetes

It's understood that higher levels of anandamide circulating in the blood are associated with diabetes. Further, CBD may be so useful because it acts as a vaso-relaxant on the endothelium. It's not clear. What we do know, it certainly does something!

In 2006, researchers in Hassadah University proved that the likelihood of a nonobese rat developing diabetes fell from 86% to 32% when treated with CBD. I have to say, potentially I may be being thick but no matter how many times I looked at the paper I can't see what they did to the creature to think that it might get ill. I don't think it says, so let's hope the average person doesn't have an 86% chance of developing type 2 too! I don't think they do!

Anyway, treatment of the mice:

Reduced:

- Levels of inflammatory cytokines
- Interferons gamma and alpha
- Production of Th1 associated cytokines
- Peritoneal macrophages

Increased:

- TH2 associated cytokines
- Pro-inflammatory markers Interleukin 4 and Interleukin 10

When compared to untreated mice.

Cannabidiol can also protect against diabetic retinopathy. Scientists at the University of Georgia, Augusta, found that CBD protects neurons in the retinas of diabetic rats from ROS by blocking tyrosine nitration. It seems likely that tyrosine nitration blocks glutamine synthase, meaning glutamine accumulates and kills neurons in the retina. Blocking nitration, CBD protects the eyes.

Stroke and TBI

The research in this area is startling and if no other section of the book encourages you to find yourself a source of CBD, then this will.

Cannabidiol, as we know, exerts strong neuroprotective effects and this also travels across to damage the brain in strokes and traumatic brain injuries. THC also protects the brain through its mechanism through the CB_1 receptor, however, a study from the Fukuoka University in 2007 showed CBD to be more useful. Over time, the CB_1 receptors become desensitized and so any benefits THC gave were short-lived. Conversely, they found that this didn't happen using CBD; the effects were neuroprotectant and antioxidant and did not generate tolerance. This seemed to happen because CBD was protecting the brain via a different avenue. Since that protection it was giving, and the increased blood flow it produced, was reversed, when they blockaded the activity of the serotonin receptor, it seems likely the benefits were being exerted via 5-HT1A.

Before we go on to rather exciting experiments from Jerusalem and Madrid, let's just clarify two things.

What is ischemia?

It's when there is inadequate blood supply to a part. Here we are obviously thinking *brain*, but it could be heart, leg, whatever.

Next:

What's an infarct?

It's dead tissue, or necrosis resulting from ischemia.

Let's start with Madrid, who are very interested in what happens when there is brain injury in a neonate. In October 2012, they wanted to examine how CBD might help a wee one with hypoxia ischemia, and if it did, how long the effects would last. This oxygen deprivation that can lead to cerebral palsy was emulated by starving mouse brains of oxygen just to 10% supply for 120 minutes (☹).

A number of tests were used to assess the damage, including histology reports and MRI, and they found that an infarct had developed.

The infarcts in the brains belonging to the mice who had been treated with the CBD were 17% smaller than those not treated. They had less excitotoxicity and less oxidative stress for seven days after (which was the end of the experiment). They found that even though there was some recovery in the histological reports the mice titrated with CBD enjoyed greater functional recovery too. In short, they got better.

Very recently, April 2017, the team then examined the effects on a neonatal arterial ischemic stroke in one of my little white furred red eyed Wistar rats. You can look up what they did to create that yourself, if you have a stronger stomach than mine! They found that by treating canna-rat with CBD it didn't really affect the size of the infarct, but that it did regain functionality much faster than those not treated. Its neuronal function was improved as ratfink got stronger and had reduced hemiparesis (weakness down one side). Its coordination was much better as was its sensorimotor function (reaching for something it can see or smell, for example).

There was a marked difference in changes in the glial cells. The CBD had modulated how many microglia had been despatched and produced and also protected the astrocyte function. Fewer neurons were lost and programmed cell death had been slowed.

Heart Disease

Here's what I've learned. When the heart is starved of blood supply or oxygen it is damaged, but part of the damage happens afterwards, as blood supply is being restored. Starved of oxygen and nutrients, the integrity of the tissues is then compromised through oxidation and perfusion injury.

In 2007, The Hadassah University in Jerusalem proved that CBD protects the heart from this through its actions at the adenosine receptor. It dramatically reduced the size of the infarct by...wait for it...

66%!

It reduced inflammation in the myocardial tissue, as well as the levels of pro-inflammatory marker interleukin 6.

In 2010, The Robert Gordon University in Aberdeen published a paper proving that CBD calmed arrhythmia and spared tissues in ischemia. Through very complex manoeuvres they also proved that CBD protected the heart in this acute stage of perfusion injury if it was administered before the ischemia took place.

You need to be using it, guys.

Just one final one that can be cross-referenced with cancer. This is a beautiful experiment that brings together scientists from all corners of the globe, from the NIH and New Jersey, from Switzerland, Taipei, and Jerusalem. The 2015 trial forms the kind of oneness that cannabis would be proud of. They came together to try to find a way to protect the heart during cancer treatment.

Doxorubicin is a chemotherapy drug and a very potent one at that. The problem is that at some doses it is cardiotoxic, so it needs to be used with great care. Its attack on the heart is very similar to that we saw before, it is oxidative and nitrative, impairing mitochondrial function in heart cells. Here we see cardiomyocytes and endothelial cells being programmed into early mass suicide.

CBD was able to balance biogenesis, re-enhancing the function impaired by the damage done by the drug, thereby protecting the heart.

Liver Disease

Another weird to thing to think about.

There are very few or no endocannabinoid receptors in a healthy liver.

Not sure why I find that odd, but I do.

By contrast, the system is distinctly ramped up in chronic liver diseases and plays a massive part in making people sicker and sicker.

In my eczema book, we talk extensively about Non-Alcoholic Fatty Liver Disease and its affects in health, especially atopic diseases and eczema. Caused by high levels of fats in the blood, type 2 diabetes, and being overweight, NAFLD can often progress to pulmonary fibrosis, developing to cirrhosis, hyper dynamic circulatory syndrome affecting blood pressure and thus the heart, then critically, heart disease cirrhotic cardiomyopathy. As the liver fails, the brain becomes addled, cognition is skewed, and the patient experiences altered consciousness, coma, and potential death. Hopefully before that happens, either a transplant can be arranged, or some other intervention to prevent deterioration.

So first of all, let's see how they are getting on with the intervention. I suppose first we want to see what's causing the fibrosis of the liver and is there anything we might be able to do about it.

The cascade causing this hardening of the liver is triggered by fat-storing cells in the perisinusoidal space of the liver. Hepatic stellate cells (HSCcs) spread, producing far too much collagen. This induces a scar matrix, and before long we have fibrosis of the liver.

Scientists at the Mount Sinai School of Medicine in New York, felt if they could bring about cell death in HSCs that might be a useful form of treatment. Could CBD help? Yes.

It brought about apoptosis…somehow…outside of endocannabinoid signalling. It cleverly found a way to elicit a stress response in the endoplasmic reticulum.

These miniscule tubules living in the cytoplasm, attached to ribosome, create lipids and proteins. Stressing them downregulated them and their production was slowed. Oddly though, this works in rat and human tissues, but not in mice!

So that's good, people might benefit, it seems. But what if there hadn't been an intervention at this point? Are we now too late?

Well as the proteins build, this can lead to bile duct ligation, putting pressure on the heart, but also causing the terrifying hepatic encephalitis.

Scientists at the Hadassah-Hebrew University Medical Faculty in 2010 found that CBD could reverse this in mice by activating the adenosine receptor A(2)A.

If we still hadn't got in, in time, and the patient is now losing consciousness, what then?

(This is terrifying, isn't it?!)

Female Sabra mice were infected with saline of thioacetamide to bring on neurological and motor impairments we would expect to see.

After two and three days, they were assessed and then...

Read fast so it doesn't sink in...

Their brains and livers were harvested so they could assess the liver enzymes in the plasma.

A luckier set of mice were given a stay of execution and were tested for cognitive function after eight days and then for levels of 5HT after 12 days.

All decreased motor activity caused by the thioacetamide was restored by CBD.

Levels of 5HT, bilirubin, and liver enzymes were all elevated by the injury and then were normalised by CBD, as was astrogliosis.

What about if we still haven't got the syringe out and the patient needs to have a transplant? Because you and I now understand way too much about what can go wrong with the body, particularly in surgery when the blood goes back into a starved organ.

Don't look. Hide your eyes, I can't look in case we got this far and hypoxic re-perfusion strikes...

Oh wait, no it's okay, we can relax. In 2011, The King Faisal University in Saudi Arabia proved that hepatic tissues are protected from hypoxic reperfusion injury by CBD.

So that's good. But my goodness how much has all this cost the National Health? All these interventions, staff resources, not to mention the emotional and physical toll it has taken on the patient's body, and indeed his loved ones too.

It's a shame we couldn't have got the cannabis out earlier.

Could we?

Yep, it seems likely that CBD will be able to attack the Non-Alcoholic Fatty Liver Disease at the source and thus gives extremely good grounds to recommend supplementation as the norm.

The Laboratory of Physiological Sciences at the NIH in 2011 found that CB_1 receptors seem to be involved in resolving fat issues in NAFLD. When assessing issues that can arise after liver transplants and hepatic surgeries, they found that CBD reduced the inflammation around the site of the injury, calmed oxidative and nitrative stress, and reduced cell death. It calmed activation of the endotoxin NF-Kb, as well as the production of tumour necrosis factor by Kupffer cells.

When blocking receptors, they found that the action was preserved at the CB_2 receptors but was halted at $CB_{1/2}$, so therefore we have our usual issue of...

How did it do that...outside of endocannabinoid signalling, we know...any more specific answers remain to be seen.

Hepatitis

Can it help?

Long answer and short answer...which would you like?

Short first then, courtesy of University of Maryland School of Medicine, Baltimore, in conjunction with Medicanja, Jamaica.

Hep C - Yes

Hep B - No

The longer answer is more interesting...unless you have Hep C of course, and the short answer was pretty thrilling I suppose, when I think about it!

The long answer concerns some cells I had never even heard of before: Myeloid Derived Suppressor Cells (MDSCs). Myeloid means coming from the spinal cord or from bone marrow and these cells are now recognised as one of the main regulating cells of the immune system.

What they do is pop up at sites of infection and control how many T Cells are allowed to operate there, suppressing the function and keeping them in check. Now, the understanding of the cells is still in its infancy, but it is known that if you can inhibit MDSCs, you have a good shot at shutting down hepatitis, my foul eczema-y skin disorder leishmaniasis, sepsis, various lung diseases, and certain types of autoimmunity.

CBD triggers suppression of MDSCs through the TPRV1 vanilloid receptors, reducing disease.

Kidney Disease

Potentially, this might be in the wrong section and should be cross-referenced with cancer because the experiment derives from concern about damage to the kidneys in patients who are using a chemotherapy drug, cisplatin. A platinum-based compound, cisplatin is one of the most powerful weapons against malignancy but it also exerts harsh effects on the rest of the body. The kidneys in particular suffer oxidative stress from ROS, but also nitrosative stress as the ROS join forces with reactive nitrogen species to destroy its tissues.

Cannabidiol reduced the injury caused by oxidative/nitrosative stress, it calmed inflammation, and prevented apoptosis where without the CBD there would have been programmed cell death. According to the trial documents, cannabidiol improved kidney function.

Since the experiment in Zhejiang University in 2009, more work has been done to assess how they might be able to take CBD forward in protecting against kidney disease.

Nausea

We know that THC exerts its anti-emetic effects through the CB_1 receptor, but that cannot be the same for CBD. A 2012 study done by the University of Guelph, Canada, (the author list is bursting with Canna-rock-star names) determined that the effects came about via an activation of 5HT1A receptors in the dorsal raphe nucleus found in the midline of the brain stem.

CBD is good, but CBDA is better in this case. That's the raw cannabidiol acid, before it is decarboxylated by heat. It is better at inhibiting nausea in rats and decreasing vomiting in shrews. Since a kindly neighbour last week called me a shrew...CBDA for me I think. But joking apart, this has extremely important treatment implications in cancer because it also successfully treated anticipatory nausea that, so far, has no treatment options available.

Imagine you had had chemotherapy, and you had been very sick. So, when you go into the treatment room for your second round, you might not need the drug at all, the scents and sounds of the room are enough to set you off. It seems this conditioned response might be helped in the future by a cocktail of THC and CBDA... For now, CBD is good enough.

But it's not just side effects to drugs that make us nauseous, of course. Many things do, not least sitting in the back seat of the car. Motion sickness is a horrible affliction affecting two of my three kids, so imagine my surprise to find scientists believe this is an eCS problem too.

They placed some willing volunteers into a flight simulator that had periods of about 22 seconds of microgravity. Now I have to say, I often question human nature, and I am wondering what possesses someone with motion sickness to volunteer for an experiment like this? Altruistic notions for the future of the human, perhaps? I hope they were paid handsomely, that's all I can say!

So, these loonies, of which there were seven out of a group of twenty-one, were subjected to the simulator doing 30 parabolas. Ace fun, if you feel good, but…ew.

Measurements were taken of anandamide and 2-AG before the flight, after 10, 20, and 30 parabolas at the end of the fight and 24 hours later.

Not surprisingly, there were higher stress scores in those who had motion sickness but there were more interesting changes in their blood samples too.

Their levels of endocannabinoids were lower.

After 20 parabolas (I'd be out of there!), levels of anandamide had dropped significantly in those with motion sickness, but in those that felt okay it had gone up. They had very high levels.

The pukers (sorry, I couldn't resist!) had very low levels of 2-AG and that didn't change throughout the experiment. When assessing the calmer bellies, scientists found their 2-AG levels had also gone up. When assessed at four hours after, there was a marked increase in the MRNA for the CB_1 receptors in the tranquil tums, but the motion sickness crew (they are bound, like brothers, now thinking *"What on God's green Earth possessed us?"*) had not had anywhere near as good expression.

So, here's an idea with no science or even reading attached to it. Two preponderances, in fact.

First…I wonder if there might also be a similar signalling error in vertigo too?

Second, I wonder if that's why I can't go on a swing or on the Waltzers, now I'm older? Perhaps, its nothing to do with age, or even just being a wuss…Perhaps my signalling's shot.

Dunno.

Let's move on.

Respiratory Distress

Asthma

In 1978, it was proven that cannabis helps asthma through the actions of Delta 1 THC. When CB_1 receptors are activated on the bronchial nerve endings, smooth muscle relaxes, dilating the bronchioles and making it easier for them to breath.

The lungs are also protected through a combined reaction of CB_1 and CB_2 receptors.

On my birthday in June 2011, The University of Hannover released results of their study into the actions of anandamide in allergic asthma. They had taken lung samples from patients with allergic asthma and placed them in a petri dish. Then they had saturated them with saline and allergens. Twenty-four hours later when examined, the levels of anandamide had multiplied four times, proving the participation of the endocannabinoid system in asthma.

Our friends in Sao Paolo wanted to understand that further and see how CBD might be able to help.

They then analysed levels of the cytokines in the serum. One would expect to see IL-4, IL-5, IL-13, IL-6, IL-10, and TNF-α all raised in asthma. The CBD reduced all levels except for IL 10, leading them to suspect it may create novel treatment options for asthma.

The Tissues

Glaucoma

We discussed, right at the beginning of the book, the obstacles placed in the way of researchers trying to find ways to treat glaucoma with cannabis. It is understood that THC ameliorates symptoms through its effects on the CB_1 receptor.

But what if THC weren't the only avenue? It's not outside of the realms of possibility, is it? We've seen how cannabis affects the body in a myriad of ways.

For example, one of the main reasons the cells die in the retina ganglion is an increased release of glutamate, and several cannabinoids have been proven to protect neurons in this situation. CBD is one. But another baddie is something called peroxynitrite, which isn't a free radical but still causes an inordinate amount of cell damage.

CBD attenuates peroxynitrite and thus, yes, might also be able to help glaucoma.

Osteoporosis/Bone Health

Okay, so you think you know the body. What if I said to you that bones are controlled by the central nervous system?

It doesn't quite compute, does it?

Yet several neurotransmitters contribute to bone density, not least, of course, calcium.

No weirder, really, than the fact that if you have your ovaries removed, then you are at higher risk of osteoporosis.

So how?

It's all down to two little cells:

Osteoblasts - form bone

Osteoclasts – resorb bone

Osteoclasts break down **bone tissue** then release minerals into the blood. It's one of the main ways calcium circulates.

Recent evidence shows anandamide and 2-AG existing in the skeleton. It looks like they are formed there, although scientists aren't sure how.

So that's the ligands...but where's the receptors?

You're gonna love this!

Osteoblasts express CB_1, osteoclasts express CB_2

So CB_1 signalling ensures there is enough bone being made and CB_2 checks that it is being processed properly when it has been finished with.

The skeleton also houses GPR55.

Problems then...

If GPR55 goes askew it creates problems in the way osteoclasts resorb bone, but bone formation is not affected. If CB_2 is skewed there is an increase in bone turnover, and somehow the cycle of production and resorption becomes unhitched. Loads of resorption, nowhere near as much production. CB_1 problems will see bone function becoming impaired, partly down to the fact that the body cannot accumulate enough bone marrow.

So clearly this CB_2 signalling is important in osteoporosis, so in 2011, scientists in Naples wanted to compare that of menopausal women with osteoporosis and those without. When they did, they found that the CB_2 receptors seems to communicate oddly with the TRPV1 channels.

Now, here's a thing to get your head around...

Osteoclasts express TRTV1 channels.

I know, I know. You just had to make the channels a billion times smaller in your head, didn't you? I did the same.

In the ladies with brittle bones, (actually, these ladies had white fur, four legs, and red eyes), they found TRPV1 upregulated. They discovered if they stimulated and stimulated and stimulated, they congregated in the plasma membrane. By response, the body went, here, have tons and tons of CB_2 receptors. It seems likely that calcium can no longer gain entry (and thus exit into the blood to moderate mood), because either the TRPV becomes desensitised or there is just far too much over-expression of the receptor and it just conks out.

Guess what? Copyscape didn't find a duplication of "conks out" in any scientific papers. How odd! But you get my drift.

What's more, when a team of scientists from Jerusalem created a mouse version of osteoporosis induced by ovariectomy, they found that balancing the CB_2 receptor rescued bone loss.

Lastly, the Bone Research Department at Tel Aviv University were able to show that CBD helped bones to heal faster by stimulating enzymes that trigger cross linking. But here's the lovely thing, when they compared it with THC they found that the psychoactive component did not do the same thing, but they also found that the CBD required the THC to potentiate the action.

So...let's mull it over.

Does CBD work at the CB_2? Yes, but very weakly. It does, however, have a strong affinity to the TRPV1 channels so that will serve us well. But we have a stronger weapon two, don't we? Certainly, I shall be adding hemp essential oil into blends for more mature ladies to use the beta caryophyllene for the CB_2. Actually, scientists have beaten us to it a bit because the School of Pharmacy at Reading already complied data of natural products that can help. Vegetables and herbs such as onion, garlic, and parsley, inhibited loss of bone density in ovariectomised rats. They also found that the essential oils of sage, rosemary, and thyme inhibited the actions of the osteoclasts, thereby increasing bone density.

Just a little aside for readers who are not aromatherapists, before you jump sidelong into that recommendation, watch your sage. This is irrelevant if she has had her ovaries removed, but if a lady has not yet gone through menopause fully, sage is going to make her bleed very, very heavily. This is only a good recommendation if she is a fully fledged and wizened crone. I look forward to my day!

Skin – Acne & Psoriasis

Considering CB_2's key action in immune response then, cannabis medicine is important for treating all manner of inflammation, from allergic reaction to psoriasis and acne.

Vetting the medicine in this field is harder, since mice and rats have fur and thus do not have the same requirement for oil on the skin as we do. So clinical trials are sparse.

CBD has been found to have extremely strong seborrheic prowess, and when assessed it was found to inhibit arachidonic acid, calm a combination of linoleic acid and testosterone, and to have used TRPV4 as a means of suppressing the proliferation of sebocytes.

In 2006, two teams from Pakistan did a lovely assessment of hemp seed oil at 3% dilution and found that both greasiness and redness were reduced in acne patients.

Since cannabinoids are also very good at inhibiting proliferation of keratinocytes that form the basis of new skin cells, it seems likely that CBD might become of interest in the future for treatment of psoriasis where there is an upregulation of K6 & K16 keratins.

Spinal Cord Injury

Well, if you, like me, were upset by the rats who were stalked by a cat for an hour, perhaps you should look away now...

Universidade de São Paulo 2012, and this time the researchers wanted to assess if CBD might help the 12,000 new cases of spinal injury per year. So naturally, they needed to injure a spine. They split the rats into five groups, then performed a laminectomy on the T10 vertebra, stripping away the lamina, the back of the vertebra that protects the spinal column. Then, on some of the groups they placed liquid nitrogen into the spinal column.

Cannabidiol was administered immediately before the injury, then three hours after, and subsequently once a day for six days after, at a dosage of 20mg/kg.

To assess the changes and hopeful recovery, they used a BBB score that measures changes in motor movement. They evaluated them just before they injured them, then on days one, three, and seven.

The CBD rodents all had higher BBB scores at the end of the week than other groups, meaning they were moving better (to run away I should think!) and the CBD also resulted in a lesser injury to their backs. The cannabis constituent had protected them and helped them to heal faster and better, leading the team to suggest that CBD might be able to help spinal injury patients.

Immunity

Antibiotic Resistance

I am surprised this area hasn't been investigated more fully yet.

In 2008, it was reported that cannabidiol, THC, cannabigerol, cannachromine, and cannabinol all potently fought the MRSA virus and won. It was concluded the success could be attributed to an interaction between the gamma subunit of the receptor and the hydrophobic molecules binding with proteins, known as their prenyl moiety. However, the *full* mechanism of their dominion over germs remains unclear, for the time being at least.

In 1976, it had already been established that CBD and THC, although bactericidal, were ineffective against gram negative bacteria (MRSA is gram positive).

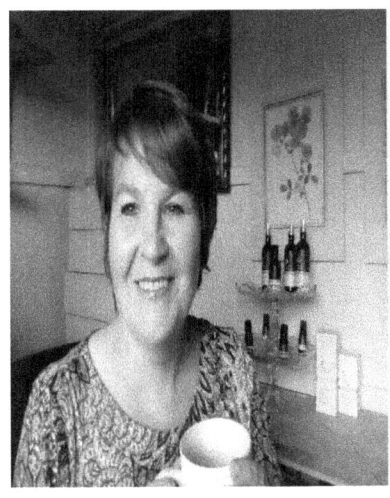

https://buildyourownreality.lpages.co/where-next/

Chapter 9 Care of the Endocannabinoid System

The following data is taken from a fascinating paper written, jointly, by G W Pharmaceuticals, the Department of Family Medicine from the University of Vermont and The Endocannabinoid Research Group, Istituto di Chimica Biomoleculare, in Napoli.

In *Care and Feeding of the Endocannabinoid System: A Systematic Review of Potential Clinical Interventions that Upregulate the Endocannabinoid System,* McPartland, Guy and Di Marzo give fascinating insights into endocannabinoid research and ways to affect the system without even going near a cannabis derivative.

Other plant species (and weirdly, shell fish too!) also interact with the endocannabinoid system. Anything that comes from outside of a cannabis plant must be differently labelled, as cannabimimetic...that is: acting *like* a cannabinoid.

Other things that interact with CB_1

Thujone

Although thujone doesn't elicit any cannabimimetic response, it does show weak binding affinity to the CB_1 receptor. The drink, Absinthe, famously contains thujone, a ketone derived from the controversial plant medicine, *Artemisia absinthium,* better known as wormwood. It was previously surmised psychoactive effects drinkers experience might come from CB_1 interaction, but in 1999 it was proven the response is caused by thujone's inhibition of GABA. Sampson and Fernandez (1939) and Steinmetz (1985) demonstrated even low doses of thujone are capable of affecting nervous tissue, hinting at the possibility the constituent may find its way across the blood brain barrier through the circulatory system.

For those less familiar with essential oil chemistry, thujone is one of the more difficult to use members of the ketone chemical group. Oils high in thujone, like mugwort, tansy (don't confuse with benign blue tansy), or thuja are traditionally contraindicated in formal aromatherapy because of their neurotoxic properties, but I confess to having a huge box full of these scary oils inherited from my late stepfather. Michael often used them to clear all manner of nasties: petrochemicals, parasites, even past life trauma. It's very interesting to see tangible evidence emerging as to why his patients always enjoyed such success.

I'm a big believer in right medicine, right place. It's why I don't believe much good comes from essential oil recipes. This becomes especially true when you think of ketonic oils, hazardous oils, and now cannabis too. I've always been fascinated by a lecture Dr. Malte Hozzel gives about ketones, because we're taught to be afraid of them when we first start our training. Their potentially neurotoxic affects correctly demand we exercise caution when using these medicines. While the owner of Oshadhi agrees with vigilance, he sees them offering a much wider perspective than most diploma courses reveal. His lecture opened up a whole new realm of healing to me, and I think it really comes into play here.

He describes ketones as disincarnators and energy givers. You and I might already recognise how they disincarnate matter, ploughing through phlegm, catarrh, scar tissue; this dissolution of resistance is a most prodigious quality of ketones. They dissolve resistance in the physical body, but they also free the mind from the shackles *of* the body. Disincarnating the mind, allowing an existence in a more spiritual realm, somehow, diffusing boundaries between realities. How strange, thujone, one of the most pervasive of the ketones might also free the imagination through CB_1. Likewise, I think of the oils I might blend with CBD if I were to treat someone who had anorexia. I'd choose tarragon because it's such a wonderful appetite stimulant but is there more going on that we have not perceived? Might its thujone disengage the mind's preoccupation with the body, then trigger the body to *gain* weight through its weak interaction with CB_1? It's already extraordinary medicine, regardless of our level of understanding, how much more will Mother Nature allow us to learn, I wonder? After all, these oils, these ketonic plants, dwell uneasily in the typical aromatherapist's box. Might they be better left as the property of the arcane?

Incidentally, in *Identification of candidate genes affecting Δ^9-tetrahydrocannabinol biosynthesis in Cannabis sativa (2009),* Marks *et al.* describe their analysis of cannabis constituents as containing 13 ketones, but perhaps I am the only one interested because I cannot find evidence of what these might be! Perhaps when everyone has left their preoccupation with terpenes affecting the scent, maybe they'll starting about ketones and phenols too. That would be interesting.

Sage of the Diviners

Salvia divinorum is a psychoactive plant used by shamanic doctors in Mexico to induce visions and disassociation. Its active constituent, Salvinorin A, is the most potent hallucinogen found in nature. Chemists are fascinated by its effects and its ketone ring seems to be a key feature its psychoactivity. In animal experiments, Salvinorin A affected rodent gastrointestinal tracts via actions mediated through the CB_1 receptor. Primarily acting as an agonist for the kappa-opioid receptor, no evidence points to Salvorin A directly interacting with either CB_1 or CB_2, but rather communicating, via a third-party relationship, through a putative CB_1-

kappa-opioid receptor subunit. It's the first interaction of an opioid receptor with anything that's not an alkaloid, ever discovered.

Not surprisingly, I couldn't find an essential oil of *Salvia divinorum* for sale. However, several shamanic websites (is that is an oxymoron...I imagined them scrying a different information superhighway?!) offer the herb with a wee dram of Salvinorin dripped on, to ramp up the effect.

It's interesting to think about thuja too, the plant used by homeopaths to treat psychosis. It contains 7.9-9.9% thujone according to Tisserand and Young (2013). Is it affecting the CB_1 receptor as it corrects the forgetful person's perception of time? I think, if I were to experiment here, and I will, I'll be using homeopathic doses of 1/15 drop for safety, but also in reverence to their medicine.

A wide range of plants contain the anthocyaniin delphinidin and cyanidin. Cyanidin, found in red berries such as cranberries, and delphinidin, which gives the blue colour to violas, have been proven to have micromolar (tinchy tiny) affinities for CB_1. Sadly, no essential oils are listed as containing these in Tisserand and Young.

Kava

Yangonin, a kavalactone found in *Piper methysticum*, otherwise known as kava, also exhibits affinity for CB_1.

Curry Powder

Levels of endocannabinoids and nerve growth factor are uplifted in certain areas of the brain when you eat curcumin in curry powder. In animal experiments, this action was halted when they used a CB_1 antagonist, suggesting that the receptor is *probably* responsible. However, studies conclusively proving the CB_1/Curcumin interaction were published, but then subsequently withdrawn, suggesting researchers perhaps found something that made them question that evidence.

Camellia

As an English woman, I feel I am well-qualified to speak on two things: cups of tea and the weather! (It's cloudy outside today, but very warm. Excellent tea party weather today!). It's time you all caught up with me and drank more tea. Epigallocatechin-3-O-gallate, the most abundant catechin in tea, exerts micromolar affinities for the CB_1 receptor. Green tea demethylates cannabinoid receptors cleaning and maintaining them. No essential oil, but of course there is a camellia carrier oil.

Kaempferol, also found in *Camellia sinensis* and many other plants, modestly inhibits FAAH. Again, I wanted to find an essential oil. I was unsuccessful, but a 2017 study by Nanjing Forestry University, China, found both kaempferol and genistin, that we'll meet in a moment, left in residues from distillation of Osmanthus fragrans essential oil "Jinqiu". To me, that implies they do not cross for some reason I'm too lazy to discover! Perchance they might be found in the CO_2 though. I don't know. It's certainly going to be worth checking GC reports.

In 1914, Lyster Dewey was enlisted to write a report about hemp as an agricultural crop for the American Government. He declared *"Hemp has no enemies"*, clearly predating prohibition. He's right, as a crop it's magnificent because insects don't seem to like it at all. It seems likely he was witnessing the effects of the natural pesticide, Falcarinol. It's a skin irritant found in several other plants apart from hemp including carrots, celery, parsnips, and parsley, and causes contact dermatitis, potentially due to its strange binding mechanism with the CB_1 receptor. A potent inverse agonist, it triggers pro-inflammatory effects in human skin. Perhaps the bugs know something we don't.

Echinacea

I doubt there is a healer on the planet who does not know the prowess of this herb. But why is it so magical? Amongst myriad other properties, several constituents from the root and herb of *Echinacea purpurea* simultaneously bind to CB_2 and inhibit uptake of anandamide. Conversely, some of its constituents *also* act as weak CB_1 antagonists, blocking the receptor. There's no essential oil, as far as I know, but it can be easily found as a maceration or a herbal extract. I'm just waiting excitedly for mine to flower in the garden.

Helichrysum umbraculigerum

Remember the South African *Helichrysum umbraculigerum* used in Shamanic rituals we looked at in the last book? Several cannabimimetic compounds have been found in that darling too.

Rhododendron

Recently, I've been introduced to rhododendron, or anthopogon oil, the most spectacular respiratory medicine. Its originating plant, Rhododendron anthopogonoides, used extensively in Chinese medicine, contains cannabinoid-like derivatives: **anthopogocyclolic acid** and **anthopogochromenic acid** metabolised from chromanes. Related compounds, referred to as "synthetic analogues of cannabinoids", have also been isolated: **cannabichromene** (CBC) type, **cannabicyclol** (CBL) type, and **cannabicitran** (CBT) type. While research is still very much in its infancy for CBL and CBT, much research has taken place into CBC. Cannabichromene interacts with the TRPV channels and their effects on pain. There is research into how it can help intestinal motility and particularly constipation, and in 2015 it was proven to be a powerful anti-acne medicine.

Liverwort

Lastly, there may potentially be another THC in a plant. Beautiful and gentle liverwort contains a molecularly very similar constituent, perrottetinenic acid. Used for centuries in herbal medicine for gall bladder, bladder, and liver problems, it's suspected that proof will be found that perrottetinenic acid binds to CB_1. Since it's not an essential oil, I know little about liverwort, so was interested to find out more. I refer to our old friend, Nicolas Culpepper:

"Description. Common liverwort grows close and spreads much upon the ground in moist and shady places, with many small green leaves, or rather (as it were) sticking flat to one another, very unevenly cut in on the edges, and crumpled; from among which arise small slender stalks an inch or two high at most, bearing small star-like flowers at the top; the roots are very fine and small.

Government and virtues.

It is under the dominion of Jupiter, and under the sign Cancer. It is a singularly good herb for all the diseases of the liver, both to cool and cleanse it, and helps the inflammations in any part, and the yellow jaundice likewise. Being bruised and boiled in small beer, and drank, it cools the heat of the liver and kidneys, and helps the running of the reins in men, and the whites in women; it is a singular remedy to stay the spreading of tetters, ringworms, and other fretting and running sores and scabs, and is an excellent remedy for such whose livers are corrupted by surfeits, which cause their bodies to break out, for it fortifies the liver exceedingly, and makes it impregnable.

Many liverworts, from the genus Radula, contain phyto-cannabimimetics.

Other things that interact with CB_2

Staying with Culpepper a moment, his words keep ringing in my ears about another herb that interacts gently with the CB_2 receptors. In speaking of "Sweet" basil, Culpepper warned we should be wary, because even rue seemed to be suspicious of basil. Even though olde medicine refers to her as "Herb of Grace", I don't think rue is a very nice gal at all. She irritates the skin and has been used as an abortifacient for hundreds of years. Nevertheless, Rutamarin in *Ruta graveolens* exerts micromolar affinity for CB_2 receptors. If you do decide to use this quite scary oil, Tisserand and Young suggest maximum dermal usage to be 0.15%.

Beta Caryophyllene

A 2008 paper by the Institute of Pharmaceutical Sciences, Zurick, Switzerland, identified beta-caryophyllene working as a cannabino-mimetic, in vivo. The terpenoid hydrocarbon and sesquiterpene acts as agonist, binding with nanomolar affinity to the CB_2 receptor. They describe how the sesquiterpene binds to the CB_2 receptor and inhibits adenylate cyclase, resulting in intracellular calcium changes that positively affect cytokine and inflammatory responses. According to *Zheng et al.* (1992), it strongly induced glutathione S-Transferase in mouse livers and intestines. Sensch *et al.* (2000), found it strongly inhibiting potassium ion fluxes. Schafer, in 1985, identified it blocking calcium channels in cardio vascular cell membrane. I'm not sure about this, but I would suspect we can say beta-caryophyllene is a cannabinoid so long as it is extracted from the cannabis plant, in all other cases, it is cannabino-mimetic.

According to Tisserand and Young, other oils containing beta-caryophyllene we can exploit are as follows. Real stars have been put into bold.

- Angelica Root 2.0-4.0%
- Angelica Seed 0.1-3.3%
- Anise (Star) – 0.1 -3.3%
- Atractylis – 2.0%
- Basil (Estragole CT) – 4.0%
- Betel – 0 -7.8%%
- **Blackcurrant Bud Absolute - 9-14%**
- **Bog Myrtle - 11.0%**
- Cade (rectified) - 6.1%
- Cajeput (Vietnamese) 0.7-2.5%
- **Camphor (Borneo) 0.3-19.1%**
- **Camphor 18.0**
- **Cangerana 28.6**
- **Catnip 6.2 – 24.6%**
- Clove Bud 0.6-12.4%
- Clove stem 3.5-12.4%
- **Copaiba 24.7-53.3%**
- Fenugreek 14.6%
- **Fern Sweet 24.5%**
- **Hemp 13.7- 19.4%**
- Hoary Basil 4.3-10.0%
- Holy Basil 1.3-1.2%
- Hop 9.8%
- Lantana 12.0%
- Lemon Basil 3.8 -4.5%

- **Pepper White 23.4**
- **Pilocarpus Microphyllus 40.6%**
- Pine Black 5.3-11.8%
- Pungent Basil 1.3%
- Thymus Serpyllum 6.0-11.2
- Winter Savoury 0-13.6%
- Wormwood (Thujone CT) 10.6%
- Ylang Ylang 1.1-21.5

Please check individual safety data for each oil before use.

You'll have noticed Copaiba, or Copal incense on the list. Extracted from the *Protium* species, a cousin species to the *Boswellia* genera, its chemical constituent pentacyclic triterpene has very high binding affinity for both CB_1 and CB_2. Nature's Gift sell a beautiful strain that they describe as having a vanilla note, and is of course extracted from a resin, just as frankincense is too. Unusually, it has a heart note, rather than the basso note we'd expect from gum oils, betraying how it especially helps chest complaint and pulmonary infections. CB_2 unlocks inflammation and fights infection and CB_1 eases the mind. Fascinating to see these oils unfurl from the endocannabinoid perspective. Previously hidden magic.

The Tahitian noni fruit, *Morinda citrifolia*, has an unidentified something that weakly binds to CB_2. ☐A patented essential oil, made from the seeds, seems to be available from only one website called "Morinda". Whether that constituent transfers over to oil though, is obviously undetermined given that we don't actually know what the constituent is. The company claims their noni seed essential oil has the capacity to improve skin health and boost absorption of other essential oils.

They have a 90-day free trial on the site. I'm gonna get myself a bottle! (I'm such a junkie, aren't I?!). Incidentally, they also have a cold press of the oil, so said active constituent might just as likely be lurking there, I suppose.

Let's move on. It's making me feel like I'm searching for Nessie!

Substrates

Earlier we spoke about the dreadful tragedy that befell the clinical trial of the drug designed to inhibit FAAH. Sometimes, I wonder if it's "better the devil you know" and perhaps sticking with plants might be a safer option. Biochanin A found in red clover and genistein from soybean both modestly inhibit FAAH.

Mastic

Mastic essential oil, *Pistacia lentiscus*, is rich with monoterpenoids and sesquiterpenoids. Rats who dined on mastic EO showed higher plasma levels of DHA, EPA, PEA, and OEA (the substrates that make arachidonic acid that produces endocannabinoids) than control rats did. However, no change was observed in levels of either anandamide or 2-AG.

Sea Buckthorn

The carrier oil, sea buckthorn, contains vaccenic acid, shown to attenuate complications observed in metabolic syndrome.

A possible explanation for the constituent's remarkable effects on dyslipidaemia, fatty liver disease, and low-grade inflammation, might be that vaccenic acid lowers intestinal inflammation as it increases production of anandamide and related N-acylethanolamines.

Khat

Many of you will be aware of the psychoactive plant, *khat*. Containing cathinone and cathine, *Catha edulis* elicits effects like amphetamine or ephedra. Effects are described by some as euphoric; they enjoy increased alertness and excitement, their ability to concentrate is much better, and their creative flow is more fluid. They feel more confident, open, friendly, and at one with the world. An alkaloid in khat, Pristimerin, potently inhibits the degradative serine hydrolase MAGL and is demonstrated to elevate levels of 2-AG in neurons in the cortex of rat brains.

I'd recommend reading *Care of the Endocannabinoid System* for yourself to glean the nuances. I'll post a link at the end of the chapter. Fundamentally though, they say eat a healthy diet, in particular organic, if you can. Meditation and massage improves endocannabinoid tone, as does moderate exercise.

Build more sources of omega-3 into your diet using oils such as hemp, camellia and fish oils. The body manufactures Anandamide and 2-AG from arachidonic acid, which in turn is built from oils and fats. Most importantly, there is a beneficial 1:4 ratio of omega-3 and omega-6.

Arachidonic acid is omega-6, thus it may seem like we should blanket supplements to increase levels of anandamide and 2-AG. However, too much omega-6 equals too much arachidonic acid, leading to an excess of endocannabinoids in the system, which as we have seen in the anxiety section might be just as damaging as a deficiency. Supplementing with omega-3 raises levels of eicosapentaenoic acid, (EPA) and docosahexaenoic acid (DHA), essential fatty acids required to fuel the ECS, as well as diffusing arachidonic acid through the tissues.

Evidence supporting this dietary change is overwhelming but not least that a deficiency in omega-3 leads to a depression of CB_1 receptors profoundly affecting neurological and physical wellbeing. Ideally, you should consume between 500-1000mg of omega-3 a day, which can be found in tuna and salmon as well as other oily fish, in seeds such as flax seed, and in massive amounts in hemp seed.

As a species, we evolved on a diet rich in omega acids – not least because hemp seed was one of the staples in our diet. However, its success as a crop began to wane, as farmers experimented with other cereals. Studies show people existed on an omega-6/omega-3 ratio of about 1:1. Western diets are now around 16:1. Suppression of omega-3 and essential fatty acids is postulated to be the underlying factor responsible for many diseases, not least because the substrate of the endocannabinoid system can no longer generate the tools needed to maintain homeostasis.

A paper by The Centre of Genetics in Washington from 2002 elucidates just how important this dietary adjustment may be:

"Excessive amounts of omega-6 polyunsaturated fatty acids (PUFA) and a very high omega-6/omega-3 ratio, as is found in today's Western diets, promote the pathogenesis of many diseases, including cardiovascular disease, cancer, and inflammatory and autoimmune diseases, whereas increased levels of omega-3 PUFA (a low omega-6/omega-3 ratio) exert suppressive effects. In the secondary prevention of cardiovascular disease, a ratio of 4/1 was associated with a 70% decrease in total mortality. A ratio of 2.5/1 reduced rectal cell proliferation in patients with colorectal cancer, whereas a ratio of 4/1 with the same amount of omega-3 PUFA had no effect. The lower omega-6/omega-3 ratio in women with breast cancer was associated with decreased risk. A ratio of 2-3/1 suppressed inflammation in patients with rheumatoid arthritis, and a ratio of 5/1 had a beneficial effect on patients with asthma, whereas a ratio of 10/1 had adverse consequences," (Simopoulos, 2002).

If you consume hemp seed, the endocannabinoid system works far more effectively. Incidentally, I say *consume* because **omega acids are not skin permeable** and so **topical application of hemp seed oil**, although useful in other ways, **has no benefits on the ECS**.

Consumption of hemp seed oil has also shown very strong improvements in multiple sclerosis sufferers. A 2015 trial in Iran included 100 patients with an extended disability score of more than six, split into three groups. The first group was supplemented with evening primrose *(Oenthera biennis)* oil and hemp seed oil, together with dietary advice, or a low saturated fat diet and hot-natured foods such as peppers and chillies (here's your TRPV!).

The second group was given olive *(Olea europea)* oil; and the third group was given evening primrose and hemp seed oil without dietary advice. After six months, the study showed significant improvements in the first and third groups and a worsening of symptoms in the second.

I'll add a codicil.

Begin with small amounts and be careful if you work in a career where you undergo drug testing. If you do, then you might be better off using the slightly less effective flax seed *(Linum usitatissimum)* oil or walnut *(Juglans regia)* oil. **_Hemp seed should not contain cannabinoids_**...and yet...

Depending on where hemp seeds are bought, sometimes there can be contamination. A report from Croatia showed that perhaps not all their local hemp seed oil was being made from industrial hemp. Some seemed to come from marijuana. Their analysis showed some samples to contain as much as 3.23 and 69.5 mg/kg of THC. This troubling discovery was deepened in June 2016 when the University of Trieste in Rome announced that they had seen the first paediatric case of cannabinoid poisoning. The child had been prescribed hemp seed oil by his paediatrician in a bid to build his immune system and he had presented with neurological symptoms. When his urine was tested, low levels of THC were found.

My daughter-in-law failed a drugs test earlier this year when she applied for a position at the fire service. Poppy seeds in the loaf she had consumed that morning showed as opiates on the test and nearly cost her her career - I'd hate to be responsible for that happening to you.

When the product was analysed it contained THC. How can one be certain? Grow your own in the garden, one would presume!

If you'd like to read the original *Care of The Endocannabinoid System* article, you can access it here:

https://www.ncbi.nlm.nih.gov/pmc/articles/PMC3951193/

Chapter 10 Spiritual Dimensions of the Essential Oil

The French 1947 Nobel Prize winner for literature, André Gide, once wrote:

"What another would have done as well as you, do not do it. What another would have said as well as you, do not say it; written as well, do not write it. Be faithful to that which exists nowhere but in yourself—and thus make yourself indispensable."

I'll begin by stating I don't conceive myself being indispensable. Quite the reverse, in fact! However, I trust the universe has a purpose for every one of us, and mine seems to be communication of a strange and unique understanding of plants. Every day I've marvelled at the temerity of writing about a sacred plant I've chosen to censor my relationship with. Goddess might have better plucked a shaman, a herbalist, or a drug dealer from our midst, all of whom surely must have more pertinent knowledge than I. When they possess substantially more wisdom to offer the world, why would She have chosen me?

Ours is not to reason why. Only to answer the call.

That said, I'd urge you to study literature written by people like Stephen Gray, Chris Bennet, and Robert Clarke, as I genuinely believe their entheogenic observations of the plant far surpass mine. So many times, I have virtually drowned under misgivings about the relevance of a trip-less book about cannabis. I don't trust censorship of plants. They grow, they belong to the Earth, so therefore they belong to the people. It's up to us how we resolve to work with them and how closely we choose to listen.

In the stillness of evening, cannabis's deep roots plunged deep into the Earth immersed in the wisdom of Gaia, absorbing Her lessons to transmit back to mankind. By day, bathed in the healing rays of the sun, her sapience photosynthesized. Processed through respiration, then capsulised into secondary metabolites for our exploitation, surely it should be up to us whether or how we choose to use them?

But some realms are sacred; knowledge of them taboo and arcane. Their secrets are the noesis of priesthoods and initiated; doctrine of the plants that take us there, recondite.

I opened the text of my book *"The Complete Guide to Clinical Aromatherapy and The Essential Oils of the Physical Body"* with a challenge for the reader:

"Let me guide you through the woodland...because I know plant medicine very well. A hedge witch, perhaps? Who knows?!"

Some of you will undoubtedly have made your own assumptions about that. But a witch, a true witch, is initiated into the mysteries. It's not only study that will take her there. She must witness the magic for herself. On her quest for mastery, she will undergo three transmutations to become third degree. A ritual takes place, projecting her through the portal to her new realm, the High Priestess escorts her to a new interpretation of life.

Likewise, a person might resolve they are ready to progress to their next stage and even initiate themselves. But the ritual is merely that. Representations of advancement. No more. No less. Any decision made by the candidate is obsolete. If Goddess disagrees you're ready, unaltered you will remain. Third degree by name, nothing more.

Ascension is earned and bestowed. It certainly isn't a right.

For me, journeying has but started. No further up the ladder than first rung. Therapist I might be, but Shaman I am not.

Not yet.

I've much more to learn in this realm before I am ready to traverse to the next.

I guess many would like to understand why I didn't smoke as I researched. The truth is psychosis lives very close to my family. I observed its evil hands snatch wonderful people away from me into Hell. I've been first party to the horror of distorted reality, frantic at my impotence to exert any change. I love my children too much to risk them standing in that same space. Marijuana echoes your presiding attention, so expecting to see demons...I suspect I almost certainly would.

If a time or place existed where I could leave that fear behind, then yes, I'd be tempted to light up. Right now, though, my intuition says keep clear. I'd be foolish to ask Her to speak, and then to blatantly ignore.

I have already made the decision that should cancer come knocking, I'll find myself a dealer. Cancer ripped the characters out of those I have loved, completely altering their view of the world. If I must be stolen into that "other place" at least with THC it might level the disease-ridden playing field a touch. I'm saving my demons for the biggest fight.

Does that diminish my understanding of the plant? Does it taint my assessments of CBD or of the essential oil? I hope it makes my observations *more* pertinent. The limits of the medicine and how it makes life tick is unconfused by the benefits of the smoke. In so doing, I remain true to Gide's advice, publishing something existing nowhere apart from me. Well, that's the plan!

What follows then is my experience of living with cannabis night and day for eight long months. My observations and journey, and mine alone. Yours may be different. That's what makes life so gloriously entrancing.

Cannabis's Effects on Thought

Now let me warn you, hempen rumination is promiscuous. Thoughts vault through space and time. Any effort to remain loyal to a subject is an insurmountable task. Dedicated focus on anything, a completely futile endeavour. She's so elated I've come to party. Deadlines, it appears, be damned!

Take my hand, she seduces, and the second I do we take flight. Soaring way above the constraints of this dimension, she breathlessly declares *"there is so much more to see"*.

Her energy was so familiar, but I knew I had not encountered it in a plant. Without ever toking up, I knew Her vibration deep in my core. Where had I seen Her? Met Her? Been wrapped in Her love? The knowledge was there; just as the answer flashed, I found it already gone. No time to grieve its passing, my mind, contentedly following her around the next beguiling twist and turn.

The most delicate breeze of concern whispered in my ear that perhaps my capacity to write had deserted me. Might I no longer be up to the job? Unfazed, I was too wasted on archaeology and science to frankly give a toss!

Conversely, what *did* concern me was potential effects the oil might exert upon my personality. Homeopathic wisdom encouraged me to wonder what parallel reality might tempt me to the other side. A mother and a wife, the risk of becoming *different* might be a dangerous thing.

Forewarned, I kept telling myself, is forearmed.

Curiosity, I reminded Alice, is what killed the cat!

Secretive, the homeopaths warned...

Did I become secretive? I don't think so, but more private? Yes.

Furtive, perhaps to outsider's eyes, although I'd convey it more as withdrawn. Discussing my work with no-one, it wasn't shame about the content, or even mindfulness that understanding me would be hard. More, I had become familiar with thoughts that flit and dart, ideas that were impossible to train. Sieve-like, it's a losing battle for the conscious mind to contain them, almost always suffering defeat. Theories last little longer than a heartbeat, before some more compelling ideation taking its place. If *I* could not form structure from them, how on Earth could anyone else be expected to? Like a child wandering off in a theme park, my brain was not being naughty, more that there was always something more "shiny" to attract my eye. With cannabis meandering is so easy - it is completely irresistible.

Now, there is a massive sense of "be careful what you wish for" here, because another reason I feel She picked the wrong person for the job, is because I am a person with zero worries in my life. How then I could I monitor effects on anxiety or distress? Without gloating, I view my life as just about as perfect as someone's can be. I have a husband who adores me and I completely worship him. We have three brilliantly, happy, healthy, and successful children. We have jobs we like and have enough money to live day to day. I've taught my brain to focus on the positive, and so when I look out of the window, all I see is flowers. Don't get me wrong, it hasn't always been this way - there have been times of hideous poverty and dreadfully ill health, but right now life *is* a garden.

So, I had no worries to weigh me down, but I feel sure that had I had, the cannabis could still have snuck us into Sleeping Beauty's Castle, or dragged me onto a roller coaster to make me giggle, because more than anything else it acts like a distractor. Try to identify the route to the present mental moment, I promise you, tracks have already been erased.

It's not *forgetfulness*; that's not what it is. It's not even scattiness...although that is damn close! It's creativity, whimsy, imagination, distraction, and being completely absorbed in the moment.

I know how that looks to an outsider, because I have viewed it though their eyes. Vexed, I have accused users of selfishness and idleness, or caring about nothing but the next puff. School-gate gossip might potentially have said the same of me as I got later and later to fetch Dex at night. Thank goodness for such lovely mates to watch my back! I haven't forgotten him, of course, I simply started to read something else...or created something else...or tested some new hypothesis and before I knew it, it was five past three!

It's just so fascinating...but when I return from school, I have absolutely no idea what the heck I was doing before I left!

One thing's for certain: whatever it was, it bore no resemblance to the morning's plan!

Now let's be clear. This isn't smoking the drug. On some days, it wasn't even using the oil, it was simply meditating on the vibration of the plant. Perhaps that's enough to tap into the THC, but I don't think so. It's just the medicine of the plant. It opens your mind to new possibilities and soaks you in fascination for what's in front of you.

Existing in this vibration for so long though made it easy for me to imagine how being around the *drug* for any length of time might expose latent problems of schizophrenia for some. Don't let your thoughts run away with you, we warn the paranoid. We frown at the jumbled and lost logic of the psychotic wondering how on Earth they ever reached conclusions they have made. How can they be so completely sure they're right, when nothing around them makes sense? Hemp essential oil has a completely sane version of the same…not yet chaotic, but running mildly, and grasping certainty at things that only *you* can perceive. I can see how the delicate balancing act tips as cannabinoid receptors become exhausted. Somehow it feels like a ballerina, whipping around pirouette after pirouette, might suddenly execute slightly wrong, twisting her ankle. From that moment on, imaginations might never be the same. Endocannabinoid keys can no longer find their locks, shadows falls and her stage becomes a very dark and scary place. Yep, I can see how it might happen, the brain just can't keep up.

Yet still, I believe it to be a thoroughly healing plant, especially our oils.

Hemp essential oil positions you to view things from a new perspective. She pivots you to face away from the sun and turns your mind to a different emotional landscape where your ego's no longer in control. Asking you to open your mind to new perspectives, hemp enables you to view quarrels and heartaches from outside. Quietly, a movie unfolds, and just like watching a potter carefully throwing a vase, you can see everything you did to bring you to that place.

The movement of the potter's thumb is so minute, so inane, it's amazing to watch as his clay crumples beneath his hands. Just the tiniest inflection can bring the world crumbing down…and it's the same in human interaction. Sometimes your part can have been so small it's impossible to extricate it as causal to someone's distress, and yet it was there. In slow motion, the junctions, the actions, and repercussions are so much easier to see. There's a slight softening of the neck, as your head drops sideways in compassion followed by a sigh of recognition of truth.

And then…it becomes so much easier to forgive.

Of course, the second you reach that conclusion, the hempen effects dissipate, reality shifts time back into normal rhythm. Moving faster…it's impossible to discern your steps…how ever did you get here?

Who knows?

Who cares?!

What matters is that you did!

Especially when matters of the heart then extend to matters of health. Reducing the fury one feels at life calms the aggression of the life force we have flowing within. Taking the foot off the accelerator gives such glorious respite to pain and inflammation. Relax inflamed minds and it eases physical inflammation too.

Calm…not sedate…it's not the same. Indeed, the effects on the nervous system are brought about by exciting and inhibiting receptors harmoniously, balancing the system. The expansion we feel in consciousness is echoed by sensations in the body. Not least by the "knowing" one feels for the fleeting second before a thought has chance to register in the mind.

The secret of how one perceives time when under the influence of marijuana is still elusive. Current research indicates it might be down to the dense population of receptors in the thalamo-cortical-striatal circuit, the area also implicated in OCD and the memory problems of Parkinson's. Marijuana somehow speeds the internal clock, dilating time, making five minutes seem twice as long. Using the essential oil is milder and subtler, but to my mind, it's still a fantastic way to build more hours into your creative day! I couldn't help but wonder if the effects of the THC have been immaculately designed to harness this power of increased thinking. Does time seem to expand as a means of accommodating the ever-flowing stream? Would this habit of drowning in a sea of fascination and allowing them to spill into non-work time be a situation better managed under the control of cannabinoids? Or would the flow have further increased and the tidal wave of words would have engulfed me entirely? I don't know.

When interviewing marijuana users, they all said the same. Time goes slower and you have more thoughts. But even without the THC I had more thoughts. Hundreds of thousands of zillions of them, so those thoughts most certainly derive from the terpenes and other essential oil components. Using the essential oil, that commodity remains intact.

Sometimes the rush from the essential oil is enough to make you want to jump out of your skin. Without reason, I've smashed open my email or Facebook tabs just to "stop the stream". It's too much, too fast, too intense. It's so akin to snatching your hand away from heat, so completely automatic, I suspect there must be some connection to the TRPV channels, but who am I to say?

Sociologist H. S. Becker suggested that the effects of marijuana must be learned. They are not spontaneous. There is a need for someone to point out how the colours are changing or the tastes are growing, for the newbie observer to first notice it. In that way, I suppose, you need to be initiated. No sooner than awareness is settled to the altered perception it is integrated, and the spiritual growth can advance. They won't have to be told again. They come to expect it.

How very astute!

I wish someone had initiated me.

Because no matter how many times I read that "intention is key", the words simply rippled over me. A key breakthrough in my work was, as ever, lying in the bath, meditating with the oil. Much of the book was already written but was flat and lack lustre. The worst part, I felt, was Ancient China (please don't tell me it still is!). Without realising it, I was focusing on how to bring it to life and my perception changed. I heard the now familiar voice saying: "I remember" and I realised that the incense burners I had seen in the Forbidden Kingdom held the key. I had knowledge to use, I just needed to be shown where to tap into it. This was the first time that my mind had not jetéed from A-Z - it had been firmly fixed on what I needed to achieve. Prior to that, I guess my brain had been saying *"There's just so much to learn"* and cannabis had got so wonderfully excited and squealed: *"I know, let me show you some more"*.

Focus is key. Not only for smoking pot, but also working with the essential oil. If you use it wondering if it will cure a tooth infection, you become more aware of every throb, the taste in your mouth, and whether the size of the abscess is changing. If you sit down to meditate on how to write a beautiful piece of music, sensory overload engulfs you (no wonder myrcene gives you couch lock, you're too overwhelmed with information to get out of your seat!). If you focus on how you can repair your relationship with your dad – and you are that specific – well, then you're going to get somewhere.

So, holding this intention is so important but in some ways, it is counter-productive. Because concentration belongs to the conscious mind, to the insistent ego, but cannabis medicine is about letting go. It's about untethering the constraints of this three-dimensional reality and its associated illusions. Rather like standing on a tight rope, sooner or later you have to loosen the grip. Balance comes from within.

So, for a moment, close your eyes and step out onto that rope. Consider the proprioceptive responses. Your heart beat changes, even the minutest muscle twitch seems enormous. There's an excitement and tightness down below as your body anticipates danger. Attention changes and you become preoccupied by the position of your feet on the rope, noticing sensations that would have gone by unheeded before. Your perception has changed, your consciousness altered.

But more, for a moment, reality shifted, didn't it? Your body reacted as if it were on the rope, without even leaving the chair, responding to the wavelengths created by your mental imagery.

In part, this is another shifting relationship with time. In this dimension, we only experience events in the present. In the past, they become a memory, and in the future, an anticipation of what can become. But cannabis moves the boundaries of time and space, and as we saw with the homeopathic medicine, cosmic ordering becomes so much easier. In conscious reality, we can *imagine* how things will be, but visualisation with the essential oil allows us to experience the reality as a physical truth of how they *feel*. If you feel something, well, then it is tangible. It exists.

Likewise, as time slows, you can tap into the moment and hold it, very similar to what we are taught with mindfulness. As the second expands, intervals open in musical cadences, allowing the listener to wander through what seems to be an enormous cavern between the notes. Noises that seemed not to exist before, caress your ear. Harmonies concealed from the uninitiated ear sing angelic praises to the gods. Doorways open to a fuller, more radiant reality where music is sweeter and life is just much…muchier! How many toke-buzzed jazz riffs, performed with supernatural speed, somehow just won't execute after the smoke has gone?

Descriptions of the fragrance of cannabis vary from bitter to fruity, from grapefruit-y to lemony or apple-y. To me CBD smells of mud, although the essential oil is a bit sweeter and more pleasant. As THC hits though, the note expands, drawing you deeper into fragrance realms usually only traversed by a more discerning "nose".

Charles Baudelaire gloriously illustrated the potent changes in sensation when he described consuming hashish marmalade, dining at the infamous Club des Hashischins.

"… a new stream of ideas carries you away: it will hurl you along in its living vortex for a further minute; and this minute, too, will be an eternity, for the normal relation between time and the individual has been completely upset by the multitude and intensity of sensations and ideas. You seem to live several men's lives in the space of an hour."

For those of you who have never read my work before, I have something called synaesthesia which means my senses are wired rather oddly. When my brain registers a fragrance, I also hear it as a sound – a musical note. Usually, when I hold a plant medicine in my hands I can hear its vibration and the music the plant creates. It threw me when I started to work with the CBD oil Dr. Pappas gave me, because I could not hear its song. That's never happened before and it made writing this book very hard. This strange quirk is a normal part of life to me. It's how I have always experienced scent, so it felt like I had been robbed of two of my senses - aroma and sound. It was very odd and distinctly unsettling. I might as well have been walking around with my eyes closed!

Dr. P had also given me some essential oil he'd distilled but when I opened my case the bottle had smashed and seeped into my shoes! So, when, some months further into the project, I purchased a replacement bottle of the essential oil, I was so relieved to hear her song. A simple chord of A Minor (C Major) resonated through my mind. It felt like home. Finally, a connection.

Then something startling took place one frosty winter's day. I had developed a dreadful cold which had then triggered toothache. Dentists and I don't share a happy history, so visits to them fill me with dread. Frankly, I would rather stick pins in my eyes than sit in their chair, so essential oils are always my first call before making the fateful appointment. To treat the infection, I reached for the essential oil in a bid to piggy back off beta-caryophyllene's effect on CB_2. Diluting it in olive oil with CBD, I rubbed some around my gums and administered it sublingually.

Lordamercy, what a vile taste. Dr. Pappas explained to me that he blended his CO_2 with vanilla and peppermint CO_2s to make his vaping mix more palatable. Good plan. I wish I had done the same. Instead I had been working with the whole extract syringe and pouring mud down my throat!

After using the blend, I trudged up the hill to fetch Dex from school. Ascending the steep hill he and I know as *Mordor*, I passed a house that perpetually emanates a stench of weed. Nothing unusual in that, there are plenty of them around here, but the effect this day was remarkable. Entering the fog, the most incredible sensation engulfed me. The disgraceful aftertaste dispersed. As it mixed with THC, it became sublime. Without warning, my music switched on. Rather than the simple A Minor chord I'd heard, a multi-layered church organ harmonic resonated through my being.

The younger me sang in a Wolverhampton church called St John's. Considered important, St John's has some astonishing artwork and is home to a most spectacular Renatus Harris organ, built in 1682. Legend has it that the premier performance of Handel's Messiah had been played upon the instrument when it was originally housed in Dublin. The music I experienced as I passed through the smoke rivalled beauty I'd heard from that instrument. The melody I knew well, but had slept unused by me for many decades. Resurrected by the cannabinoids around my gums the *Libera Me* from Fauré's Requiem blasted through my aura. The words familiar from singing in so many funerals...

Libera me Domine, de mort aeternera – Free me from death.

Just as fast, the breeze stole the smoke. The fleeting overture was gone. Mysterious, never repeated and indeed, it did feel divine.

Explanations elude me because it can't be the cannabinoids active here, or I wouldn't be triggered by essential oils. It can't be something as simple as terpenes, because again, I can hear the music of other oils, but there are terpenes in CBD. I wonder if it's the intact nature of the oil, but again, not all molecules travel across... Who knows, perhaps I am just a little odd! (The bookies tell me they are offering very short odds on that one!)

In his article, *Mr X*, cosmologist Carl Sagan speaks of his quite electrifying musical experience when smoking grass. He describes how his perception of the music was somehow deepened by the weed, how it enabled him to separate out each instrument's part and listen to its melody independently. Now, I've always done that as second nature, and had assumed other people could too! When researching how cannabis interacted with music, suggestions abounded of users experiencing music synesthetically, as barriers between senses somehow diffused inside the brain.

I wonder if it might somehow be to do with the frequency I am vibrating on? One theory posed by mind-body-spirit expert Teal Scott is that people experience the highs and lows of marijuana differently based on their vibration at any time. It amplifies emotional outlook, raising those feelings of those already elated and plummeting those who feel low. Experts agree that enjoying marijuana at its best should be done when you are fairly wide awake or you will just end up falling asleep! Likewise, smoking when life seems mean serves only to drag you lower.

Grass magnifies intention, so whatever is foremost in your mind becomes the focus of your altered perception. Feeling anxious of bad trips almost certainly ensures they happen (although marijuana-fuelled anxiety attacks can happen for any number of reasons). Those operating on a high vibration are lifted higher, stretching out into the cosmic connection drawing back enlightenment and vision. A lower vibration might not be so kind. I wonder if it is this realignment of vibration that shifts me off the frequency I would ormally inhabit. Whatever it is, hemp certainly changes me at the most energetic level.

And how we want to change is fundamentally important, because cannabis is never about *me*, but always about *the other*.

Pushing the curtain of the conscious mind aside, She whispers, but what about *them*? How do *they* hurt? Where is *their* pain? Removing the shackles of the ego, the mind takes on a gentler, far more benign outlook, releasing anger, resurrecting a soft and gentle heart, and connecting the user with the most serene and loving cosmic ray.

8 p.m. one Tuesday, the phone rang and recognition kicked in. I knew Her. Of *course*, I did. What's more, in her essay *"Who is She?"* Kathleen Harrison had already let me in on the secret, but I had ignored her cue.

She writes: *"The window in my mind opens to my beloved Big Sister. Here She is; I can count on Her. She always shows up when I ask. She knows me. We are old companions. We chuckle at the joy of getting together again. I am so very grateful to have this beautiful wise Big Sister in my life, she helps me to know what to take seriously and what to let go of. I feel so fully alive in every cell. She is a gift from nature to us, a gift from the mystery itself."*

Yes! That *is* how I knew Her.

She was my sister...not just the biological one, but She is embodied by that effervescent feeling that engulfs you, embracing those whom you have known and loved for ever. Those women who know your secrets. Those you trade confidences and memories with and howl with laughter as you reminisce. She is the girl you never need to explain *why* to...the one who simply *knows*. The one who, when she speaks, you listen, no matter how hard the truth. The one who always holds you in her love and would come running whenever you called, even if it was 2 a.m.

The caller that evening had been my most beloved step sister, who does *exactly* what cannabis does, mentally and verbally leapfrogging from one subject to the next. She almost speaks in shorthand, she zips about so fast. Often describing her as "unable to speak in straight lines", I never cease to be amazed how much conversational ground she can cover in just a few seconds. She'll speak of people I'm expected to know, but have never met or even previously heard of. She throws in health service jargon and abbreviations for good measure, without giving her audience a moment to catch their breath! I have never yet had a conversation with Angela that has not made my head spin!

Many of you will recognise "Jelly" from my Facebook page. She is the closest Goddess ever came to creating a fairy godmother. Every second with her is exhausting and you howl with laughter and squeal with delight as she regales another tale from childhood and then potentially she will teach you to "wang a wellie" across a cricket pitch, hauling off her boots in middle of a muddy field, in the pouring rain, and donkey daring you to throw yours even farther than hers.

Often, she has been seen clad head to toe in pink (hat, rosy sunglasses, wellington boots, teamed with bright pink fishing net and bucket), heading off to the river in the hope of catching newts. Incidentally, this picture wasn't taken for the book, it's just one of many pictures of her dressed like a fairy lying around! That should be telling, in itself!

Now, she (we!) are older, her focus has shifted a tad to breeding rare Ayam Cemani chickens and mucking about with goats! Life is one spectacularly glorious Adventure to Ang, and it's exactly the same with hemp.

Her effervescent energy is contagious and without fail every time I see her I am reduced to an uncontrollably idiotic giggling wreck.

For me, there is no medicine like it.

Neuroscientists and psychologists would have their work cut out elucidating what parts of the brain we trigger when we are nostalgically guffawing. Rolling about on the floor. How can it be that memories flood back so quickly? What strange biology takes place as the forty something women observe their fifteen-year-old selves and bear witness to previously hidden syntaxes taking place? So easy to spot jealousy, when you view them from a far.

The observer...

Sagan described that too...

Recognising Her now, I'd like to try to identify the work she was sent here to do. Which divine being is active within the plant?

The Archetype of Cannabis
Aaah...

Now there *is* a question!

The Ancient Egyptians burned roses to summon Isis to their side. The presence of Artemis filled tombs and temples as she answered Helichrysum's call to protect in battle. When the ancients called to Her, who was it arrived at their side?

Culpepper places hemp's rulership under Saturn and I entirely agree. That is correct, but the archetype, the god/goddess holding the mysteries? Kali Ma, Daoism's Hemp Lady, Krishna, Shiva, are all known to answer the cannabis smoke. But none of them really seem to carry the medicine of the plant.

It's so strange how this book has developed, and at times it has seemingly written itself. It's been impossible to keep track of what has been note taking and what has found its way onto the page. Mid-March, becoming increasingly frustrated with the lack of progress in understanding the archetype of such a powerful and strange plant, I was close to knocking it on the head. The plant was shielding her magic and I had, frankly, had enough! Lying in the bath one Thursday evening, I asked for insights to write this section of the book. Next morning, I woke and suggested a visit to Hereford Cathedral to mum, to sneak a peek at the famous ancient chained library. Completely the opposite of what I had planned for the day, mum, looking bemused and bewildered, agreed we should jump on the train.

The library, tucked out of the way, is difficult and awkward to find inside of the cathedral. I felt so nervous as I approached, and yet I felt entirely as if I'd come home. Amongst the books, I had no understanding of why I was in the right place, but I absolutely knew that I was. The whole day, I felt like I would burst into tears of joy.

Being around old books isn't unusual for me, as you can imagine. But I was so moved by these extraordinary tomes dating from the 15th century onwards. Every book is turned with its spines facing inwards and each is connected to the shelf by its original chain. The books are enormous, all carefully written or printed onto thick pieces of paper and then bound with leather. The oldest book in the library, the Hereford Apostles, dates to 800AD. Also, housed there is the Mappa Mundi, a 13th Century map of how the medieval world saw our lives in both geographical and spiritual terms. Painted onto calf skin, the map is bizarre with all manner of strange creatures the painter had encountered on his travels to Jerusalem. The library smells dusty, solemn, and entirely sacred. This truly is hallowed ground.

When we went out into the body of the cathedral, I couldn't fail to be entirely awestruck by the dimensions of the huge transept. The enormity and grandeur of the building is spectacular. I stood in reverence in front of the tomb of St Thomas. I gazed around me at some of the most glorious glass windows you've ever seen. I felt a kind of emptiness and envy that I might never feel the sensation of devotion these people must have had to be able to build such monumental constructions.

Outside of the cathedral is a working stone mason's yard and the cathedral is bursting with symbology of the Freemasons; their work, powerful testimony to why they have become such a powerful organisation. Their astute knowledge of sacred geometry; their powerful use of stone. I didn't understand why, but I was aware that I had learnt something incredibly important there that afternoon.

Within five minutes of sitting at my desk on Monday, I understood what I had learned. I had visited the archetype of cannabis, Seshat.

Let me introduce you to the ancient Egyptian goddess of writing – Seshat.

Isn't she glorious?

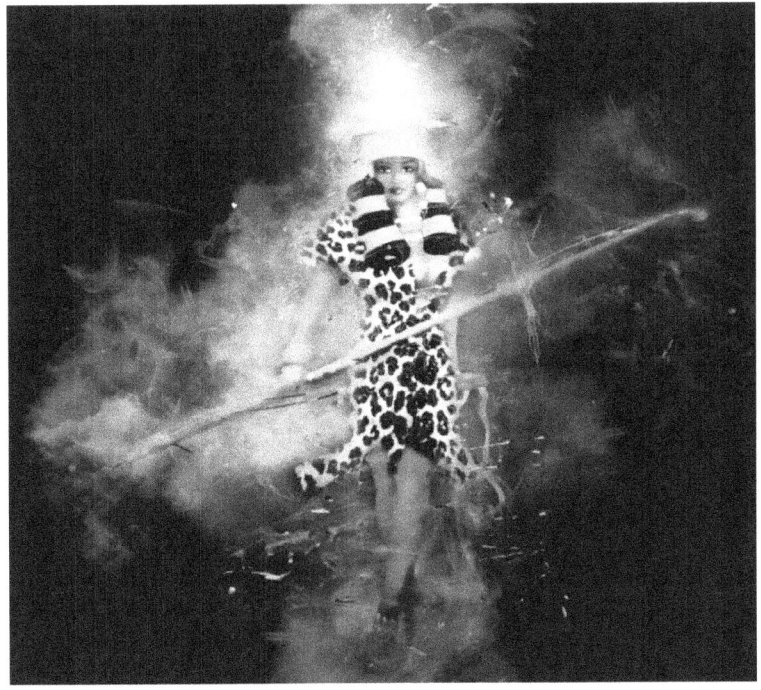

The goddess of writing, of sacred geometry and librarians, amongst many other titles, Seshat is keeper of the records of time. An extremely ancient goddess, by the fourth dynasty she was already beginning to lose her power. Originally, Seshat had been a great goddess, fully worshipped, with her duties being carried out by priests and officials.

If you believe such things, some say she was an Ascended Master from before the fall of Atlantis, had roamed the Nubian deserts, and then had been adopted by the Ancient Egyptians. She was a powerful and revered goddess. There is no evidence she was ever celebrated as her own cult, and yet there is evidence of her everywhere, most of all in the buildings and constructions of the Ancient Egyptians.

Most certainly in the early dynasties she had been celebrated, but eventually her role seemed to change. Then, it seemed to be that she served the pharaoh, and she is the Goddess of the Kingship. She is an incarnation of Nephthys, whom you may remember from the rose book. Nephthys was the sister wife of Set, who had tricked Osiris into climbing into an ornate coffin and trapped him to do away with him after Osiris had become so beloved by his people. When Isis had struggled to find Osiris, Nephthys had stepped in to help her. She was a sky goddess and, like Isis, a sorceress. Nephthys is Seshat.

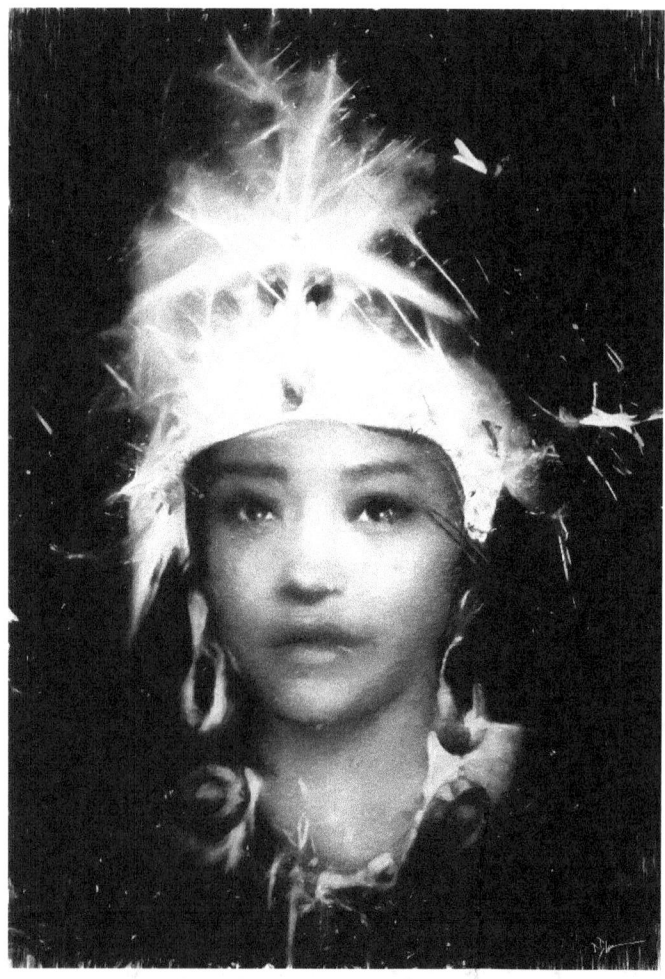

She is one of the most glamorous of the Goddesses. Tall, willowy, and slender with a full and ample bosom, she is always depicted wearing a long leopard-skin dress, tapering outwards at the base. Some have suggested illustrations might be showing legs of a leopard hanging down. Her most striking attribute is a headdress with a seven-pointed star or flower. Many interpret the star as being an illustration of the hemp leaf. It seems to me the seven-pointed star could likewise show the fan-shaped form of papyrus, but either way, as papyrus too would represent paper, this is in perfect alignment with her title **Ruler of Scribes**.

Over time, her head dress changed slightly and it seemed as if, by the 12th Dynasty, the original meaning may have been forgotten. Later in history we see her being referred to as *"she who wears two horns"*- **Sefekh aubi**, as her head dress seems to be a moon (might possibly have been in reverence to Thoth, who was a moon god), or perhaps a bow or the horns. This may have been an aspect of Seshat, or an epithet of her as an actual goddess.

Very little has been written about Seshat. Her birth was recorded on the Palermo Stone, a fragment of basalt which records the births of the kings from the first to the fifth dynasty. Most of what we know about her comes from illustration.

She had three very important functions:

- She records the length of the pharaoh's life
- She helps him to calculate the position, alignment, and geometry of the buildings he created in his lifetime
- She records all accomplishments of his reign.

Writing

She is known as the *"Original One, who originated writing at the beginning"*. She is said to have invented writing and is known as the female scribe, the record keeper, the lover and consort of Thoth (the keeper of records). Thoth is described as giving and teaching writing to man. Both Seshat and Thoth are seen as representing the Divine masculine and feminine principles of wisdom. In the most prosaic sense, we can see how Seshat was the female, yin creatrix of the writing, but it was Thoth who was active in teaching it and spreading it over the Earth.

She is Goddess of Architecture, Goddess of Construction, of astronomy and mathematics. She is known as Great Lady of the House of Books, Lady of Architects, building and surveying. She is known as Mistress of the House of Books where it is imagined she took care of Thoth's tomes and spells. She rules census and accounting, wisdom, knowledge, and writing. She is the Goddess of History.

There have been many discoveries of Egyptian depictions of women *holding* writing brushes, so we know that woman knew how to write (it was an extremely egalitarian society in many ways), but to date, only Seshat has been found as being depicted in the actual process of writing.

Time

She has many names. The pyramid texts call her *"She who reckons the life; Lady of Year, Lady of Fate."* She defines the archetype of female librarians and of civil engineers.

Depictions of Seshat always show her holding a cord, the hemp rope she uses for measuring, as well as a palm staff. We see her notching the years of the pharaoh's life onto the staff. The time she bestows belongs to gods far older than the sun god, Ra. The years belonged to the most ancient of the Egyptian deities to

Tatanen and Atum, and later Ra, who replaced Atum as god of the kingship. It is interesting that we see her noting the staff, therefore counting. It seems that Seshat was counting time even before the Egyptians were writing.

There are many versions of her name. As Seshat, her name means *"Female Scribe."* Alternative Names: Safkhet, Sesat, Seshet, Sesheta, and Seshata. Safkhet means seven. Indeed, she has a very profound relationship with the number seven and in many instances in Egyptian sources we hear how the time she extends to the pharaoh is measured in instances of seven years, other times she signifies their longevity.

Ancient Egyptian literature tells us she said to Amenhotep III *"I give the millions of years of life and prosperity."*

By the period of the New Kingdom, she was involved in the Heb-Sed festival of any pharaoh who had reached 30 years. She was invited as a means of renewing the vigour of the pharaoh, who it was seen as having so far cheated death.

The Book of the Dead relates: *"Thou shalt renew thy youth, thou shalt flourish again like Aah-Thoth when he is a child."*

I found it interesting to discover that, on ascension to the throne, each king would express a desire to have many Sed festivals. Thirty years was a generation, each festival a renewal of his energy to continue cosmic building which, after all, was his main responsibility before the gods.

Recording

In some artwork, we see Seshat writing on the branches of the Tree of Life. This was an intricate record of everything that happened in life, the Divine Order, The Plan.

Present at the birth of the pharaoh, it was her duty to record all subsequent events. She recorded the speeches of crowning ceremonies, and by the time of the Middle Kingdom, she was also responsible for inventory of foreign captures and goods gained in military campaigns.

Measurement

The most important function of the pharaoh was to maintain cosmic order and part of the success of this was in his construction of temples in worship to the gods. Seshat is always found in an important ritual known as Pedjeshes (Pedj - to stretch; shes - cord), or The Stretching of The Cord. This ritual is believed to have taken place before any of the temples or tombs were built and was a means of connecting the physical plane with the mysteries of the other realms. Egyptologist George Hart explains: *"as early as dynasty II, she assisted the monarch in hammering the boundary poles into the ground for the ceremony of stretching the cord. This is a crucial part of the temple foundation ritual."* Aligning the pyramids to north, south, east, and west, she aligned them to the stars. The hemp cord was fundamental in creating the sacred geometry that would connect this world with the other.

This text is taken from the Temple of Edfu:

"I take the stake and I hold the handle of the mallet. I hold the cord with Seshat."

There are many depictions of this ritual. In them, she is always stood facing the King and each is seen with a peg in one hand and a mallet in the other. A short hemp rope is looped between two pegs.

Another version says:

"I hold the peg. I grasped the handle of the mallet and grip the measuring cord with Seshat. I turn my eyes to the movement of the stars. I direct my gaze to the bull's thigh. (Meskhetiu; The modern-day constellation of the plough). *I make firm the corners of the temple."*

A priestess took the form of Seshat and acted out the invisible mastery of the Goddess. Meanwhile, Seshat invisibly aligned the temple to the celestial bull's head while she connected the other peg to her home place, opening the sacred geometry to the gods.

It is said her home place exists betwixt the bull horns of Taurus, inhabiting a great celestial junction within the eight-pointed cross. Some scholars say the leg is Pleiades. The following quote is taken from the walls of the Temple of Hathor in Dendera.

"The living God Thoth - nourished by the sublime goddess in the temple - the sovereign of the country - stretches the rope in joy (align with it) - with his glance - towards the "ak" of the bull's thigh constellation - he establishes the temple house of the ministers of Dendera, as it took place before."

In her book *Akashik Cosmic Connection* Amanda Romania describes how she met Seshat in meditation and then came to witness her on many of the inscriptions she saw when travelling around Egypt.

She writes: *"In meditation, I asked Seshat to share her past life connected to this time in history. I saw Rameses II in a past life with his court, and an Oracle bought forward, who wore the robe and star headdress of Seshat. I watched the Oracle begin to draw out lines and energy spots on a papyrus map, which way a building should be facing, and where the energy connected to the stars. She appeared almost lost in a dream and again and again I would see a connection to the Great Pyramids and that of a bright star, the dog star we know as Sirius, in the night sky. It was as if she knew the collective energy in the timeline matrix, connected with this location could give great insight that could be used upon the planet."*

It is interesting that no temple has ever been found in Seshat's name, but in the very foundation laying she becomes part of every Egyptian temple. Of course, being the keeper of records and female scribes, she is also responsible for the written works each temple produced too.

Death

Seshat has an important relationship with death. The Coffin Texts explain that *"Seshat opens the door of heaven for the deceased"* and was thus a friend of the dead. To understand this, is it is vital to comprehend that the Ancient Egyptians believed this world was a carbon copy of the other world. Thus, when a person died, they would need house to live in, which Seshat provided for them. On the journey to the after-life they would encounter many puzzles and mysteries they needed to decipher, and these were housed at Per Ankh. Per Ankh was a physical place, a library of higher learning, a scriptorium, a printer's workshop, as well as a spiritual publisher and distributer of lessons. Seshat opened the house of life "Per Ankh" for the deceased.

She wears a leopard skin, which was also associated with the funereal priests and the old gods. Her dress may be the reason we know so little about her. The radical Pharaoh, Akhenaten, found sem priests and their leopard skins obnoxious, reminders of the old religion he sought to eradicate. In his efforts to obliterate all memory of it, many depictions were destroyed, which might explain why so many illustrations of Seshat and the leopard skin dress has been chiselled out of Egyptian art. Strangely, the Sadhus of India, also cannabis smokers, also roam wearing little more than a leopard skin too!

Interestingly, while the Ancient Egyptians used hemp for their ropes to lift the blocks of the pyramids, the death shrouds of their mummies were still made from flax.

This association with funereal priests is also closely aligned to the god Set, who found a way to cheat death. So, just as Set outwitted mortality, so does the pharaoh, attaining immortality through his tomb.

But the pharaoh could also escape the year of his death by using a substitute from foreigners in the country, and putting him to death by fire. Another title Seshat held was *"Controller of the Foreigners of Upper and Lower Egypt"* and she ruled the census of foreigners. Perhaps it may have been she who found suitable new pharaohs or substitutes from the unlucky.

As the keeper of records, Seshat also represents genealogy. It is she who keeps the genetic story of DNA.

As the goddess of Measure, Celestial Alignment, and Harmony, Seshat also governs the relationship between sound in space. In his book, Spirit in the Sky: The High Wisdom of Ancient Egypt, John Anthony West explains the name and symbology of the Seshat also directly implies her connection to wavelength and to harmonious music. He writes:

"Seshat, also called Sefhet, which means seven, is the female counterpart of Thoth, therefore mistress of measure, and always attends the foundation ceremonies of the temples. Her emblem is the seven-petalled flower. Seshat is found on the earliest inscriptions. Thus, it is clear that the correspondence between seven (harmony) and measure was known to Egypt from the onset. [. . .]

"Phenomena tend to completion in seven stages, or are complete within their specific stage. There are seven tones in the harmonic scale. It is the harmonic scale, and the human function of hearing, that give us direct access into the process of growth, of creativity manifesting itself. It is for this reason -- not chance or superstition -- that led the Pythagoreans explicitly, and the Egyptians implicitly, to employ the harmonic scale as the perfect instrument for teaching and demonstrating the workings of the cosmos.

"Consider a string of a given length as unity. Set it vibrating; it produces a sound. Stop the string at its midpoint and set it vibrating. It produces a sound one octave higher. Division in two results in an analogue of the original unity. [. . .]

"Between the original note and its octave there are seven intervals, seven unequal stages which, despite their inequality, the ear interprets as 'harmonious.'"

So, what can we learn from her?

In the Book of Thoth, Seshat is named the *"Mistress of the Sustenance of the Foremost of the Chamber of Darkness"*, this probably tells us more about her than any other name. For she is found in the first space between our conscious and unconscious mind. She lives in the darkness as we close our eyes and as we lay half asleep in the morning. She is the space where we need to withdraw from normal life to reflect and contemplate our lot. She is the space of reflection where that which is hidden, speaks back.

Of course, this is the very chamber most people wish to access as they light a joint. They fervently want to draw back the curtain to this dimension and see what lies behind. For behind that curtain, of course, is dusty, sombre, and full of records. It houses the knowledge of what once was, what is now, and everything that can come to pass.

The Akashic records have become somewhat diluted thanks to the Internet. It has become the stuff of knowledge of past lives and little more, but in fact, it is the space where every answer to every question inhabits. Consider it the Internet without the cats!

On meditating with hemp essential oil (not the CO_2, you notice), I felt the solar plexus open quickly and effortlessly, which is not what I expected to perceive. The solar plexus chakra is the gateway that houses the ladders to the Akashic records, I reached them easily without a modicum of help from THC.

But, of course, the solar plexus has so much more meaning and use attached.

First, remember it is a physical place; a ganglion of nerves branching out into the digestive system. They reach from the sympathetic nervous system, right into the pit of your stomach. If you feel sick and nervy, and you have a bad feeling in your gut, it's active intuition of something bad going to happen.

But it is a psychic and spiritual centre, home to the subtle energies of the third chakra.

Emotionally and spiritually, this is, I feel, the most powerful of all the chakras when you are thinking about balanced personality. Coiled energy, kundalini, pushes up through the chakras in a sacred rhythm drummed by the development of our selves. The deep resonance of the pelvic chakra beats out our connection with our tribe. As the energy pushes up to the sacral, the lessons of one's interaction with others play out. The energy strives to meet with consciousness, up through the chakras to the crown, but will often falter at the solar plexus as the individual struggles to find equilibrium within their self.

For this is the centre of self-esteem and of self-worth. The place where energy demands you become independent and live in your power. Where you make your own mistakes, but feel comfortable asking for help. You are the helper without becoming the drudge. The strange thing is, when you think of so many of the illnesses we are going to see cannabis helping, there is an element of becoming dependant – Alzheimer's, Huntington's, Parkinson's, ALS, cancer - but on the opposite side we have those where isolation becomes the pain: in schizophrenia, autism, and PTSD.

So just as we might ask when does personality end and neurological damage begin, we might also ask which came first. Did fear of losing one's identity affect the chakra, or is that an internal manifestation of solar plexus dis-ease? Is the invisibility we feel due to some endocannabinoid imbalance, or does our chakra need infusing with more yellow? As it loses it vibrancy, feeling invisible is a key feature of solar plexus imbalance. Or is that psychosis, depression...or even autism?

When the solar plexus is jammed wide open, the body becomes furiously yang. The patient is angry, judgmental, fiercely competitive to a nasty degree. They're over bearing, pushy, chaotic...in fact...they are goddamn [p]sychotic... Has anyone checked if it's snowing?

But if it's not vital enough, kundalini doesn't have to project them out of their shell. These are the drudges the world is taking advantage of. Unable to bathe in their own rainbow they crave the colours other people project. Constantly chasing approval, they do too much, smile too much, and never complain, but my Goddess they expect you to be thankful. They're not happy people. They're martyrs slowly and silently waving goodbye to themselves inside. And while they can't quite put their finger on what's wrong, they have this overwhelming sensation they'll wake up and they'll just be gone, and no-one will even notice.

Pre-occupation drives them further and further into decline. It's harder to take part in things, and they project their dislike of themselves outward, mistaking it as other people's distaste. They avoid social situations, worrying they will be out of place. While people do miss them, in some ways it's a relief. Their loved ones enjoy respite from perpetually having to say the right thing. They can act more freely without having to acknowledge, re-acknowledge, and appreciate again. It's like a breath of fresh air not having to worry about hurting their feelings every time they have taken something the wrong way.

They are missed, but the hole they left behind is not necessarily empty. Colleagues and lovers feel very differently, no longer feeding the voracious hunger of their energetic vampire. They feel like they've got their lives back.

And I've said it before - loneliness is a dangerous thing. It's very hard to come back from.

Unless, of course, you've got a bottle of hemp essential oil and then it's a doddle!

No...

Not quite a doddle, but much easier. Meditation with focus on the solar plexus gently frees kundalini upwards to the challenges of the heart chakra, those of love.

Uranus and Neptune
When we seek details of planet rulership to help us understand plant medicines better, we can always rely upon the meticulous note-keeping of our friend, Nicholas Culpepper, to give us insights into how the plant was seen five hundred years ago. I like to think of him roaming in the countryside, collecting plants to suit each patient he treats. In hemp, his recommendations do not disappoint. He lists it as being under the ***warming, stabilizing*** influences of ***Saturn*** building

foundations you can trust. His assessment is mainly based on hemp being used to make strong ropes and being a good medicine for wind.

I agree.

But by today's understanding of how cannabis medicine is used, it's an incomplete story, to say the least. As seems to be my wont lately - I couldn't just let the rulership lie. I needed to pick at it like a scab, because it simply doesn't sit right with me. Well, not in terms of CBD and the essential oil, at least.

In 2017, we know so much more about cannabis. By next Tuesday we will know even more and by the next Sunday probably lots more than that, because cannabis has garnered a revolution gathering more momentum with every passing hour. Rather than possessing the dull, long and chronically slow vibration of Saturn, cannabis medicine sparks electrical energy, polarizing people in its wake.

Changes in people's perceptions of cannabis remind me of how the ancient Greek religions originated differently from other faiths. Not bestowed by some omnipotent deity, their religion came from the people, built by the mathematicians, the poets, the authors of the time. Cannabis medicine has a dynamic we've never seen the like of before. Building Her message from the inside; She refuses to wait for the establishment to catch up. She squeals in delight to witness the enthusiasm and innovations of ordinary men, sick to death of their disease and loving it every time someone utters the phrase:

"I wonder if that would work for me?"

I'm convinced that the chronic element of Culpepper's Saturn assessment is correct, but only partly so. An understanding of Saturnic medicine, when using cannabis, will serve you very well, but I don't intend to elucidate it again. It is very clearly delineated in the spikenard book for all to review. Suffice it to say, it has strong connections to chronic illness and is a warming medicine to the psychological lessons from a very chilly planet.

And yet...

On March 13th, 1781, two hundred years after Culpepper assessed his flatulent rope, William Herschel and his sister, Charlotte, recorded a new planet in the sky. Previously when people had noticed it they had supposed it might be a comet. When status was finally declared to be a planet, rulership of the house of Aquarius was changed. Previously ruled by Saturn, Uranus was made co-ruler. Thus, not all medicines remain true to Saturn's effects. There's more modern aspects of Aquarian rulership available to us.

Psychoactive drugs are usually classified under the nebulous power of Neptune, so perhaps cannabis should fall here, but again, for CBD this doesn't seem to work. Mum (aromatherapist, Jill Bruce, author of the astrological aromatherapy handbook: Garden of Eden) and I had quite a heated debate over this. We pondered whether cannabis should fall under a dual rulership of Uranus and Neptune. After deep, deep, deep reflection I have placed the generic cultivars, *Cannabis sativa/indica/ruderalis* under joint triple rulership of Uranus, Saturn, and Neptune.

One of the main concerns I had writing this book was a fervent belief that if the chemical structure of a plant is changed, then so is the essence of the plant and, therefore, so is the essential oil. It never even occurred to me I had yet to form an opinion about CO_2's!

My initial concerns about Culpepper's plant being different to the one I was using were further complicated by the fact he was using industrial hemp, where I was working with THC-less marijuana. Was it the same plant if neither of us needed to be worried about THC? Or, perhaps the gap wasn't as wide as I envisaged it to be.

Here's my quandary.

While Saturn's medicine is about constriction, Uranus's medicine is about breaking free. Saturn is about the existing status quo, where order and form is crystallised. Uranus is about transformation into something different. Saturn is to do with warming the bones, strengthening the teeth, enabling the mind to sustain through long protracted illnesses, and it slows chronic decline. So yes, in some ways, it does speak of cannabis.

But if CBD oil were placed under Uranus, it would speak of the genius of the people, creating a revolution against the establishment. It would speak of the radical thinking of brilliant minds who looked at something they loved, but saw its limitations. It would speak of time spent alone, scratching their heads about how they could improve. Uranus bears testimony to the inventiveness of breeding a plant high in CBD.

Placing it under Uranus would bear quiet witness to a medicine gently holding the disassociated and the withdrawn. It would celebrate the uniqueness of those who feel isolated, alienated, or just who are *different* in some way. Most of all, it speaks of a medicine aligned to electricity running through the network of receptors of the mind and the depolarised cells of the physical body.

There is very little written about the medical astrology of Uranus, but luckily for me, what *is* written, is brilliant in its intensity. This illustrates another dimension of Uranus energy, which pours out of every piece of writing I have found about cannabis; genius. When I began the process, I came into the cannabis research with same mindset as I has with my other books, especially those on the single notes. I'd held a certainty, that anything I read would be overly hyped and needed to be checked back to source. In short, the chances were anything I found would be crap!

After a while, in any research project, you start to recognise sources you can trust, those who may have a nugget of truth but polished it to make it shine, and those whose assertions are simply laughable. I haven't always got it right, but I have developed a fairly reliable ABCD (aromatherapy bullshit and crap detector!).

With essential oils data, this is always the case, and *of course* it exists in cannabis medicine too, but to a much smaller degree. Google's algorithm is extremely canny when it comes to cannabis searches, and it tends to weed out the trouble makers. What's more, check out the comments sections and it is policed intensely by other cannabis activists who will undoubted comb my book meticulously too. Make a mistake, they come down on you like a ton of bricks. The power is, most definitely, with the people.

But there is more, because for the main part, people writing about cannabis are talented researchers through and through. This need for individualism from conservative medicine may have made them into rebels, but every one of them most certainly *does* have a cause, and they take it extremely seriously. Detail in their work is meticulous and all of it deliciously lyrical to read. Genius runs through the syntax of pretty much every piece of research I have read. History has been carefully, respectfully, and lovingly elucidated and the science is gloriously exciting to read. It has been a breath of fresh air, after years of reading essential oil spin. The hardest part was the duo of Seshat and Uranus whispering in my ear, urging me of the importance of accurate details, but just as important is that the work is your own. Where, they demanded, was the creative element that made it my own? Dig deeper for innovative genius, to create a legacy belonging to you and you alone.

Not much pressure then?!

It's felt like a very difficult line to tread.

My love for Saturnic medicine goes *way* back. Funnily enough, I'd been hoping to find an oil under Neptune rulership for a long time. I was eager to learn its medicine better.

When I started to try to match cannabis to mum's suggestion of Neptune, I was excited, but the yen very swiftly deserted me. Neptune is *diff-i-cult!*

It is nebulous and sifting and you never seem to grasp it in your hands. It speaks to an understanding of the collective unconscious, to a greater understanding of music and the arts, and a potent elixir that brings dreams. In fact, I think mum's right. It speaks to marijuana.

Of all planetary medicines, any falling under Uranus must surely be the most transformative. The planet was discovered as Britain choked on the smog of the Industrial Revolution and coincided with the influences of the romanticism movement. So it takes on the cultural references of the period of the Revolution, challenging the status quo, but also freedom of expression and most of all, individuality. It questions authority and traditional ways of doing. On the corporeal level, we imagine explosive problems; ones that cramp, cause spasm or seizure, and of course, affect the electrical circuitry of the system.

It is a breakthrough planet, both in the microcosm and the macrocosm, expressing awareness and perception of the self and how one relates to others on the mental plane, but also in a wider societal context. Its medicine forces individuals into a new awareness of how to relate on both social levels but in particular as part of the group dynamic. Uranus *rules* groups and especially societies and clubs with any kind of humanitarian or progressive ideals. Uranus loves democracy and always demands power to the people.

It's a strange contradiction, isn't it? How can a planet rule individuality and isolation but also be associated with the collective? Part of understanding that is to recognise that rather than being an explicit definition, the story of the archetype is a thread, an evolving theme. It explains the natural order of life.

One can see the process as five distinct stages. The first, where the newcomer has found a new reason to be interested. In our case, perhaps it is a new diagnosis or physical decline in health. To educate themselves and to feel more secure about the future, they venture out to find support (Saturn, you note. They need to find stability and be reassured). For a while they find the group very beneficial and glean huge amounts of reassurance from it. As part of the agreement with them, they abide by its rules and expectations. Uranus demands the collective agree to minimum standards and its members concur: minimum standards are good and we can be assured of quality of service when we are here. Life trundles on well, until, after a while, certain things begin to niggle. There will be the odd irritation here, a snarky remark there, and pretty soon, Uranian influence feels like the group no longer serves. The member feels they have outgrown it and can see its flaws. He becomes critical until eventually he thinks this is a waste of time. These guys are holding me back and he wanders off into the wilderness, leaving the others behind.

Eventually, he thinks, the *others* were the problem. I reckon I could do it better. And he starts to think of ways he could do something better himself. He designs, he engineers, and eventually he comes up with a solution. So then he needs to test it. Well, don't get me wrong, not all ideas are fantastic and work, but if it does, then a Uranian development is remarkable. Then, we see another Uranian paradox because Uranus rules equality, but here the opposite is true. A hierarchy has formed as the Uranian left the group, feeling the other members were primitive. Thus, he set himself apart. Then, when he created his magical mastermind, he has all the reason in the world to consider himself superior, because he has proved to everyone that he *is*. But to survive in his ivory tower he can go one of two ways. He can separate himself off even more, becoming terrified of how people might look to level the playing field, or he can bend to Uranian will.

Uranus is always about progress. It's about looking to the future, raising the bar so life can be better for the next generation. If our pioneer can take his discovery to the masses, everyone benefits. This truly is the story of Rick Simpson oil and then CBD. I can almost see Uranus peering over Simpson's shoulder, into his cauldron whispering *"Go on my son, let's prove those doctors wrong..."*

What's interesting is we're not created equal, are we? We are all born in different times in different places. We are brought up with different social conditionings and values. If there were no time and space, then yes, we would be equal, and *that* is Neptunian medicine. What does marijuana teach us? In a place where time and space have no dominion, then we are one. Here though, in this reality, we are limited by the constraints of the Saturnian disease and, can only be liberated by Uranian CBD.

More than anything, Uranus represents the unexpected, unusual, or drastic. You can feel a Uranian transit coming in your horoscope as Saturn/Capricorn limits you and you have this hideous sense of being trapped. You feel whichever way you turn, there is no way out. It's not just frustrating, it feels soul destroying, but then somehow, you break through. Fascinatingly, cannabis medicine seems to be choice taken at the end of your tether. It's "last chance saloon", when nothing else seems to make a difference. CBD is often a desperate measure, bringing about drastic change.

Uranus had initially felt right to me, because the planet rules revolution and anarchy, both of which seemed most appropriate for the oil. The moment I picked up a copy of Jeffery Wolf Green's book *Uranus – Freedom from The Known*, I knew I had struck gold. As I went down the list of part brain and body parts influenced by Uranus, I felt CBD's magic crackling in my hands.

Anatomical correlations
The brain in general with specific co-rulers:

- Hindbrain or primary brain in co-rulership with Pluto, Mars, and the moon
- Midbrain: with the moon
- Inner brain: with Venus and Neptune

- Left hemisphere also ruled by mercury
- Right hemisphere with Jupiter
- Cortex, in addition to Saturn
- Frontal light lobes and parietal lobes co-ruled with Venus and Neptune
- Occipital lobe with the moon
- Temporal lobe with mercury
- Brainstem with Pluto and Neptune

Within the brain:

- Medulla
- Limbic system with Neptune, moon, and Pluto is general co-rulers
- Amygdala with the moon, Pluto, and Mercury
- Cingulate gyrus with the moon
- Fornix with Saturn
- Para-hippocampal gyrus with Saturn
- Hypothalamus with the moon
- Thalamus with Neptune
- Hippocampus
- Basal ganglia with Jupiter
- Synapses
- Neurons
- Axons
- Sacs
- Receptors with Venus and Neptune
- Sheath that can have myelin within it, that is then co-ruled with Saturn
- Neurotransmitters with Mercury and Neptune in general with specific correlations like acetylcholine, which is then co-ruled with Mars, GABA co-ruled with Saturn, and serotonin co-ruled with Saturn and the moon

Physiological correlations - Uranus

The types of neurotransmitters also correlate with specific physiological substances:

- Dopamine
- Serotonin
- GABA
- Acetylcholine

Additional anatomical correlations - Uranus

Entire central nervous system with co-ruler Mercury

- Sympathetic and parasympathetic systems co-rulers the moon and Mercury
- Sheathing on various nerves throughout the body co-ruled with Saturn
- Lungs and bronchial tubes

- Trachea co-ruled with Saturn
- Structure of the nose co-ruled with Saturn and Venus
- *"With the co-ruler Mercury, it correlates with the very nature of thought: thinking. As a result, it correlates with the messaging taking place within the entre physical body that is ultimately traceable to the various areas within the brain itself."*
- *"Uranus also correlates with what are called Free Radicals, strokes, dehydration, stress and tension, and the full spectrum of neurological disorders. It correlates to the physical action of bursting when an existing restriction within the body has reached an extreme that then triggers this bursting action."*

In her *Dictionary of Medical Astrology*, Diane L. Cramer builds on this and moulds her attributions around the idea of limitation and then explosive break free from it.

- Abnormality
- Abortion (spontaneous with the moon)
- Accident-prone/Dyspraxia/Clumsiness – Mars/Uranus
- ADD – Sun Moon relationship with Uranus
- Agitation
- AIDS (Ruled by Neptune but in cases of survival the emphasis is Uranus)
- Alzheimer's
- Cardiac arrhythmia
- Cerebral palsy
- Contortion
- Contraction
- Contrariness
- Convulsions
- Cramps
- Crohn's disease (8th House Mars and Uranus)
- Crippling disease
- Cruelty
- CT scan
- Electrical accidents
- Electrical procedures
- Electrical therapies (Saturn, Neptune, Uranus)
- Electrolytes
- Electromagnetism
- Emotional illness (moon Saturn/moon Uranus)
- Emotionalism
- Emotional shock
- Endocrine disorders
- Epilepsy
- Healing powers
- Hearing aids
- Heart block (Saturn/Uranus)
- Heart disease
- Heart block (Saturn/Uranus)
- Heart failure
- Heart palpitations
- Heart valves
- Muscle spasm
- Multiple sclerosis
- Organ regeneration
- Parkinson's

- Prostate disease
- Scar tissue
- Schizophrenia
- Skin sensitivity
- Sexually transmitted disease
- Spasmodic actions and spasm
- Spastic colon
- Speech defects
- Spinal problems (Mars/Uranus & Uranus/Neptune)
- Squinting (Mercury in stressful alignment to either Mars or Uranus)
- Stammer (Mercury/Uranus)
- Stillborn (Uranus/Neptune)

The nervous system, per se, falls under the rulership of Mercury. Uranus, rather than holding dominion over a specific bodily system, rules kinetic process (think of the machines tirelessly bringing coal to the surface of the mine - it chugs on and on and on!). So, where Mercury sends the messages from synapse to synapse, Uranus controls the processes, making it *automatic*. Likewise, keeping digestion churning and the old ticker ticking…

The planet's orbit totals 84 years; by the time someone experiences a return, they have already lived a long and eventful life. Half way through its cycle, it will come into opposition and, of course, you will feel its subtler energies throughout your life. Transiting slowly, it stays in a sign for seven years, so it has a long slow effect on the psyche. Its influence in each sign will probably last about a year, with two or three moments in that time where crises of consciousness feel very difficult as you wobble beneath its stare.

Understanding Uranus Medicine in the Birth Chart

The strongest effect of Uranus is felt around the age of 42, the beginnings of the midlife crisis. The maturation lessons have been learned and assimilated during the long and arduous Saturn return at the age of 29.

Years later, Uranus peeks through the clouds and mocks how old and predicable you have become. If you look back at ancient mythology, you'll find Saturn and Uranus always fighting. They despise each other's faults. Accordingly, Uranus waits until Saturn has completely crystallised the form of your life, and then comes in and says:

"Too late, old guy, time has moved on. This no longer serves our purpose, it's time to strip out the psyche and create something new."

It wants to know:

"How did you allow things to get to this? This is so far from your path. Don't you remember …" it disrupts *"actually, what you always wanted to do was…"*

"Why did you let that fall by the wayside? What have you achieved?"

How does this compare to the broad outline the soul had in mind when it incarnated? If the path of the physical and mental bodies is outside of the plan, the soul seems to use Uranus as a hired gun to smack you right back where it wants you to be. In other words, when the universe seems to be kicking your ass, I'd suggest seeing were Uranus was when the strange twists and turns seemed to start.

Augmenting the mischievous mental sprite, often its arrival coincides with kids leaving home to go to uni, and sadly with divorce. Suddenly, the ground seems to fall away and we see the patient spiralling into depression and anxiety screaming the familiar mantra...

"Who the hell am I?"

We've all been there. I'm sure you can pinpoint yours where you suddenly feel the overwhelming certainty that something is missing. Unrealised dreams from the past suddenly hold a huge amount of importance and there is a deep yearning for change. This need for transformation manifests itself as restless energy and we can see how thought processes might become disturbed; for disturbance is what Uranus prides itself upon. Visualise its Tarot counterpart and you will see the lightning bolt shattering the tower, destroying the structures of the ego, our reality structures and dependencies on our familiar attachments. Cannabis medicine throws a life belt when everything else has been swallowed by an earthquake of uncertainty and panic.

Remember Uranus rules the house of Aquarius and thus perception of one's own interaction with others; but it also co-rules Capricorn too. One step further along body-mind awareness is Capricorn's objective understanding of just how far you've come.

Might these be the astrological creators of mind body disease? One can only wonder at the impact of dissatisfaction and frustration on the carnal viscera of our lives. Many body-mind practitioners will tell you, Chronic Fatigue Syndrome especially, is usually conjoined with a loss of purpose and direction, and an underpinning loss of spirit. In her book *When the Body Speaks the Mind*, Deb Shapiro explains: *"It's as if the desire to participate and enter into life has drained away, leaving you without intention or motivation."* If Ethan Russo always had this correct, and CFS, fibromyalgia, and migraines all come from an endocannabinoid deficiency, a dose of Uranian medicine might be just what the body needs, after all, Uranus's favourite mantra is: *"There is no greater loss than a life not lived."*

So, these afflictions, that rob us of our wellbeing, seem to indeed come like lightning bolts from the blue, but actually with Uranus there is always a trend of clues being missed. They were there but Saturn has drawn the curtains to shield you from the view and its only in hindsight you can see where the strange signposts might have been giving you hints. In retrospect, it is easy to kick yourself for things you have ignored.

In times of revolution there are always three separate groups in any society. There are those fervently against the status quo and vying for change. There are those conservatives appalled by the crass stance being taken against how things have always been, and then the third group is apathetic and cannot be galvanised into change. It takes energy of a gargantuan size to move the cycle of nonchalance around to change, but it can be done.

Could a planet, four times the size of Earth and the coldest in space, change their outlook?

I'm not sure.

But I bet cancer, epilepsy, or autism could.

Those would be sure things to move you from zero interest in plant healing whatsoever, to becoming an expert on the mechanics of high CBD hemp.

In the context of this book, I contemplate the element of the slowness of Uranian progression through the astrological chart, affecting change through entire generations at a time. This seems entirely poignant, as our generation feels so uneasy about replacing twentieth century marijuana *conditioning* with twenty-*first* century medical *evidence*. I feel sure younger generations will accept it far more readily than us. Will they be like our seven-year-olds, blasting their way around the Internet while the rest of us need to Google *"what the hell's a browser?"* Might Dex's peers develop second nature of mind body integration, monitoring effects of diet and lifestyle on the endocannabinoid system, in the same way as our generation polices E-numbers?

I wonder. It would be nice to think it *could* be true!

Speaking of children, another dimension of Uranus is contrariness, and it made me giggle to discover the very best way to get a child with a predominating Uranus to do something, is to tell them to do the exact opposite, and that certainly seems to match with the fight for the emancipation of CBD here in England. I am not sure people were that excited about it until restrictions on it were applied!

Interpretation about Uranus relies on the understanding that it is the higher octave of Mercury. Mercury rules thinking and thought processes, but Uranus takes that one step further. It rules ingenuity, and new and conventional ideas. Discoveries and individuality. For me, Karen Charboneau-Harrison described it gloriously: where Mercury is the maths professor, Uranus is Einstein intuitively making sense of the universe. And likewise, where we have marijuana ruled by

Neptune and its irrational intuitive function, CBD also works in the same way as rational Mercury but with a bit more intuition. Where Neptune rules dreams, Uranus is a vision made incarnate. It is that strong **a-ha** moment, and it is the corresponding energy as the house of Aquarius…it no longer thinks or imagines…Uranus *knows*.

There's that awkward line again.

What is inspired genius and what is the rantings of a mad man?

How does one discern the ramblings of the inner voice from the proclamations of schizophrenia, and how often have the two been confused?

You know, Uranus irritates the pants off Saturn; he is a threat to the neat and orderly life of Cronus. Ipso facto, Saturn always seeks to quash Uranian energy, he tries to regain law and order. Internally, Saturn forces are always going to be hostile to Uranus's desire for change, and the more it tries to impose restriction, the more violent the Uranian outbursts are likely to be. It's very difficult stuff, and yet Uranian energy is so important. Personally, it allows us to re-invent ourselves but on a social and political level it garners change. It heralds new dawns. It breaks down walls and it demands that things transform.

But remember the rule of three. You have those revolutionaries pushing us forward, but there are those who like the Saturnian world just the way it is. It's worked for them this long, so why in heaven's name does it need to change? And just as internally, the logical mind demands the intuitive keeps its messy ideas to itself, so society will now ostracise the Uranian baby…again. Even if you do find Uranian propulsion is enough to ignite some kind of change, you can expect Saturn's retribution from the wider society as a backlash to a road less trod.

Activists are set apart, made to feel different, and who knows, in the silence of isolation, perhaps they might resolve the theory of everything, find a way to make a mute child speak or even find a cure for cancer. Ironically of course, if there is a Uranian transit (or worse opposition) happening to someone with a strong Uranus aspect in their chart, all they will crave in these times is for Saturn to win the battle and for a little peace and quiet!

Might Uranus be the Shaman? Certainly, it is the awakener and the magician, with radical thinking and just being…well, different. And often, we're talking different, for difference *sake*. If the rest of the world starts to dress like Alice Cooper, Uranian guy dons a shirt and tie!

There's an interesting paradox to this icy planet, because even though Uranian medicine wants to be different, to stand out and alone, it's not because he hates people, but more because he loves them so very much. Uranian medicine yearns to integrate us all like sisters and brothers. Where mercury is able to be more analytical and rational with its rulership of the higher mind, Uranus is the instrument of soul consciousness. At its highest vibration, Uranus allows us to quieten our mind and focus on consciousness of the here and now.

Chapter 11 Cannabis in Aromatherapy

Hemp Seed Oil (Carrier Oil)

We'll start with eating it first - even though that's not aromatherapy - because I experienced quite an event I'd like to share.

You know that feeling you get when people keep talking and your brain say's *"I've got to say something, because they are wrong"*? You know that kid, at the back of the class, who always has to disrupt with *"But Miss..."*?

Yep, I had my hand up all through the Chinese history section and the "Eating the seeds makes you see devils..." passages, because I told you these were probably historical mistakes, because there's no THC in the seeds, and so why would you see devils? Hemp seed is not psychoactive. Scholars, experts, and wise men, all tell us so. And I am sure they are correct. In fact, I am entirely *certain* that they are.

Some small samples have been found that contain THC, but I'm not sure that's where the demons come from. Because I had this dream...

Well, not a dream, a nightmare.

To be truthful people, it was THE nightmare to end all nightmares. I should explain I don't dream that much, or rather I don't remember them, because when I was nine I was so disturbed by nightmares I was having every night I was sent to a child psychologist. She taught me strategies to control them, which I still use today. They are very helpful in a job like mine! So, me and dreams don't really happen.

During March, my mind became extremely pre-occupied by this book, Aimée started at a new university course to become a paramedic, and most of all I was very distracted by Bronze Age day at school. Dex had to dress up as a Bronze Age Celt and I'd asked if I could go along to help out and hear their talk because I know very little about the era of the Scythians. His costume was made and I was very excited.

I dreamt a man came up from the fires of hell to stop me going to Bronze Age day. He'd been set three labours to ensure I didn't get there. The first was he flailed off all his skin. I was running as fast as I could, but he kept coming. Every time I looked back at him he had less and less skin, and more viscera on show, until finally there was nothing at all. He had carefully peeled away everything except a thin strip of white flesh around his eyes and lips.

I was terrified and managed to wake myself up...I wasn't hanging around to find out what the other two labours were. I wanted to go to the toilet to break the dream, but we have a downstairs bathroom in the cottage. I was petrified to leave the room, so I stood for ages, in front of the closed door, in the dark.

I managed to wake the dog with my weirdness, so she made me go downstairs with her unreliable bladder/manners. The flagstone floor in the kitchen is so cold, it's like torture, but I still felt as though the fire was following me and I realised *I* was on fire...not literally, but my temperature was sky high.

I sat on the loo and closed my eyes. He was still there, vivid...scary as hell. I made myself a cup of tea and ate a brioche to see if it was hunger or thirst that was the cause. But he was still there.

And I *couldn't* escape him.

I went back upstairs, shoved Darrell over and clung to him in bed, and told him I was running from a nightmare...running...*that's* how vivid it was. For three days, the image would not leave me. It did not dissipate. It was behind my eyelids the whole time.

So luckily, mum had been staying the night and so I am able to tell you it was Friday night/Saturday morning because I can remember telling her about the weird dream, still very afraid of it. This is useful, because I can verify exactly what I did the next day too.

In the afternoon, I took Dex to his drama class and mum and I went for afternoon tea at Ludlow Castle. We spoke at length about the headache I had been complaining about since the previous afternoon. We wondered if it might have been the cream in the mushroom stroganoff I'd eaten the day before. I discussed how I felt that I now seemed to be going through the menopause. I was having hot flushes, so fierce I had been stripping clothes off in all manner of unusual places. I was like a furnace and they had come on, out of nowhere. My nan went through the menopause at 40 and I am physically like her in every way, so it is kind of a family expectation that it might happen to me. Consequently, we didn't really question how weird it was.

Skip forward to Sunday afternoon. Mom's gone home and I am editing and revising...and bored. So, I decide to get some of the Medieval research done to get a good start on Monday. Easiest, is always to start with Galen...

And there it was *"[Cannabis seed] heatens efficiently because of its characteristic that it heats the head, if it is ingested in too much quantity in a short time, and sends hot in meantime pharmaceutical fumes to it."*

What had I done on Friday morning? I had been experimenting with making hemp milk from the seeds and drunk two smoothies made with it.

He also writes *"In the same way agno castus seed and the cannabis seed are not only pharmacological but painful to the head."*

There is *almost* certainly no psychoactive component in your hemp seeds but I don't think THC was the problem, I think the furnace of *heat* detonated the nightmare.

Either way, I promise you people...

I saw...and still can see, as I write...a demon.

And it was **_not_** good.

Topical Use

So that's eating the seeds, but that's not aromatherapy, so what are hemp seed oil's properties when used topically? Its main mechanism is drying and heating, clearly, and it makes it a superlative oil for mopping up suppurated or weeping wounds, especially for eczema.

I was amazed by how fast it healed my winter legs. I love woolly tights but my eczema really doesn't, and whilst I can control it well throughout the year, peeling off hosiery at the end of the evening leaves me itching, scratching, and irritated. A simple treatment of the carrier oil, with no essential oils added, left the skin soft, moisturised, and calm by the next morning. The cracked and dry skin, which normally requires tons of calendula oil, looked cared for and presentable, which is a winter first for me!

In his book, *Carrier Oils for Aromatherapy and Massage* (4th Edition), Len Price cites the uses of hemp seed oil for eczema, but also for psoriasis, and I would concur whole heartedly after having seen a friend smile broadly from ear to ear at its effects. Psoriasis is a strange disease that tends to congregate in geographical areas, and I must say I see very little of it here in the countryside in Ludlow. Perhaps it's the cleaner air, because it contrasts starkly with the state of people's skins, where I used to live, near junction 10 of the M6, one of the busiest motorway intersections in Europe. A friend from Walsall came to visit, covered in thick scales of psoriasis. After using hemp seed ointment for a week, her lesions had lost much of their redness and, she reported, appeared about half their size. Rate of improvement slowed a bit after about a fortnight, but still continued. I'd also suggested taking vitamin B to fuel and cleanse her liver which will have influenced her good results a good deal. Nevertheless, the change in her condition was impressive.

Perhaps we can attribute skin care dimension to the oil's anti-oxidant abilities. These would certainly preserve the skin well. In August 2016, a team from Messina University, Italy, found a certain strain of hemp seed oil called Finola, displaying the same astonishing anti-oxidant potential we've come to expect from other cannabis medicines too. I suspect all strains would demonstrate the same, if tested.

I have experimented with hemp seed a lot, over the last few months, and found it works spectacularly on any condition where moisture is involved; for example, bronchitis and phlegm, runny noses, greasy skin, and so on.

Dioscorides described Romans eating hemp seeds to calm diarrhoea and that medicine still holds true. In fact, consuming too much of it will give you chronic constipation. Believe me, I know, that was another delight of the demonic weekend.

I do suffer for my art you know!

Topical application of the carrier oil is warming and cosseting and you can almost feel the heat of Bedouin campfires that carried cannabis for so long. It chases away chills, but also sadness. It is a gentle and soothing balm. I'll use it as a carrier for spikenard and ginger next time we have a tummy upset here.

I have found hemp seed oil responds to the same rule as all cannabis medicines. It works best in small amounts with other oils. Certainly in cooking, blending with other oils helps to dilute the sensation of sucking the bottom of a lagoon, but blending with other topical carriers radically changes their vibration. As a carrier oil, it seems to work as a synergist, and, just like hemp essential oil, boosts the effects of other oils. In particular, I like to blend hemp seed oil with evening primrose oil, camellia oil and borage oil to further exploit their own inherent fatty acids. What I adore is each seems to exhibit the same benign, laid back, sunny disposition as the hemp medicines do.

CBD Oil

I'm not going to write tons. We've hear enough about this magical elixir. This brief synopsis is taken from a 2009 CBD literature review. It cited CBD as being:

- Anxiolytic
- Anti-psychotic
- Anti-epileptic
- Neuroprotectant
- Vaso-relaxant
- Antispasmodic
- Anti-ischemic
- Anti-cancer
- Anti-emetic
- Anti-bacterial
- Anti-diabetic

- Anti-inflammatory
- Stimulant of bone-growth

You know enough of the medicine now for me to skive off citing the benefits. It will all be repetition now. Let's take some time to think about the essential oil.

Hemp Essential Oil
I think I'm in love.

Not with the fragrance.

It's vile.

That is unless you put her with something else and then she is utterly transformative. Immediately, you get that same *"It's not about me, it's about them"* feeling and she disappears, opening up the nuances of the other oils. If you buy some based on this book, I tell ya, blend it with rose and melissa and you will just drift to heaven; its sublime.

It's a middle note but I have found it tends to drift toward top if you don't have a heavy anchor like vetiver or galbanum weighing her down. There is no point telling you what it blends with, because out of 100-odd mixes, I didn't find her clashing in any. She is completely versatile.

The oil itself does smell like cannabis, but it's somehow cleaner.

It opens with a very strong herbaceous bitterness that softens out to a kind of citrus floral like a grapefruit petitgrain, for example. Perfumers might enjoy adding it to fougère blends and aldehydic chypres. On its own it almost has a green note, but just like everything with cannabis, the second your mind locks onto that, it's gone. She's a blender, without doubt. I can't see her working as a single note.

Physical Medicine
We'd be stupid not to exploit our knowledge of beta-caryophyllenes effects on CB_2, so the long story cut very short, is hemp essential oil is best used to treat ailments derived from CB_2 dysfunction. That covers a huge range.

Inflammation
- Liver disease
- Problems in the gut - IBS, Crohn's, diarrhoea, constipation
- Allergies and atopic reposes like asthma, hay fever. and eczema
- Psoriasis and dermatitis
- Rheumatism, arthritis, osteoporosis

- Diabetes

Symptoms of neurological inflammation
- Schizophrenia, Parkinson's, Huntington's
- Symptoms of autism

Pain
Infection

The medicine would also say cancer and tumours. I'll be using it now alongside CBD for these, even though I have always avoided using oils during cancer treatments before. I think the medicine outweighs any traditional concerns that essential oils might make cells proliferate and grow. My instincts say cannabis is stronger. Whether you choose to use that way can only be your choice and yours alone.

Emotional and Spiritual Medicine
Emotionally, hemp essential oil is like a blanket. She's like the teddy you always took to bed. You can sob and sob and she won't let go and when you've finished crying, the ache has gone. She creates productive tears.

I mentioned before how she seems to whisper, *"I remember"*. That happens in so many ways. Mostly though, she connected me to my past. I miss my dad so much and when I have hemp around me I can hear his words. I know what he'd say if he were sitting here now and that's such a comfort.

In meditation, it's almost as if you are in a TARDIS. You can focus on a moment you want to recall and it's there, clear as day. But you watch it as if there are mirrors reflecting every element at play. It's so easy to see events take a turn when they evolve like this. Why did that argument start? Why won't she forgive me? Why didn't that book sell? I can see answers with laser precision under her light.

Is seeing the future in hemp's remit too? I feel sure for many people it will be, but I chose not to look. A clairvoyant, I suspect, would feel like their abilities were ramped up a hundred-fold on her scent.

Manifestation? In my limited experience, it brought about incredible changes I desired, and a couple that I didn't, potentially because I kept worrying about them. Can we attribute that to hemp? Prove, no. Suspect, yes - I think it has.

What most definitely happens is she filters through consciousness. I sleep and without fail when I wake next morning my head is full of what I asked the night before. It's almost as if she leaves books open on my desk for me to read before I open my eyes. By the time I greet the morning I always know how to create something bigger and better than yesterday. I know where to look for sources and how to do it.

She's quirky and creative. Like I said in her spiritual section, she doesn't like things to be the same. She craves - nay, demands - originality, twisting and turning your ideas to discover how to make them catch light in the most pleasing way. If it's been done before, look out. She's easily bored and she is like a naughty toddler and will find something else to do when she is. Come play with me, and see what's over here, she entices and I promise you, you will, as she leads into cerebral quicksand fascinating you and absorbing every aspect of your being. Anything is easier than doing some work! I can almost see the paint being thrown in Holi as she cries *"make it colourful, make it bold"*. If you're going to work with her, be determined and firm about what you want to create and set some boundaries because cannabis medicine, as she is, she's going to break them down. At least that way, you'll give yourself half a chance.

If an essay needs to be written, she's a brilliant ally to have, but trust me, plan it first. Clearly define your headings and then ask her to help you with each point in turn. Restrict the areas she can show you and how fast she can fly, or you will write and write and realise half the work has absolutely nothing to do with question at hand.

Oh! You noticed that in the book too, did you? Hmm, it took me a long time to learn!

Be aware of the myrcene. It's not the THC that keeps people slobbing about on the couch. It's our pal hanging out in the essential oil. Get off your arse and stretch. Meditate while walking in the trees. Let hemp speak to you out in the air. She sounds different when you've had a shower! Trust me, this oil is so deliciously relaxing, you won't want to move because you've got far too many interesting things to think about.

Get physical and do.

Find some active yang to compliment her cerebral yin.

Create, procreate, bake, shag, dance, sing, spin, orgasm, breathe, sigh, giggle, languidly stretch, dream, write poetry, make music, visualise, manifest, play, eat, heal, reminisce, lose all resistance, forgive, let go.

Make love.

Make happiness.

Make cannabis medicine.

Chapter 12 Resources

Where to buy High CBD Hemp CO2

A few resources to help you make the medicine.

I was first introduced to the medicine by Dr. Pappas when he was with Roxanne Benton at her Aromamatrix stand at the NAHA Conference. She is the retail distributor for Alchemy Products, a cannabis production company for whom he has consulted.

She stocks many CBD products and other aromatherapy goodies here:

https://aromamatrix.com/collections/apothecary

Since Roxanne does not stock CBD syringes, I'm giving you this link. Clearly, I have not tried any of the other US ones and so cannot give recommendations, but…

https://www.buyhempcbdoil.com/shop/plus-cbd-gold-oil-oral-applicators/

UK therapists: I really like the whole plant extract from CBD Brothers.

http://cbdbrothers.com/product-category/whole-plant-extracts/

Create a Carrier

I made some nice carrier by decarboxylating flowers (baking on a 115°C under some foil for forty minutes) and then diffusing into olive oil for six hours in the slow cooker. Most recommendations say use coconut oil because the oil welcomes the cannabinoids better, but I found it difficult working with the solid oil when decanting into ointments. Decarboxylating is important to change the CBDA in the raw flowers to CBD.

Once they are decarboxylated, they can be used in cooking too, so obviously brownies, but I like mine better in pasta sauce and pizza!

I bought my flowers on Amazon. Look for them listed as Hemp Tea.

You'll know by now that cannabinoids cannot come through steam, but they can be stripped if you boil them vigorously. Hence tea, but also bhang if you fancy trying the recipe in the Indian history section. I found it delish.

Recipes

I'll begin with my usual apology to those readers who have come here expecting an overall synopsis of how to use and blend essential oils. It is not here, because it can be found in depth in my free book The Complete Guide to Clinical Aromatherapy and Essential Oils for the Physical Body.

Find it at: https://buildyourownreality.lpages.co/freebook/

I'll send it straight to your inbox.

Please recall that most of the clinical trials say CBD will improve an existing medicine you are taking.

Do not stop taking anti-depressants, anti-psychotics or any other meds, without talking it through with your doctor.

Now, I wanted to do a range of recipes that address presenting symptoms of each case. Genuinely, I think recommendations of oral CBD is a good plan, but of course that is something each therapist should address individually since I cannot see our UK insurances touching it with a barge pole at the moment.

With that in mind, each recipe here touches all bases; it has topical administration of CBD, it has hemp essential oil to stimulate the CB2 receptor if inflammation or infection seems to be involved, and I have used hemp seed oil as a base unless I see a better carrier oil option. Clearly, if you want to use a liquid CBD alternative to the paste I used, that works too. I found one squirt to be equivalent to two drops of the lovely CO_2 select oil Dr. Pappas gave me.

You'll notice that *Helichrysum italicum* turns up a lot. Not that surprising since most of us love it, but something has been playing my mind since about a month into the book. Remember the dreadful trial that went wrong? Well, perhaps they are trying to make a drug which you and I already have in our toolbox?

See if you come to the same hypothesis as me.

- Anandamide is derived from arachidonic acid
- So therefore: arachidonic acid makes anandamide (over simplistic but, in essence, correct)
- FAAH breaks down anandamide

Now, do you remember in the *Helichrysum* book we learned that *Helichrysum* prevented degradation of arachidonic acid? I had no idea how important that would be when I wrote it. Goddess may have been preparing me for this book longer than I thought! But that's what it does.

If *Helichrysum* maintains levels of arachidonic acid, thus also keeping anandamide supplied, might this be how *Helichrysum* alleviates pain? Dunno...but my bottle seems to be going down very quickly since I thought of it.

Acne

We'll start with the amazing power of *Helichrysum*, ideally one from Corsica for the elevated levels of Neryl acetate to protect the complexion from scarring. Likewise, the jasmine protects the skin but has a cooling property, reducing redness and inflammation. Tea tree kills any underlying infection.

I like jojoba and rosehip as carriers for acne. In fact, jojoba is not a lipid but rather an oil, so it absorbs through the skin without clogging the pores. Rosehip seems counter intuitive, since it is a heavy oil, but it seems to work very subtly on the sufferer's psyche. Acne patients often develop a sense of *"Don't look at me"* for obvious reason and their personality turns inwards. Rosehip neutralises that, a little, as the medicine says, *"See me"* and lets their character radiate past the skin. It's a powerful and confidence building medicine in addition, of course, to rosehip's scar-protecting properties. I've just added a smidge of wheatgerm oil to preserve the blend a little and to boost it with some vitamin E.

- 25ml (1fl oz) Aqueous Lotion
- 1 tsp Hemp Seed Carrier Oil – *Cannabis sativa*
- 1 tsp Jojoba Carrier Oil – *Simmondsia chinensis*
- 1 tsp Rosehip Carrier Oil – *Rosa rugosa*
- 5 drops Wheatgerm Oil – *Triticum vulgare*
- One squirt High CBD Hemp Oil – *Cannabis sativa*
- 3 x *Helichrysum* – *Helichrysum italicum*
- 3 x Jasmine Absolute - *Jasmine grandiflorum*
- 1 x Tea Tree – *Melaleuca alternifolia*

Method of Use: Blend together and keep in a 50ml (2oz) dark glass jar. I like to store this in the fridge, not for any reasons of longevity (although they do exist) but the chill of the cream is so refreshing and cooling to hot angry skin.

Use morning and evening after cleansing and toning the skin.

Safety: The rosehip and jasmine make this blend unsuitable for use during pregnancy.

ADD & ADHD

I struggled for some time as to whether I should group these together, since I am aware there is no hyperactivity element with ADD. However, I think in both cases I would use vetiver to bring the concentration into play.

- 25ml (1 fl oz) Hemp Seed Oil – *Cannabis sativa*
- 1 squirt high CBD Hemp Oil – *Cannabis sativa*
- 1 x Neroli – *Citrus aurantium*
- 1 x Hemp Essential Oil - *Cannabis sativa*
- 1 x vetiver – Vetiver *zizanioides*

Method of use: Blend and stroke into the back at bedtime to calm and induce sleep.

Alternatively, mixing the hemp essential oil, neroli and vetiver into an evaporator, or even an aromastick would be great to use during the day.

When I was writing the vetiver book, I had to think about kids and concentration a lot, because a lot of the research pertains to that. I made some pencils soaked in the oils.

Take an unvarnished pencil, then with a cotton bud stroke it along the wood.

These are great for kids at school, because they have the fragrance with them all day. Don't worry if they are pencil nibblers, I am! The lead will do them more harm than the oils and it actually tastes quite nice!

Addiction

To treat the anxiety of withdrawal. Both rose and spikenard have sections about how well the oils have performed in this area in my books. While the effects of essential oils are cumulative, getting stronger the more you use, you might want to change it up now and then, so I've listed a couple of blends. In the first, lemon is refreshing and uplifting, motivating you with a positive outlook for success. In the second, it's a more clinical attack on the neurotransmitters playing games in your head.

- 25ml 1 fl oz Hemp Seed Oil – *Cannabis sativa*
- 1 squirt High CBD Hemp Oil – *Cannabis sativa*
- 1 x Lemon – *Citrus limonum*
- 1 x Rose Otto – *Rosa damascena*
- 1 x Hemp Essential Oil - *Cannabis sativa*
- 1 x Spikenard – *Nardostachys jatamansi*

Method of use: Whack it on as often as you need it.

Again, the oils blended into an aromastick are a great thing to have with you to sniff as craving grips you.

Safety: Do not use the massage oil during pregnancy, but the aromastick would be okay.

Cravings

Blend into an evaporator or use in an aromastick

- 1 x Hemp Essential Oil - *Cannabis sativa*
- 1 x Grapefruit – *Citrus paradisi*
- 1 x Black Pepper – *Piper nigrum*
- 1 x Rose Otto – *Rosa damascena*
- 1 x Spikenard - *Nardostachys jatamansi*

Withdrawal Symptoms

Just as you can have nicotine patches, you can buy aroma patches to put on your arm. You can make them simply by taping gauze to your arm. The black pepper, grapefruit, and lemon might be a bit much in the larger quantities you need to put onto the skin, so this time I've added uplifting bergamot, calming valerian, and marjoram to bring your central nervous system into line.

- 1 tsp Evening Primrose Oil
- 3 x Hemp Essential Oil - *Cannabis sativa*
- 3 x Bergamot – *Citrus bergamia*
- 3 x Marjoram – *Origanum majorana*
- 1 x Valerian – *Valerian officinalis*

Blend and soak the gauze or follow the instructions for your brand of aroma patch. Cover well with cling film, if home-made, to protect your clothes from oil. There are no cut and dried rules saying it has to go on your arm; I hide mine under my frock and attach it to my tum!

Alzheimer's Disease

All of these are written as massage oils, but just using the essential oils in a diffuser or on a cool flannel work just as well for emergency medicine. The sense of smell is a beautiful means of communication for these people who might otherwise be locked away from us. Dementia patients respond very happily to scent.

Agitation

- 25ml 1 fl oz Hemp Seed Oil – *Cannabis sativa*
- 1 squirt High CBD Hemp Oil – *Cannabis sativa*
- 1 x Hemp Essential Oil - *Cannabis sativa*
- 1 x Rose Otto – *Rosa damascena*
- 1 x Clary Sage – *Salvia sclarea*
- 1 x Melissa – *Melissa officinalis*

Method of Use: This is lovely for a hand massage, but it could be shoulders or feet as well. It's just a very gentle treatment that, if used regularly enough, will become a peaceful anchor, conditioning the brain to relax when they perceive the smell.

Contraindications: Both possible contraindications would not apply of the person were old, but if the illness has been cruel enough to steal someone younger, the clary sage and rose would be contraindicated during pregnancy. That scenario is a nightmare I hope you'd never have to contemplate.

Clary sage is a very interesting and helpful oil for the hormones, but since it mimic oestrogen, I'd be careful of using it on anyone you suspect of being peri-menopausal protecting them from further mood imbalance

Aggression

- 25ml 1 fl oz Hemp Seed Oil – *Cannabis sativa*
- 1 squirt High CBD Hemp Oil – *Cannabis sativa*
- 1 x Neroli – *Citrus aurantium*
- 1 x Roman Camomile - *Anthemis nobilis*
- 1 x Valerian – *Valerian officinalis*

Contraindications: None

Anxiety

Likewise, this could be blended as a massage oil, but I am a big believer in surrounding someone with a garden of calm. This room spray is a lovely little spritz that care assistants can use to fragrance the room even if you can't be around. The vodka dilutes the oils so they bled into the refreshing rosewater.

- 25ml 1 fl oz Rosewater

- 1 tsp Vodka
- 1 x Lavender – *Lavandula angustifolia*
- 1 x Myrrh – *Myrrhis communis*
- 2 x Hemp Essential Oil - *Cannabis sativa*

Method of use: Decant into a spray bottle to spritz as and when required.

Appetite Stimulant

- 25ml (1 fl oz) Hemp Seed Oil – *Cannabis sativa*
- 1 squirt High CBD Hemp Oil – *Cannabis sativa*
- 1 x Tarragon - *Artemisia dracunculus*
- 1 x Sweet Orange – *Citrus x sinensis*
- 1 x Violet Leaf Absolute – *Viola odorata*

Method of Use: Daily massage morning and evening, or simple apply onto the wrists to let the oils get into the system and do their work. To my mind, this is probably the most important dimension of the treatment so there is no reason why you can't add a couple of more calming oils (lavender, geranium, neroli, etc.) to make this a master blend that you use as their complete therapy if you are worried about how you are going to fit all these massages in!

Contraindications: None.

Arthritis

I have a jar of this looking forlornly from the shelf to give my hands relief when I have finished typing this book. It seems pointless using it now if I'm not going to rest them! The juniper dissipates the uric acid and since it is diuretic it cleans the toxicity right from the joints. Davana is a new discovery to me this year, thanks to Christine Goans, and has become my go-to oils for aches and pains. I've added tamanu to provide relief to the neuralgic pain that often accompanies sending pain signals to the brain.

- 50ml (2oz) Blank Ointment
- 1 tsp Hemp Seed Oil – *Cannabis sativa*
- 1 tsp Tamanu Carrier Oil- *Calophyllum inophyllum*
- 1 squirt High CBD Hemp Oil – *Cannabis sativa*
- 1 x Hemp Essential Oil - *Cannabis sativa*
- 2 x Lavender - *Lavandula angustifolia*
- 1 x Juniper – *Juniperus communis*
- 2 x Davana – *Artemisia pallens*

Method of use: Massage into the affected part five times a day for the first two weeks, then morning and night.

Safety: Not suitable for patients with kidney disease nor in the first sixteen weeks of pregnancy.

Asthma

When I inhale this blend, I can see Julie Andrews running across the Alps singing *"The hills are alive...!"* It's so fresh and light. Monarda is one of my personal favourite oils for breathing problems, strengthening the system, and relaxing the bronchial tubes. Frankincense opens the airways and slows the breathing but comforts the distressed too, calming the person and easing exacerbation stress. Ravensara calms allergies and reduces underlying infection.

- 50ml Aqueous Lotion
- 25ml 1 fl oz Hemp Seed Oil – *Cannabis sativa*
- 1 squirt High CBD Hemp Oil – *Cannabis sativa*
- 1 x Hemp Essential Oil - *Cannabis sativa*
- 1 x Monarda – *Monarda fistulosa*
- 2 x Frankincense – *Boswellia carterii*
- 2 x Ravensara - *Ravensara aromatica*

Method of use: Rub a fingerful over the chest five times a day for the first fortnight, then twice a day thereafter. If there is a particularly reactive day, use as and when required.

Safety: Do not use in first 16 weeks of pregnancy.

Atherosclerosis

A gently fortifying and cleansing blend, easing pressure on the heart. Very few words for a whole lotta medicine!

- 50ml Aqueous Lotion
- 1 tsp Hemp Seed Oil – *Cannabis sativa*
- 1 squirt High CBD Hemp Oil – *Cannabis sativa*
- 1 x Hemp Essential Oil - *Cannabis sativa*
- 3 x Rose Absolute - *Rosa damascena*
- 3 x Melissa – *Melissa officinalis*
- 3 x *Helichrysum* – *Helichrysum italicum*

Method of use: Spread over the chest three times a day.

Contraindications: Unsuitable for use during pregnancy.

Autism

I've thought a lot about children on the spectrum because of course I have one of my own, albeit at the very mild end. I've tried to help with several dimensions of the illness, but if course these are symptoms which could just as readily apply to any condition. I've use the essential oil because of the strange signalling at CB_2.

Vetiver, as I have said in other sections, is grounding, but it really helps to focus the attention. Geranium, I recall very clearly being used in case histories written by three headmistresses from special needs schools when I was a tutor for the IFA. They regaled many changes in autistic children including the sense of release it brought to one little boy who used to repeatedly smash his head against a wall.

Potentially, I should have a whole other section of recipes for the carers of all the conditions, but the same thing really applies with all, long chronic stress. Geranium in particular is a wonderful balancer, ensuring the carer maintains a sense of me, not only a sense of them, which is the remit of hemp.

I've used citruses to lift and balance the serotonin levels and juice a little happiness. Because of that, please check the dates on bottles. Sensitive skin easily reacts to oxidised monoterpenes in expressed oils.

Aggression

- 25ml 1 fl oz Hemp Seed Oil – *Cannabis sativa*
- 1 squirt High CBD Hemp Oil – *Cannabis sativa*
- 1 x Hemp Essential Oil - *Cannabis sativa*
- 1 x Geranium – *Pelargonium graveolens*
- 1 x Vetiver – *Vetiver zizanioides*
- 1 x Lemon – *Citrus limonum*

Withdrawn

In my video course, I have quite a long lecture about lavender oil and its effects on social anxiety disorder. There was a lovely clinical trial which watched the brain waves on an electroencephalogram after inhalation of lavender oil. Over time, the brain activity moved from the right side of the brain, which is reclusive, to the more open and welcoming left side.

- 1 x Hemp Essential Oil - *Cannabis sativa*
- 3 x Lavender – *Lavandula angustifolia*
- 1 x Patchouli – *Pogostemon cablin*
- 1 x Mandarin - *Citrus reticulata*

Method of use: Burn in an evaporator or add to a smelly stick. These oils would be lovely in a bath, before story time and bed.

Safety: No contraindications.

Frustration

Bath Salts

I find frustration can last for several days, rather than being a here and gone thing, so I keep bath salts at the ready. Magnesium is deliciously calming and really takes the edge off anxiety.

- 100g (4oz) Sea Salt
- 25g (1oz) Epsom salts
- 6 x Hemp Essential Oil - *Cannabis sativa*
- 6 x Holy Basil - *Ocimum sanctum*
- 10 x Ylang Ylang - *Cananga odorata*
- 4 x May Chang – *Litsea cubeba*

Method of Use: Mix the salt and oils and place in a jar. Give them a good shake. There is enough for about eight baths. Throw the salts under a warm tap, then agitate the water for them to dissolve.

Safety: No contraindications of use.

Insomnia

Peace, perfect, perfect peace.

If the no-sleeping-lark has been going on for a while, perhaps add a drop of marjoram to bring the body clock into line. Again, this blend of essential oils would be lush added into sea and Epsom salts for a winding down on a massive scale. Hop is an expensive oil, so if it's not in your box, some lavender would do.

- 10 ml Grapeseed Oil - *Vitus vinifera*
- 1 squirt High CBD Hemp Oil – *Cannabis sativa*
- 1 x Spikenard – *Nardostachys jatamansi*
- 1 x Mandarin – *Citrus reticulata*
- 1 x Hop – *Humulus lupulus*

Method of use: Massage and body work bring their own magic in these situations but, if they won't submit, the soporific fragrance will have them nodding off in no time.

Contraindications: Do not use in the first 16 weeks of pregnancy.

OCD

Obsessive compulsive disorder comes up a lot in my clary sage book because trials show treating men with oestrogen can calm their OCD. Clary sage mimics oestrogen, and since oestrogen is thought to be the neurotransmitter of worry, it's an interesting dynamic. Spikenard asks us to face our deepest fear letting go of our repetitive trait.

If you've not come across yuzu yet, you have a rather nice surprise coming. It's a Japanese citrus performing better in clinical trials for depression than even bergamot is.

I've made a massage oil to absorb through the skin because I wanted to exploit the CBD, but in some ways, I think an aromastick or evaporator would be better without it in the blend. Then, of course, you need to find another way to administer the cannabinoid and so orally might be the best way.

- 25ml (1 oz) Aqueous Lotion
- 1 squirt High CBD Hemp Oil – *Cannabis sativa*
- 1 x Spikenard – *Nardostachys jatamansi*
- 3 x Clary Sage – *Salvia sclarea*
- 1 x Yuzu - *Citrus ichangensis x Citrus reticulata var. austere*

Method of use: Rub a fingerful into the wrist five times a day for the first week and then decide your own level based on urges and anxiety. There is no way you can overdose. The body will just rid excess through waste.

Safety: Not suitable for use during pregnancy. Clary sage does not work with alcohol so beware that you do not drink for twelve hours after use. Also, if you think you may be perimenopausal you might find the clary sage makes your hormones become even more odd, in which case omit this oil and use lavender instead. The lavender substitution would work for pregnancy too, after 16 weeks.

Chronic Cystitis

I've ramped up the hemp essential oil here to really get the immune system kicking in. The others are just urinary and soothing really. Make the massage oil, but use the essential oils in a sitz bath too, to really soothe the burning.

- 10ml (2 tsp) Tamanu - *Calophyllum inophyllum*
- 10ml (2 tsp) Hemp seed oil – *Cannabis sativa*
- 5 ml (1 tsp) St John's Wort - *Hypericum perforatum*
- 1 squirt High CBD Hemp Oil – *Cannabis sativa*
- 6 x Hemp Essential Oil - *Cannabis sativa*
- 1 x Bergamot FCF – *Citrus bergaia*

- 2 x Cypress – *Cupressus sempiverens*
- 2 x Spikenard – *Nardostachys jatamansi*

Method of use: Massage morning, noon, and night into lower abdomen and back until four full days have past, after the last symptoms of infection.

Safety: Not suitable during the first 16 weeks of pregnancy. Strictly speaking there are no other contraindications but a couple of things to be mindful of. St John's Wort is wonderful for anything to do with the water works but interacts oddly with a lot of pharmaceutical drugs. Check any you are taking against interactions with it first. Also, I've used bergamot FCF, to ensure no photosensitivity, but if you have standard oil be careful of sunlight for 12 hours after use.

COPD

If this is you, I suggest cross-referencing with two of my books. *The Aromatherapy Bronchitis Treatment*, which is entirely about COPD, and my *Monarda* book focuses a lot on lung medicine. I discovered monarda when I was searching for an oil rich in both thymol and geraniol, after uncovering a nugget of research saying these constituents healed lung scarring. What ensued was a love affair, and my garden is full of the plant that I use to make tea when my lungs are not doing too well. After having a blood clot in the left one in 2008, I can become compromised in the winter with coughs and colds and monarda chases the bugs away. Frankincense slows the breathing and opens the airways.

I've added a little melissa, because she's a stalwart anti-allergenic. As we push TH1 disease over to TH2, it's important we don't undo the good work if an allergic reaction occurs.

This recipe is enough to make you a 2-ounce cream to use morning, noon, and night for about two months.

- 25ml 1fl oz Aqueous Lotion
- 5ml (1 tsp) Hemp Seed Oil – *Cannabis sativa*
- 5ml (1tsp) Borage Oil – *Borago officinalis*
- 5ml (1tsp) Sea Buckthorn
- 1 squirt High CBD Hemp Oil – *Cannabis sativa*
- 1 x Hemp Essential Oil - *Cannabis sativa*
- 3 x Monarda – *Monarda fistulosa*
- 1 x Frankincense – *Boswellia carterii*
- *1 x* Lemon Balm - *Melissa officinalis*

Method of use: Blend together in a dark glass pot. Use morning, noon, and night over the chest, neck, and upper back, if you can reach there. If not, even rubbing into the inside of your wrists, where you can see the blue veins, will give you good enough access to the blood supply to make a good difference.

Diabetes

- 10ml (2 tsp) Hemp Seed Oil – *Cannabis sativa*
- 10ml (2 tsp) Rosehip Oil – *Rosa rugosa*
- 5ml (1 tsp) *Centella - Centella asiatica*
- 1 squirt High CBD Hemp Oil – *Cannabis sativa*
- 1 x Hemp Essential Oil - *Cannabis sativa*
- 1 x Holy Basil – *Ocimum sanctam*
- 2 x Rose Otto – *Rosa damascena*

There is a great deal of research about diabetes in my Holy Basil book, not least the bunnies who had diabetes retinopathy who gained their sight after eating the herb. Incidentally, you might find it interesting to know that The Strong Silent One, my husband, has reversed his type two diabetes by giving up carbohydrates. He lost 10% of his body weight in a period of three months and got his blood glucose levels right down.

One of the reasons rose is one of my go-to oils here is, during times of stress, cortisol increases the fat cells around the waist line by four-fold. Rose reduces cortisol levels. Again, this is in the rose book.

Centella performs very well in anti-anxiety trials, also helping the cortisol issue, but also increases elasticity in the skin, guarding against the flabby belly as your improved diet gets the weight off.

Method of use: Blend and massage into the abdomen daily.

Safety: Do not use in pregnancy.

Depression

Use this in as many permutations as you can. In the bath, as a massage oil, in an aromapendant, on the pillow, and take your CBD orally.

- 5ml (1 tsp) Hemp Seed Oil – *Cannabis sativa*
- 10ml (2 tsp) Apricot Kernel - *Prunus Armeniaca*
- 10ml (2 tsp) Camellia Carrier Oil – *Camellia sinensis*
- 1 Squirt High CBD Hemp Oil – *Cannabis sativa*
- 1 x Hemp Essential Oil - *Cannabis sativa*
- 2 x Rose Absolute – *Rosa damascena*
- 1 x Geranium Egypt – *Pelargonium graveolens*
- 2 x Yuzu - *Citrus ichangensis x Citrus reticulata var. austere*

Method of Use: *As many ways as you can in as many different ways! Surround yourself with a garden.*

Cancer care

Until now I have always said do not use essential oils during cancer, but if you are taking the CBD oil, use it topically too. That said, I still feel your biggest benefits are going to be using the oils to affect the emotions, inspiring positivity, and ensuring the serotonin works hardest to kick cancer cells into touch.

Nausea Inhaler Stick

- 1 x Mandarin
- 1 x Spearmint
- 1 x Ginger

Anxiety Inhaler Stick

- 1 x Rose
- 1 x Yarrow
- 1 x Myrrh

Cancer Skin Care

Whilst boswellic acid does not cross through distillation to bring its cancer-fighting properties to this blend, its magic comes from its comforting aspect and how it nourishes the skin. The cream is light and indulgent, making the patient feel pampered and calm. It is a big mix, to use the smallest dose of essential oils during chemotherapy.

Ensure you read the preparation instructions first. Because it is an oil and water mix, its success is going to depend on the order you add ingredients.

- 125g (5fl oz) Aqueous Lotion
- 125g (5fl oz) Shea Butter
- 1tbs Hemp Seed Oil
- 1 squirt High CBD Hemp Oil
- 6 tbsp. Rosewater
- 2 x Rose Absolute
- 1 x Frankincense
- 3 x Hemp Essential Oil

Directions: Prepare your aqueous first, stirring in the rosewater.

Now do your carrier oils, blending your CBD into the hempseed oil. Blend these into the shea butter, mixing well. Add the aqueous mix to the shea. Finally, add your essential oils. Gorgeous!

Methods of Use: Use morning and night.

Safety: For clarity: according to Tisserand use of essential oils is best avoided during the month immediately after chemotherapy treatment. This is a mild blend with far more powerful medicine than the essential oils. I am happy for you to use your discretion when to start and stop. Not suitable for use during pregnancy.

Dermatitis

Whilst I have been writing this book I have been creating an enormous mosaic in the garden to cover a very ugly 5ft across sewage pipe that we have used as a planter. It was one of those jobs that was a good idea at the time, not least because I have to sit on the floor to do it. My hands keep reacting to the concrete. This cream is so soothing and has calmed them down so much. Calendula is my absolute favourite skin care oil, even repairing skin damaged by radiotherapy.

- 50ml (2 fl oz) Blank Ointment
- 1 tsp Hemp Seed Oil – *Cannabis sativa*
- 1 tsp Calendula – *Calendula officinalis*
- 1 tsp Evening Primrose – *Oenothera biennis*
- 1 squirt High CBD Hemp Oil – *Cannabis sativa*
- 1 x Hemp Essential Oil - *Cannabis sativa*
- 1 x Geranium – *Pelargonium graveolens*
- 1 x Myrrh – *Commiphora myrrha*

Method of use: Use five times a day for the first week then morning and night, or as and when needed.

Safety: The myrrh makes this unsuitable for pregnancy at all. If you take out the myrrh, I would be happy for you to use it after 16 weeks gestation.

Diverticulitis, Crohn's, IBS, and Coeliac Disease

In all these conditions there seems to be a signalling issue with CB_2, so we'll use hemp essential oil for many reasons including their relating pain. CBD has a chat with zonulin about letting a few less toxins through the mesh of the gut. Jasmine, marigold (Calendula), and spikenard are well known Ayurvedic anti-inflammatories for these conditions.

- 50ml (2fl oz) Aqueous Lotion
- 1 tsp Hemp Seed Oil – *Cannabis sativa*
- 1 tsp Calendula Carrier Oil - *Calendula officinalis*
- 1 squirt High CBD Hemp Oil – *Cannabis sativa*
- 4 x Hemp Essential Oil - *Cannabis sativa*
- 1 x Neroli – *Citrus aurantium*
- 1 x Jasmine Absolute – *Jasminum officinale*

- 1 x Spikenard – *Nardostachys jatamansi*

Method of Use: Massage onto the lower abdomen and back three times a day.

Contraindications: Not suitable for use in pregnancy.

Dystonia

Here I focused on calming the twitching and tics.

- 25ml (1 fl oz) Hemp Seed Oil – *Cannabis sativa*
- 1 squirt High CBD Hemp Oil – *Cannabis sativa*
- 1 x Hemp Essential Oil - *Cannabis sativa*
- 1 x Neroli – *Citrus aurantium*
- 1 x Valerian – *Valeriana officinalis*
- 1 x Spikenard – *Nardostachys jatamansi*

Method of use: Massage into the body, as often as possible.

Use 3 drops each of neroli, valerian and spikenard in the bath, and also use the oils on an aromapendant or inhaler stick.

Safety: Do not use in first 16 weeks of pregnancy.

Epilepsy

This is a heavy blend, but gloriously effective. The effects of CB_2 on epilepsy remain largely unexplored even though CBD seems to exert beneficial effects there. I've added the essential oil in, just in case!

- 50ml (2fl oz) Aqueous Lotion
- 1 tsp Hemp Seed Oil – *Cannabis sativa*
- 1 squirt High CBD Hemp Oil – *Cannabis sativa*
- 1 x Hemp Essential Oil - *Cannabis sativa*
- 3 x Rose Otto – *Rosa damascena*
- 3 x Vetiver – *Vetiver zizanoides*
- 3 x Spikenard – *Nardostachys jatamansi*

Method of Use: Rub a fingerful into the back of the neck three times a day for very fast access to the brain and to relax the neck and shoulders.

Contraindications: Not suitable for use during pregnancy.

Hashimoto's Disease

Here, cannabis definitely acts as if it were under Saturn's rulership, working with spikenard to sustain the system and to fortify against the long trials of having such a disease. Spikenard also has the benefit of thickening thinning hair and calming joint pain. Boost the thyroid with black spruce. Rose is laxative and eases the ongoing constipation many people experience. It settles the hormonal system and eases depression. Hemp essential oil reduces hyperalgesia.

- 50ml (2 fl oz) Aqueous Lotion
- 1 tsp Rosehip – *Rosa rugosa*
- 1 tsp Camellia – *Camellia sinensis*
- 1 squirt High CBD Hemp Oil- *Cannabis sativa*
- 1 x Black Spruce - *Picea mariana*
- 1 x Hemp Essential Oil- *Cannabis sativa*
- 1 x Spikenard- *Nardostachys jatamansi*
- 1 x Rose Otto – *Rose damascena*

Method of Use: Rub into the chest and throat to activate the throat chakra, three times a day.

Contraindications: Not suitable for use during pregnancy.

Hepatitis

This is interesting because CBD is working here, but *Helichrysum* is the star of the show being able to treat both B and C in test tubes and also proven in human studies. Application is weird because I am going to suggest rubbing it up and down the outside of the right calf. This is the liver meridian, activating points to further boost the healing. All of the oils are hepatic.

- 25ml (1 fl oz) Hemp Seed Oil – *Cannabis sativa*
- 1 squirt High CBD Hemp Oil – *Cannabis sativa*
- 1 x Hemp Essential Oil - *Cannabis sativa*
- 2 x Helichrysum – *Helichrysum italicum*
- 1 x Eucalyptus – *Eucalyptus globulus*
- 2 x Camomile maroc – *Ormenis mutlicaulis*

Method of use: Apply three times a day, rubbing a fingerful up and down the outside of the right calf.

Safety: I doubt this applies, but apply onto the back rather than the leg if it is for a child under the age of six, (please, Goddess, I hope not). Just a precaution of how eucalyptus slows wee one's respiration.

Herpes

This is a weird recipe that defies all dilution standards. Science shows the adrenals being one of the first organs affected during herpes so mandarin supercharges their power to overturn the attack.

- 50ml (2fl oz) Aqueous Lotion
- 1 tsp Hemp Seed Oil – *Cannabis sativa*
- 1 squirt High CBD Hemp Oil – *Cannabis sativa*
- 1 x Hemp Essential Oil - *Cannabis sativa*
- 1 x *Helichrysum – Helichrysum italicum*
- 10 x Mandarin – *Citrus reticulata*

Methods for use: The adrenals are small glands that sit atop the kidneys. We apply this cream over the lower back for past access. Apply three times a day.

Contraindications: Do not use in first 16 weeks of pregnancy.

High Blood Pressure

Blood pressure is executed via CB_1 and CB_2 receptors. To be fair though, this recipe is overkill for the purposes of the recipe. Clary sage and ylang ylang are perfectly capable of doing this job on their own in an aromapendant! If you add CBD too that will be a kickass treatment!

- 1 x Hemp Essential Oil- Cannabis sativa
- 1 x Clary Sage – Salvia sclaria
- 1 x Ylang Ylang – Canaga odorata

Method of use: Use in an aromapendant and wear around the neck for three or four hours. Any longer and the ylang ylang becomes nauseating.

Safety: No contraindications.

Insomnia

This blend could have any number of oils, rose, or violet leaf for their hypnotic qualities for example, or camomile to soothe. But, I like marjoram's gentle effects on the CNS, aligning the body clock for a longer term solution. *Valerian officinalis* would work nearly as well, but I have found *wallichi* something a little bit special for insomnia.

- 25ml (1 fl oz) Hemp Seed Oil – *Cannabis sativa*
- 1 squirt High CBD Hemp Oil – *Cannabis sativa*
- 1 x Hemp Essential Oil - *Cannabis sativa*
- 1 x Spikenard- *Nardostachys jatamansi*
- 1 x Valerian Root– *Valerian wallichii*
- 1 x Marjoram – *Origanum majora*

Method of Use: Massage into the neck and shoulders at tea time, then keep applying periodically up to bed time.

Safety: No contraindications.

Lyme's Disease

There is a lot of success associated with CBD and Lyme's disease for the associated neuropathic pain, but also the underlying bacterial problems. The essential oil of course can improve both of these further. Spikenard treats the muscle pain and mandarin fights the debilitating fatigue. Rosemary is a specific for nerve pain, but it can potentially be neurotoxic. Omit rosemary if there are issues with high BP, epilepsy, or psychosis.

- 50ml (2fl oz) Aqueous Lotion
- 1 squirt High CBD Hemp Oil - *Cannabis sativa*
- 1 tsp Sea Buckthorn - *Hippophae rhamnoides*
- 1 x Rosemary – *Rosmarinus officinalis*
- 1 x Spikenard – *Nardostachys jatamansi*
- 1 x Mandarin – *Citrus reticulata*
- 1 x Hemp Essential Oil – *Cannabis sativa*

Method of Use: Massage into the most painful parts, applying three times a day.

Contraindications: Not suitable for use if the person has epilepsy or is suffering from psychosis.

Headaches and Migraine

As with application in hepatitis, rub up and down the outside of the right calf twice a day. Rub on the back of the neck during an attack, to let the painkilling actions of cinnamon and nutmeg get speedily to the brain.

I would also recommend taking daily doses of Vitamin B complex (one tablet is usually enough) to fuel the liver, as well as one vitamin C tablet daily to help the B absorb. Up the vitamin B to every four hours during an attack.

- 50ml (2fl oz) Aqueous Lotion
- 1 tsp Hemp Seed Oil – *Cannabis sativa*
- 1 squirt High CBD Hemp Oil – *Cannabis sativa*
- 1 x Hemp Essential Oil - *Cannabis sativa*
- 3 x Eucalyptus- *Eucalyptus globulus*
- 1 x Cinnamon - *Cinnamomum verum*
- 1 x Nutmeg - *Myristica fragrans*
- 1 x Rosemary - *Rosmarinus officinalis*

- 1 x Sweet Basil – *Ocimum basilicum*
- 1 x Spikenard - *Nardostachys jatamansi*

Contraindications: Not suitable for children or use during pregnancy

PTSD

It's a long road ahead, but celery promotes the oxytocin required to keep the emotional bonding with one's loved ones intact. Rose is anti-depressant and helps process the memories through the hippocampus. I have added cistus and labdanum to deal with the trauma but it is a big recipe so if you wanted to buy the oils bit by bit, I think buy those two last. It's a very strong mix without them. Think of this as the premium brand!

- 50 ml (2 fl oz) Aqueous Cream
- 1 squirt High CBD Hemp Oil – *Cannabis sativa*
- 1 tsp Grapeseed Oil- *Vitus vinifera*
- 3 x Rose Absolute - *Rosa damascena*
- 1 x Cypress – *Cupressus semperivens*
- 1 x Labdanum – *Cistus Labdanum*
- 1 x Celery Seed- *Apium graveolens*
- 1 x Hemp Essential Oil - *Cannabis sativa*

Method of use: Rub a fingerful into the back of the neck five times a day.

Contraindications: Not suitable for use in pregnancy.

Sarcoidosis

We can move the TH1 infection across to TH2, thus easing the sarcoidosis, but that could exacerbate allergies, so I have added Melissa and ravensara to calm those down. Myrtle and monarda ease the cough. In all cases the hemp essential oil is calming the infection and the pain, reducing swollen lymph glands, easing redness and soreness, and calming that soul-destroying cough.

Again, I'm going to suggest a strange method of application. Straightforwardly, rub into the chest, but also rub into the locations of any scar tissue. This will give the CBD a chance to protect against granuloma.

- 50ml (2fl oz) Aqueous Cream
- 1 squirt High CBD Hemp Oil – *Cannabis sativa*
- 1 tsp Sea Buckthorn Oil
- 1 x Melissa - *Melissa officinalis*
- 1 x Ravensara – *Ravensara aromatica*
- 5 x Hemp Essential Oil - *Cannabis sativa*
- 3 x Myrtle – *Myrtis communis*

- 2 x Monarda – *Monarda fistulosa*

Method of use: See instructions at the beginning of the recipe. Use five times a day for the first week then morning noon and night.

Safety: Not for use in the first 16 weeks of pregnancy.

Pain

Here the essential oil really comes into its own to supercharge the painkilling effects of CBD. Remember, although CBD is effective at the TRPV channels and the GPRs18, 55, and 119, it only shows weak binding affinity to CB_2. Since this is the largest expression of pain, we utilise all resources we have at our disposal. Our secret weapon in the beta caryophyllene is in the essential oil to boost the receptor further.

Fibromyalgia

If you are a fibromyalgia sufferer I'm going to suggest you read my sweet basil book as there is a great deal of research in there into linalool's effects in inflammation in fibro. Spikenard and yarrow are like liquid anaesthetic being stroked into the limbs, thanks to yarrow's azulene.

- 50ml (2 fl oz) Aqueous Lotion
- 1 tsp Hemp Seed Oil – *Cannabis sativa*
- 1 squirt High CBD Hemp Oil – *Cannabis sativa*
- 4 x Hemp Essential Oil - *Cannabis sativa*
- 2 x Sweet Basil (Linalool) – *Ocimum basilicum*
- 1 x Spikenard – *Nardostachys jatamansi*
- 1 x Yarrow – *Achillea millefolium*

Method of Use: Use five times a day on the most painfully affected parts.

Safety: Do not use in the first 16 weeks of pregnancy.

Joint pain

The Helichrysum I'd suggest using here is different from in skin care. I'd recommend you seek out the Croatian Helichrysum instead. I can't give you any science. I just find it more anti-inflammatory. I've added juniper here to flush out any toxins from the joints.

- 50ml (2 fl oz) Aqueous Lotion
- 1 tsp Hemp Seed Oil – *Cannabis sativa*
- 1 squirt High CBD Hemp Oil – *Cannabis sativa*
- 2 x Spikenard – *Nardostachys jatamansi*
- 1 x Helichrysum – *Helichrysum italicum*
- 2 x Roman Camomile - *Anthemis nobilis*

- 1 x Hemp – *Cannabis sativa*

Method of Use: Use five times a day on the most painfully affected parts.

Safety: Do not use in the first 16 weeks of pregnancy.

Muscle Pain

- 25ml (1 fl oz) Aqueous Lotion
- 1 tsp Hemp Seed Oil – *Cannabis sativa*
- 1 squirt High CBD Hemp Oil – *Cannabis sativa*
- 1 x Ravensara – *Ravensara aromatica*
- 1 x Davana - *Artemesia pallens*
- 3 x Geranium – *Pelargonium graveolens*
- 4 x Lavender – *Lavandula angustifolia*
- 4 x Hemp Essential Oil – *Cannabis sativa*

Method of Use: Use five times a day on the most painfully affected parts.

Safety: Do not use in the first 16 weeks of pregnancy.

Nerve Pain

- 25ml (1 fl oz) Aqueous Lotion
- 1 tsp Hemp Seed Oil – *Cannabis sativa*
- 1 squirt High CBD Hemp Oil – *Cannabis sativa*
- 1 x Rosemary – *Rosemarinus officinalis*
- 2 x Yarrow – *Achillea millefolium*
- 1 x Roman Camomile - *Anthemis nobilis*
- 4 x Lavender- *Lavendula angustifolia*
- 6 x Hemp Essential Oil – *Cannabis sativa*

Method of Use: Use five times a day on the most painfully affected parts.

Safety: Do not use in the first 16 weeks of pregnancy.

Muscle Cramps

- 25ml (1 fl oz) Hemp Seed Oil – *Cannabis sativa*
- 1 squirt High CBD Hemp Oil – *Cannabis sativa*
- 1 x Hemp Essential Oil - *Cannabis sativa*
- 1 x Geranium – *Pelargonium graveolens*
- 1 x Roman Camomile – *Anthemis nobilis*
- 1 x Clary Sage – *Salvia sclarea*

Method of Use: Massage into the affected area as and when needed. Safety: Keep away from alcohol for 12 hours after using the clary sage. They really don't mix well and can cause hallucinations.

Leg Weakness

This blend brings the strengthening medicine of *Helichrysum* oil and the grounding medicine of vetiver (both have their own books should you want to understand this more deeply), but vetiver in particular is very good at helping integrate the spirit more readily into the physical body, aligning the two. Frankincense restores elasticity to the tendons and joints.

- 10ml (2 tsp) Borage Carrier Oil - *Borago officinalis*
- 10ml (2 tsp) Hemp Seed Oil – *Cannabis sativa*
- 5 ml (1 tsp) Sea Buckthorn - *Hippophae rhamnoides*
- 1 squirt High CBD Hemp Oil – *Cannabis sativa*
- 1 x Hemp Essential Oil - *Cannabis sativa*
- 1 x Frankincense – *Boswellia carterii*
- 1 x Helichrysum – *Helichrysm italicum*
- 1 x Vetiver – *Vetiver zizanioides*

Method of Use: Massage twice daily into legs.

Safety: Not suitable for before 16 weeks of pregnancy.

Spasticity

I've have no idea why ginger seemed to work, but I kept hearing "fluid." Normally I'd associate that with moisture but I suppose it does apply to movement too.

- 25ml (1 fl oz) Hemp Seed Oil – *Cannabis sativa*
- 1 squirt High CBD Hemp Oil – *Cannabis sativa*
- 1 x Hemp Essential Oil - *Cannabis sativa*
- 1 x Spikenard – *Nardostachys jatamansi*
- 2 x Roman Camomile – *Anthemis nobilis*
- 1 x Ginger – *Zingiber officinale*
- 2 x Clary Sage – *Salvia sclarea*

Meditation blends

When I asked on my Facebook page what recipes people wanted me to include, one lady asked for a meditation blend that won't send you to sleep. I can't do that I'm afraid, but I will remind you of the rule of using cannabis. Use it when you're wide awake or you really will fall asleep!

Remember too, She is waiting excitedly to get you to party. Manage Her well. Specific questions with very small outcomes.

Use in evaporators, or just a bowl of warm water in front of you as you think.

Help Me See My Part in [xxx] So I can forgive.

- 1 x Holy Basil
- 1 x Hemp
- 1 x Jasmine

What's my purpose in life? What are my innate abilities and how can I use them best to serve mankind?

I believe everyone was brought to the planet to do a job. Part of being happy is understanding and delivering that function. I think these essential oils might help you perceive yours, or at least light up clues over the coming days. Watch for reminders, especially of things that come very naturally to you.

- 1 x Monarda – *Monarda fistulosa*
- 1 x Thyme-*Thymus vulgaris*
- 1 x Hemp essential oil – *Cannabis sativa*

What's Causing My Obstacles to Success With…

I can't really explain this blend, it's just the one that works for me!

- Fennel - *Foeniculum vulgare*
- Hemp Essential Oil – *Cannabis sativa*
- Benzoin - *Styrax benzoin*

World Healing

Lofty, I know, but it was part of my deal with Her for teaching me Her song.

I've found using this once a week, rather than asking a question, seems to make Her happier to impart her knowledge. It seems like a happy trade and I feel blessed She feels fit to ask me to repay my dues.

Visualise the globe with everyone holding hands around. Visualise the sun coming through you like a radio transmitter, then focus it toward the globe through you heart chakra.

- Hemp Essential Oil – *Cannabis sativa*
- Sweet Orange – *Citrus x sinensis*
- Aniseed - *Pimpinella anisum*

Before we conclude: You might be interested to see how I felt when I started. It's an interesting contrast. I filmed my doubts about this book back in Dec 16, four weeks into the project.

https://buildyourownreality.lpages.co/in-the-beginning/

Conclusion

It's 4.30am and the moon is twenty minutes away from full as I write these final words of the book. It feels like the universe and I are in tune. Although my hands hurt like crazy, I feel quite bereft to be putting away my oils. I feel like I am waving au revoir to someone I love. It's heartfelt and exquisitely painful, but we have too long been in each other's space. It's time to take a break.

I feel like a different person. Like I've been initiated into an unknown space. I'm aware I can never unknow the strange biological system of which doctors seem reluctant to tell. If I went into my GP's office, I wonder, how much of this science would they even *know*? Is it the stuff of medical practice, or are the drug companies keeping it taboo?

It worries me, I'll confess. When a plant doesn't just heal, but controls the very system required for health, how can it be right to place its future in politician's hands? They have closed maternity wards in my town, that's how much they care! Might prohibition happen again, now we understand the potency of this cure? Let's hope not.

It's very hard to conclude this book, just like it was difficult to start! In some ways, there is so much to say, in others, words just won't cut it. How can you describe the relief as the heart chakra finally relaxes in grief, or perceive its healing effect? What phrases do justice to a peaceful night's slumber after months of terror filling your dreams? How can one convey the loosening of the knot in your stomach as your terminal child gets better? Perhaps that's why scientists never persisted with making endocannabinoid names pronounceable because with cannabis, language simply fails.

There's an existential perspective we haven't even touched on in the book, but just as the glia link hands, so do we with cannabis. A brotherhood of man connected by one plant.

In Jean Paul Satre's novel *Huis Clos*, the story is set in hell, but it resembles the real world we find ourselves in when someone we love is ill. We become tortured by the pain of others. Just as with cannabis, the theme of "the others" is integral to the works of Sartre. Throughout his lifetime essays he contemplates how other people can condemn us, define us, withhold love from us, murder us — in short, take the power away from us to live life as we wish.

But "the others" cannot rob us of our freedom, and this is the central notion in Sartrean existentialism. Funnily enough, Sate has a name for the hideous anguish that engulfs us when confronted with the infinite meaningless of universe. He calls it nausea. Man, exerts Satre, has the power to use his freedom to fight off "nausea." Just as cannabis locks to CB_1 receptors to reduce nausea, I'm challenging you to take up Satre's call. Build cannabis medicine from the inside, be a warrior to drive the medicine forward as a force for good.

Do it gently, proudly, and firmly.

As you sniff your hemp essential oil, remember the old prayer Desiderata. There is much knowledge that applies with this oil.

Go placidly amid the noise and haste, and remember what peace there may be in silence.

As far as possible, without surrender, be on good terms with all persons.

Speak your truth quietly and clearly; and listen to others,

even to the dull and ignorant; they too have their story.

Avoid loud and aggressive persons, they are vexations to the spirit.

If you compare yourself with others, you may become vain and bitter,

for always there will be greater and lesser persons than yourself.

Enjoy your achievements as well as your plans.

Keep interested in your own career, however humble;

it is a real possession in the changing fortunes of time.

Exercise caution in your business affairs, for the world is full of trickery.

But let this not blind you to what virtue there is;

many persons strive for high ideals,

and everywhere life is full of heroism.

Be yourself. Especially do not feign affection. Neither be cynical about love;

for in the face of all aridity and disenchantment it is as perennial as the grass.

Take kindly the counsel of the years, gracefully surrendering the things of youth.

Nurture strength of spirit to shield you in sudden misfortune.

But do not distress yourself with dark imaginings.

Many fears are born of fatigue and loneliness.

Beyond a wholesome discipline, be gentle with yourself.

This has been a long and arduous book. I want to thank you all for being so patient with me, whilst I have taken so long. Thank you for all the messages and interaction on Facebook and email. Thanks especially go Christine Goans, moderator of the Essential oils and herbs Facebook page, who has been such a dear friend to me since the first day I posted up my free book. One lady attacked me quite viscously and immediately sought to derail it by posting a spiteful review on the British site (even though she was American) to be sure I saw it. Christine waded in, protected me, and fought off all comers. It was a kind and generous thing to do. She is a healer without compare when it comes to herbs and I am grateful for all the resources she has sent me whilst I have been writing. Christine also suggested I should write more about different strains of cannabis because clearly, different chemotypes have different strengths. I would have loved to but there simply wasn't enough room in the book. I can, however, recommend you go over to the App Store, and download the Leafly app, which is fantastic for recommending strains.

Tina Jones won't thank me for telling you what she did to make me smile so much, but there is a pot of a very clever sometin' sometin' in my fridge that she concocted in her kitchen, despite great angst about what she was doing. She bravely called me on the phone and inspired me to do the same. It's thanks to Tina you can now make your own cannabis carrier oil. I'd have never have worked it out for myself.

Sandra Shuff and Liz Fulcher rescued me in Utah, at the NAHA conference, from an evening alone in my hotel room and took me around Salt Lake City. I laughed so much that night and met someone with as much love for old books as I have. You two are dear, dear women and I love you both lots. Dr. Robert Pappas, of course, since without his generosity of time that first day, and the oils he gave me, this book wouldn't exist. For the inspiration, Dr. P., I owe you. For the many hours of torturous hard work and sleepless nights, you wanna hope I don't decide to get my own back! Many thanks for all the support.

Clinical trials and snippets came from the most unusual sources. Most interesting was one from Nancy Sherry Baker of the Bard's Apothecary (love her app!) explaining that the status of cannabis has now changed, and medical cannabis is now recognised at kosher at Passover. Even my daughter, who never has any interest in my work, started tagging me in cannabis posts, and one of my husband's colleagues started to send me news posts. Aims and Nick, hopefully you will read this and know how much that meant to me. It's very easy to feel like you are invisible working in a shed. To know that people who know me care enough about what I am doing to make efforts to help, makes all the difference in the world.

My illustrator, Robert Elsmore, has been tested to breaking point with videos and physiology slides. As ever I appreciate your reliable artistry, Rob. Thanks for all you've done. And to Nikki, for editing out seven or eight thousand typos without complaint.

As ever, Mum and Darrell deserve medals. Mum has become adept at keeping her voice level when, every time she asks, *"How's your book coming?"* I really appreciate the lack of a raised eyebrow at the same answer *"nearly there"* over and over again. I didn't really realise how hard things had become until the waning computer lost some work on Uranus and I broke down in tears saying *I don't think I can do this anymore"*. A very large arm belonging to a warm bald man reached round me and said *"I know that. But I know you can."* You were right. I don't think I would have reached the finish line without your words.

A large thank you must surely go to the providers of the site Project CBD. Their relentless researching and care of their database made researching an impossible task bearable...at least some of the time.

But the largest thanks must be to you for buying the book and reading the book this far. It makes me proud that you didn't give up. If you liked the book, please leave a review and tell your friends. It makes all the difference, and I am sad enough to read them all.

So, what next?

Sleep.

No typing for a couple of weeks...

Then we'll see. Yarrow, melissa and violet all seem exciting...

Watch this space.

In the meantime...

CANNABIS TRAINING

As a bit of a bonus, I have added in a little mini course for you. Personally, I find it damn near impossible to put down a book and then translate that into my own needs and situation. It takes me a lot of time and more than a few mistakes.

FREE bonus training
Click:

https://buildyourownreality.lpages.co/start-working-with-cannabis-oils/

The benefit, (apart from seeing inside the Secret Healer's Shed) is it is a little taster course of my Cannabis Healing Courses.

Professional Training

Your Cannabis Life
For talented essential oil amateurs and people who want help integrating CBD and hemp essential oil into their daily lives.

Your Cannabis Practice
For professional therapists who would like to use the cannabis oils in their therapy. Here in the UK, you are only insured to use oils which you have a certificate from training in. I do not know of any training here that covers hemp essential oil here, so this will allow you to use it on your patients. The course also covers CBD, but for obvious reasons, in the UK, still cannot be included into insurances at this time.

Cannabis Future
A mastermind group for professional therapists who would like to create a best practice model for using these oils. I believe it's the therapy of the future and I want to ensure we use it to the best of our potential.

Cannabis Medicine Support
Not everyone wants to study and I get that. If I wanted a pianist at my party, the last thing I would want to do is practice the 10,000 hours it takes to become an expert. I'd just go and find someone who could prove they were up to the job Hopefully this and my other books have proved I am that.

Do you feel you need some extra help?

Because let's be honest, we all need it from time to time, especially if we, or someone we love is sick. In the past, I have offered basic support for free, but as I write more books and gain more readers, it is becoming unfeasible. I've put a system together that hopefully helps me to serve you better.

I offer a full consultancy service from one to one coaching over skype, with full case history, vitamin and essential oil therapies. Bespoke treatment formulae are created and sent to you as they need them. Journals and care plans provided. It's your personal therapist on demand.

Check out my new gig on fiverr that will help you buy with confidence.

https://www.fiverr.com/elizabethstarns/l-will-check-your-essential-oil-blending

Perhaps you don't need the premium package. Maybe you know what oils you want to use but want reassurance you've picked safe ones. Again, I can help. Click the same link.

Finally…

Are you a newcomer to aromatherapy and feel a bit bewildered or excited to learn more? Please feel free to get acquainted with a few basic oils.

The Secret Healer's Introduction to Aromatherapy

93 videos about the fundamentals of aromatherapy and in-depth information on 15 different oils.

(Not cannabis oils, incidentally!)

Find the course at:

https://beta.ofcourse.co.uk/course/aromatherapy-essential-oils-advanced

Normally priced at £199, please use discount code **TEACHER_ELIZA82** to get it for £35 (around $50) as a little thank you for all your support

Other Books by The Secret Healer

Book 1:- The Complete Guide to Clinical Aromatherapy & Essential Oils for the Physical Body (Free to download)

Book 2:- Essential Oils for Mind Body Spirit

Book 3:- The Essential Oil Liver Cleanse

Book 4:- The Professional Stress Solution

Book 5:- The Aromatherapy Eczema Treatment

Book 6:- The Aromatherapy Bronchitis Treatment

Book 7:- 50 Easy Recipes for Dry Skin

Book 8:- 75 Easy Christmas Aromatherapy Recipes

The Secret Healer Oils Profiles

1: Monarda – A Native American Medicine

2: Vetiver – An Ayurvedic Medicine

3: Holy Basil – An Ayurvedic Medicine

4: Rose – Goddess Medicine

5: Sweet Basil – The Oil of Empowerment

6: Clary Sage- Natural Estrogen?

7: Spikenard- A Woman Washes Jesus's Feet. Was It our Oil of Aromatherapy?

8: Helichrysum – For The Wound That Will Not Heal

Business Training for Professional Aromatherapists

Sales Strategies for Gentle Souls

About the Author

Elizabeth Ashley is an international speaker for the International Federation of Aromatherapists and the UK Director for the National Association of Holistic Aromatherapists. She is a prolific writer of professional articles, in particular for the IFA magazine Aromatherapy Thymes, Aromatika.hu, NAHA Journal and Holistic Therapist. She qualified as an aromatherapist in 1993, and then passed her Advanced Aromatherapy Diploma in 1994. She has been practicing aromatherapy for almost 25 years.

In 1999, she fell into a whole new career in the aggressive commercial sector of recruitment consultancy. There she discovered her father's second-hand car salesman genes had passed along and found she had quite the gift of the gab! More than that, she discovered she could sell...and then some.

In 2008, Elizabeth fell ill during pregnancy, with a blood clot in her lungs. The pulmonary embolism prevented her from working and she started to write. Very quickly, she gained her first contract as a ghost writer...a recipe book for cheese cakes!

In 2010, she was published professionally for her work on Galbanum - (*Ferula Galbaniflua*) oil in the Aromatherapy Thymes, journal of the International Federation of Aromatherapists, and on Tuberose (*Polianthes tuberosa*) oil by the New Zealand Register of Holistic Therapist.

In 2011, she was seconded on a consultative basis to Walsall Independent Treatment Centre, designed to be a rainbow bridge between traditional and complementary medicines. There she became aware of the rumblings of change in healthcare. Her book *Sales Strategies for Gentle Souls* explains the connotations of this.

Many of her books are aimed at helping qualified aromatherapists to expand their healing repertoire and build their businesses. She also writes for people who have an interest in essential oils and want to learn how to heal. Her in-depth essential oil profiles chart the healing properties of plants from the most arcane depths of historic folklore up to the scientific lab trials of today.

She lives in Shropshire with her husband and youngest son, kept company by their Staffordshire Bull Terrier, Bella, and many shoals of tropical fish! Her elder son and daughter have graduated from university this year (2017) and make her prouder than anything ever could. Elizabeth Ashley is The Secret Healer.

Disclaimer

by SEQ Legal

(1) Introduction

This disclaimer governs the use of this eBook. By using this eBook, you accept this disclaimer in full. We will ask you to agree to this disclaimer before you can access the eBook.

(2) Credit

This disclaimer was created using an SEQ Legal template.

(3) No advice

The eBook contains information about aromatherapy and the use of essential oils. The information is not advice, and should not be treated as such.

You must not rely on the information in the eBook as an alternative to qualified medical advice from a health professional. If you have any specific questions about any medical matter you should consult an appropriately qualified professional.

If you think you may be suffering from any medical condition you should seek immediate medical attention. You should never delay seeking medical advice, disregard medical advice, or discontinue medical treatment because of information in this eBook.

(4) No representations or warranties

To the maximum extent permitted by applicable law and subject to section 6 below, we exclude all representations, warranties, undertakings, and guarantees relating to the eBook.

Without prejudice to the generality of the foregoing paragraph, we do not represent, warrant, undertake or guarantee:

> that the information in the eBook is correct, accurate, complete, or non-misleading;

> that the use of the guidance in the eBook will lead to any particular outcome or result; or

> in particular, that by using the guidance in the eBook you will heal disease or work in any way as a cure for illness.

(5) Limitations and exclusions of liability

The limitations and exclusions of liability set out in this section and elsewhere in this disclaimer: are subject to section 6 below; and govern all liabilities arising under the disclaimer or in relation to the eBook, including liabilities arising in contract, in tort (including negligence), and for breach of statutory duty.

We will not be liable to you in respect of any losses arising out of any event or events beyond our reasonable control.

We will not be liable to you in respect of any business losses, including without limitation loss of or damage to profits, income, revenue, use, production, anticipated savings, business, contracts, commercial opportunities, or goodwill.

We will not be liable to you in respect of any loss or corruption of any data, database or software.

We will not be liable to you in respect of any special, indirect or consequential loss or damage.

(6) Exceptions

Nothing in this disclaimer shall: limit or exclude our liability for death or personal injury resulting from negligence; limit or exclude our liability for fraud or fraudulent misrepresentation; limit any of our liabilities in any way that is not permitted under applicable law; or exclude any of our liabilities that may not be excluded under applicable law.

(7) Severability

If a section of this disclaimer is determined by any court or other competent authority to be unlawful and/or unenforceable, the other sections of this disclaimer continue in effect.

If any unlawful and/or unenforceable section would be lawful or enforceable if part of it were deleted, that part will be deemed to be deleted, and the rest of the section will continue in effect.

(8) Law and jurisdiction

This disclaimer will be governed by and construed in accordance with English law, and any disputes relating to this disclaimer will be subject to the exclusive jurisdiction of the courts of England and Wales.

(9) Our details

In this disclaimer, "we" means (and "us" and "our" refer to) [*The Secret Healer)*] of [*4, SY8 1LQ)*].

References

Adinolfi B1, R. A. (2013, 10). *Anticancer activity of anandamide in human cutaneous melanoma cells*. Retrieved from Pubmed: https://www.ncbi.nlm.nih.gov/pubmed/24041928

Alapoet, S. E. (2011, 04 11). *Worth Repeating: Cannabis Found In Ancient Shaman's Tomb*. Retrieved from Toke of tThe Town: http://www.tokeofthetown.com/2011/04/worth_repeating_cannabis_found_in_ancient_shamans.php/

Ali A1, A. N. (2015, 07). *The safety and efficacy of 3% Cannabis seeds extract cream for reduction of human cheek skin sebum and erythema content*. Retrieved from Pubmed: https://www.ncbi.nlm.nih.gov/pubmed/26142529

Álvaro-Bartolomé M1, G.-S. J. (09, 2013). *Dysregulation of cannabinoid CB1 receptor and associated signaling networks in brains of cocaine addicts and cocaine-treated rodents*. Retrieved from Pubmed: https://www.ncbi.nlm.nih.gov/pubmed/23727505

Ancient Cannabis Book. (Unlisted). *Cannabis in Ancient Hebrew History*. Retrieved from Ancient Cannabis Book: http://antiquecannabisbook.com/chap2B/Hebrew/Hebrew.htm

Andrei, M. (2015, 05 29). *Archaeologists find 2,400 year old gold bongs used for cannabis and opium*. Retrieved from ZME Science: http://www.zmescience.com/science/archaeology/gold-bongs-scythian-29052015/

Antique Cannabis Book. (Unlisted). *A Short Geographical History - India*. Retrieved from Antique Cannabis Book: http://antiquecannabisbook.com/chap2B/India/India.htm

Antique Cannabis Book. (Unlisted). *Indian Materia Medica*. Retrieved from Antique Cannabis Book: http://antiquecannabisbook.com/chap2B/India/IndianMateraMedica.htm

Appendino G1, G. S. (2008, 08). *Antibacterial cannabinoids from Cannabis sativa: a structure-activity study*. Retrieved from Pubmed: https://www.ncbi.nlm.nih.gov/pubmed/18681481

Arata, L. (2004). Nepenthes and cannabis in ancient Greece. *PhilPapers*.

Ashton CH1, M. P. (2005, 05). *Cannabinoids in bipolar affective disorder: a review and discussion of their therapeutic potential*. Retrieved from Pubmed: https://www.ncbi.nlm.nih.gov/pubmed/15888515

Ashton CH1, M. P. (2011, 08). *Endocannabinoid system dysfunction in mood and related disorders*. Retrieved from Pubmed: https://www.ncbi.nlm.nih.gov/pubmed/21916860

Aso E1, 2. A.-B. (2016, 10). *Delineating the Efficacy of a Cannabis-Based Medicine at Advanced Stages of Dementia in a Murine Model*. Retrieved from Pubmed: https://www.ncbi.nlm.nih.gov/pubmed/27567873

Aso E1, F. I. (2014, 03). *Cannabinoids for treatment of Alzheimer's disease: moving toward the clinic*. Retrieved from Pubmed: https://www.ncbi.nlm.nih.gov/pubmed/24634659

B1., L. (2007, 08). *The endocannabinoid system and extinction learning*. Retrieved from Pubmed: https://www.ncbi.nlm.nih.gov/pubmed/17952654

Bab I1, S. R. (2011, 08). *Skeletal lipidomics: regulation of bone metabolism by fatty acid amide family*. Retrieved from Pubmed: https://www.ncbi.nlm.nih.gov/pubmed/21557736

Bab I1, Z. A. (2009). *Cannabinoids and the skeleton: from marijuana to reversal of bone loss*. Retrieved from Pubmed: https://www.ncbi.nlm.nih.gov/pubmed/19634029

Bachhuber MA1, S. B. (10, 2014). *Medical cannabis laws and opioid analgesic overdose mortality in the United States, 1999-2010*. Retrieved from Pubmed: https://www.ncbi.nlm.nih.gov/pubmed/25154332

Baiula M1, B. A. (2015). *Role of nociceptin/orphanin FQ in thermoregulation*. Retrieved from Pubmed: https://www.ncbi.nlm.nih.gov/pubmed/25812480

Bakas T1, v. N. (2017, 05). *The direct actions of cannabidiol and 2-arachidonoyl glycerol at GABAA receptors*. Retrieved from Pubmed: https://www.ncbi.nlm.nih.gov/pubmed/28249817

Banerjee SP, S. S. (1975). *Cannabinoids: influence on neurotransmitter uptake in rat brain synaptosomes*. Retrieved from Pubmed: https://www.ncbi.nlm.nih.gov/pubmed/168349

Bátkai S1, P. P.-H.-W. (2004, 10). *Endocannabinoids acting at cannabinoid-1 receptors regulate cardiovascular function in hypertension*. Retrieved from Pubmed: https://www.ncbi.nlm.nih.gov/pubmed/?term=Endocannabinoids+acting

+at+cannabinoid-1+receptors+regulate+cardiovascular+function+in+hypertension

BBC. (2005, 06 15). *Timeline Th Use of Cannabis*. Retrieved from Panorama: http://news.bbc.co.uk/1/hi/programmes/panorama/4079668.stm

BE1., A. (2014, 09). *Seizing an opportunity for the endocannabinoid system*. Retrieved from https://www.ncbi.nlm.nih.gov/pubmed/25346637

BE1., M. (2013, 03). *Cannabinoids and hallucinogens for headache*. Retrieved from https://www.ncbi.nlm.nih.gov/pubmed/23278122

Bedse G1, R. A. (2015). *The role of endocannabinoid signaling in the molecular mechanisms of neurodegeneration in Alzheimer's disease*. Retrieved from Pubmed: https://www.ncbi.nlm.nih.gov/pubmed/25147120

Benet, S. (1975). Retrieved from https://www.degruyter.com/view/books/9783110812060/9783110812060.39/9783110812060.39.xml

Bennet, C. (1995, 07 15). *The Scythians – High Plains Drifters*. Retrieved from Cannabis Culture : http://www.cannabisculture.com/content/1995/07/15/986

Bennet, C. (1996, 05 01). *Kaneh Bosm: Cannabis in the Old Testament*. Retrieved from Cannabis Culture: http://www.cannabisculture.com/content/1996/05/01/1090

Bennet, C. (1998, 09 01). *Marijuana and the Goddess*. Retrieved from Cannabis Culture : http://www.cannabisculture.com/content/1998/09/01/1374

Bennet, C. (Unlisted). *Marijuana in The Bible*. Retrieved from Patients for Medical Marijuana: https://patients4medicalmarijuana.wordpress.com/marijuana-info/marijuana-in-the-bible/

Bennett, C. (2010). *Cannabis and the Soma Solution*. Trine Day.

Bera, E. B.-E.-X. (2008, 11 01). *Phytochemical and genetic analyses of ancient cannabis from Central Asia*. Retrieved from Journal of Experimental Botany: https://academic.oup.com/jxb/article/59/15/4171/518859/Phytochemical-and-genetic-analyses-of-ancient

Bergamaschi MM1, Q. R.-S. (2011, 05). *Cannabidiol reduces the anxiety induced by simulated public speaking in treatment-naïve social phobia patients*. Retrieved from Pubmed: https://www.ncbi.nlm.nih.gov/pubmed/21307846

Bergamaschi MM1, Q. R.-S. (2011, 05). *Cannabidiol reduces the anxiety induced by simulated public speaking in treatment-naïve social phobia patients.* Retrieved from Pubmed: https://www.ncbi.nlm.nih.gov/pubmed/21307846

Bermudez-Silva FJ1, C. P. (2012, 01). *The role of the endocannabinoid system in the neuroendocrine regulation of energy balance.* Retrieved from Pubmed: https://www.ncbi.nlm.nih.gov/pubmed/21824982

Bidwell LC1, H. E. (2014, 02). *Childhood and current ADHD symptom dimensions are associated with more severe cannabis outcomes in college students.* Retrieved from Pubmed: https://www.ncbi.nlm.nih.gov/pubmed/24332802

Bifulco M1, M. A. (2008, 06). *Endocannabinoids in endocrine and related tumours.* Retrieved from Pubmed: https://www.ncbi.nlm.nih.gov/pubmed/18508995

Bíró T1, T. B. (2008, 08). *The endocannabinoid system of the skin in health and disease: novel perspectives and therapeutic opportunities.* Retrieved from Pubmed: https://www.ncbi.nlm.nih.gov/pubmed/19608284

Bisogno T1, D. M. (2008). *The role of the endocannabinoid system in Alzheimer's disease: facts and hypotheses.* Retrieved from Pubmed: https://www.ncbi.nlm.nih.gov/pubmed/18781980

Blake DR1, R. P. (2006, 01). *Preliminary assessment of the efficacy, tolerability and safety of a cannabis-based medicine (Sativex) in the treatment of pain caused by rheumatoid arthritis.* Retrieved from Pubmed: https://www.ncbi.nlm.nih.gov/pubmed/16282192

Bluett RJ1, G.-G. J. (2014, 07). *Central anandamide deficiency predicts stress-induced anxiety: behavioral reversal through endocannabinoid augmentation.* Retrieved from Pubmed: https://www.ncbi.nlm.nih.gov/pubmed/25004388

Bluett RJ1, G.-G. J. (2014, 07). *Central anandamide deficiency predicts stress-induced anxiety: behavioral reversal through endocannabinoid augmentation.* Retrieved from Pubmed: https://www.ncbi.nlm.nih.gov/pubmed/25004388

Brenneisen, R. (Unlisted). *Chemistry and Analysis of Phytocannabnoids and other Cannabis Constituents.* Retrieved from Medical Genomics.

BROSIOUS, E. G. (n.d.). *7 types of cannabis oils.* Retrieved from Extract.Suntimes : http://extract.suntimes.com/information-resources/10/153/21941/easy-guide-7-types-cannabis-oil-photos/

Brown, D. T. (2003). *Cannabis: The Genus Cannabis*. CRC Press.

Campos AC1, F. F. (2012, 11). *Cannabidiol blocks long-lasting behavioral consequences of predator threat stress: possible involvement of 5HT1A receptors*. Retrieved from Pubmed: https://www.ncbi.nlm.nih.gov/pubmed/22979992

Campos AC1, G. F. (2009, 11). *Evidence for a potential role for TRPV1 receptors in the dorsolateral periaqueductal gray in the attenuation of the anxiolytic effects of cannabinoids*. Retrieved from Pubmed: https://www.ncbi.nlm.nih.gov/pubmed/19735690

Campos AC1, M. F. (2012, 12). *Multiple mechanisms involved in the large-spectrum therapeutic potential of cannabidiol in psychiatric disorders*. Retrieved from Pubmed: https://www.ncbi.nlm.nih.gov/pubmed/23108553

Campos AC1, O. Z.-A.-G.-V.-R. (2013, 07). *The anxiolytic effect of cannabidiol on chronically stressed mice depends on hippocampal neurogenesis: involvement of the endocannabinoid system*. Retrieved from Pubmed: https://www.ncbi.nlm.nih.gov/pubmed/23298518

Cannabis and Time Perception. (n.d.). Retrieved from https://en.wikipedia.org/wiki/Cannabis_and_time_perception

Cannabis. (Unlisted). Retrieved from Spoken Sanskrit: http://www.spokensanskrit.de/index.php?tinput=Cannabis&link=m

Carlini EA, C. J. (1981). *Hypnotic and antiepileptic effects of cannabidiol*. Retrieved from Pubmed: https://www.ncbi.nlm.nih.gov/pubmed/7028792

Carter GT1, A. M. (2010, 08). *Cannabis and amyotrophic lateral sclerosis: hypothetical and practical applications, and a call for clinical trials*. Retrieved from Pubmed: https://www.ncbi.nlm.nih.gov/pubmed/20439484

Carvajal C1, D. Y. (2006, 04). *Neuropeptide y: role in emotion and alcohol dependence*. Retrieved from Pubmed: https://www.ncbi.nlm.nih.gov/pubmed/16611091

Castillo A1, T. M.-R.-O. (2010, 02). *The neuroprotective effect of cannabidiol in an in vitro model of newborn hypoxic-ischemic brain damage in mice is mediated by CB(2) and adenosine receptors*. Retrieved from Pubmed: https://www.ncbi.nlm.nih.gov/pubmed/19900555

CCICannabinoids, V. o. (Director). (2012). *https://www.youtube.com/watch?v=jznQfMj9RWM* [Motion Picture].

Ceprián M1, J.-S. L.-O. (2017, 04). *annabidiol reduces brain damage and improves functional recovery in a neonatal rat model of arterial ischemic stroke.* Retrieved from Pubmed: https://www.ncbi.nlm.nih.gov/pubmed/28012949

Chagas MH1, Z. A.-P. (2014, 11). *Effects of cannabidiol in the treatment of patients with Parkinson's disease: an exploratory double-blind trial.* Retrieved from Pubmed: https://www.ncbi.nlm.nih.gov/pubmed/25237116

Chasteen, B. J. (2016). *Getting High: Marijuana through the Ages.* Rowman and Littlefield.

Chhatwal JP1, D. M. (2005, 03). *Enhancing cannabinoid neurotransmission augments the extinction of conditioned fear.* Retrieved from Pubmed: https://www.ncbi.nlm.nih.gov/pubmed/15637635

China Wood Store. (Unlisted). *Magu - Goddess of Cannabis.* Retrieved from https://www.chinawoodsstore.com/magu-priestess-of-cannabis/

Christelle M. Andre*, J.-F. H. (2016, 02 04). *Plant of a Thousand Molecules.* Retrieved from Frontiers in Science: http://journal.frontiersin.org/article/10.3389/fpls.2016.00019/full

Chronology of Hemp. (Unlisted). Retrieved from Hemphasis.

CJ1., H. (2014, 10). *Stress regulates endocannabinoid-CB1 receptor signaling.* Retrieved from Pubmed: https://www.ncbi.nlm.nih.gov/pubmed/24882055

Clarke2, X. L. (n.d.). *The cultivation and use of hemp (Cannabis Sativa L) in Ancient China.* Retrieved from http://www.druglibrary.org/olsen/hemp/iha/iha02111.html

Cleversley, K. (2002, 01 01). *Cannabis ruderalis.* Retrieved from entheology.com: http://entheology.com/plants/cannabis-ruderalis-weedy-hemp/

Coderre AM1, Z. A. (2010, 06). *Assessment of upper-limb sensorimotor function of subacute stroke patients using visually guided reaching.* Retrieved from Pubmed: https://www.ncbi.nlm.nih.gov/pubmed/20233965

Consroe P, B. M. (1982). *Effects of cannabidiol on behavioral seizures caused by convulsant drugs or current in mice.* Retrieved from Pubmed: https://www.ncbi.nlm.nih.gov/pubmed/6129147

Consroe P, W. A. (1977). *Cannabidiol--antiepileptic drug comparisons and interactions in experimentally induced seizures in rats.* Retrieved from Pubmed: https://www.ncbi.nlm.nih.gov/pubmed/850145

Consroe P1, L. J. (1991, 11). *Controlled clinical trial of cannabidiol in Huntington's disease.* Retrieved from Pubmed: https://www.ncbi.nlm.nih.gov/pubmed/1839644

Crippa JA1, D. G.-A.-S.-P.-F. (2011, 01). *Neural basis of anxiolytic effects of cannabidiol (CBD) in generalized social anxiety disorder: a preliminary report.* Retrieved from Pubmed: https://www.ncbi.nlm.nih.gov/pubmed/20829306

Crippa JA1, D. G.-A.-S.-P.-F. (2011, 01). *Neural basis of anxiolytic effects of cannabidiol (CBD) in generalized social anxiety disorder: a preliminary report.* Retrieved from Pubmed: https://www.ncbi.nlm.nih.gov/pubmed/20829306

Crippa JA1, D. G.-A.-S.-P.-F. (2011, 01). *Neural basis of anxiolytic effects of cannabidiol (CBD) in generalized social anxiety disorder: a preliminary report.* Retrieved from Pubmed: https://www.ncbi.nlm.nih.gov/pubmed/20829306

Crippa JA1, D. G.-S. (2012, 01). *Pharmacological interventions in the treatment of the acute effects of cannabis: a systematic review of literature.* Retrieved from Pubmed: https://www.ncbi.nlm.nih.gov/pubmed/22273390

Crippa JA1, H. J.-d.-S. (2013, 04). *Cannabidiol for the treatment of cannabis withdrawal syndrome: a case report.* Retrieved from Pubmed: https://www.ncbi.nlm.nih.gov/pubmed/23095052

Crippa JA1, Z. A.-A.-M. (2004, 02). *Effects of cannabidiol (CBD) on regional cerebral blood flow.* Retrieved from Pubmed: https://www.ncbi.nlm.nih.gov/pubmed/14583744

Crippa JA1, Z. A.-A.-M. (2004, 02). *Effects of cannabidiol (CBD) on regional cerebral blood flow.* Retrieved from Pubmed: https://www.ncbi.nlm.nih.gov/pubmed/14583744

Culpeppers Complete Herbal. (n.d.). Retrieved from http://www.complete-herbal.com/culpepper/hemp.htm

Cunha JM, C. E. (1980). *Chronic administration of cannabidiol to healthy volunteers and epileptic patients.* Retrieved from Pubmed: https://www.ncbi.nlm.nih.gov/pubmed/7413719

da Silva JA1, B. A. (2015, 07). *Dissociation between the panicolytic effect of cannabidiol microinjected into the substantia nigra, pars reticulata, and fear-induced antinociception elicited by bicuculline administration in deep layers of the superior colliculus: The role of CB1-cannabi.* Retrieved from Pubmed: https://www.ncbi.nlm.nih.gov/pubmed/25841876

Dachun Xu, P. U. (1993). *Forgotten Traditions of Ancient Chinese Medicine.* Churchill Livingstone.

de Bitencourt RM1, P. F. (2013, 01). *A current overview of cannabinoids and glucocorticoids in facilitating extinction of aversive memories: potential extinction enhancers.* Retrieved from Pubmed: https://www.ncbi.nlm.nih.gov/pubmed/22687521

De Laurentiis A1, F. S. (2010). *Endocannabinoid system participates in neuroendocrine control of homeostasis.* Retrieved from Pubmed: https://www.ncbi.nlm.nih.gov/pubmed/20134190

de Mello Schier AR, d. O.-C. (2014). *Antidepressant-like and anxiolytic-like effects of cannabidiol: a chemical compound of Cannabis sativa.* Retrieved from Pubmed: https://www.ncbi.nlm.nih.gov/pubmed/24923339

de Mello Schier AR, d. O.-C. (2014). *Antidepressant-like and anxiolytic-like effects of cannabidiol: a chemical compound of Cannabis sativa.* Retrieved from Pubmed: https://www.ncbi.nlm.nih.gov/pubmed/24923339

de Mello Schier AR, d. O.-C. (2014). *Antidepressant-like and anxiolytic-like effects of cannabidiol: a chemical compound of Cannabis sativa.* Retrieved from Pubmed: https://www.ncbi.nlm.nih.gov/pubmed/24923339

De Petrocellis L1, L. A. (2011, 08). *Effects of cannabinoids and cannabinoid-enriched Cannabis extracts on TRP channels and endocannabinoid metabolic enzymes.* Retrieved from Pubmed: https://www.ncbi.nlm.nih.gov/pubmed/21175579

De Petrocellis L1, L. A. (2011, 08). *Effects of cannabinoids and cannabinoid-enriched Cannabis extracts on TRP channels and endocannabinoid metabolic enzymes.* Retrieved from Pubmed: https://www.ncbi.nlm.nih.gov/pubmed/21175579

Deiana S1, W. A. (2012, 02). *Plasma and brain pharmacokinetic profile of cannabidiol (CBD), cannabidivarine (CBDV), Δ^9-tetrahydrocannabivarin (THCV) and cannabigerol (CBG) in rats and mice following oral and* *intraperitoneal administration and CBD action on obsessive-compulsive behavi*. Retrieved from Pubmed: https://www.ncbi.nlm.nih.gov/pubmed/?term=Plasma+and+brain+pharmacokinetic+profile+of+cannabidiol+%28CBD%29%2C+cannabidivarine+%28CBDV%29%2C+%CE%94%E2%81%B9-tetrahydrocannabivarin+%28THCV%29+and+cannabigerol+%28CBG%29+in+rats+and+mice+following+oral+and+i

Delfin Rodriguez-Leyva1, 2. a. (2010, 04 21). *The cardiac and haemostatic effects of dietary hempseed*. Retrieved from Pubmed: https://www.ncbi.nlm.nih.gov/pmc/articles/PMC2868018/

Deng L1, N. L. (2017). *Quantitative Analyses of Synergistic Responses between Cannabidiol and DNA-Damaging Agents on the Proliferation and Viability of Glioblastoma and Neural Progenitor Cells in Culture*. Retrieved from Pubmed: https://www.ncbi.nlm.nih.gov/pubmed/27821713

Deng L1, N. L. (2017, 01). *Quantitative Analyses of Synergistic Responses between Cannabidiol and DNA-Damaging Agents on the Proliferation and Viability of Glioblastoma and Neural Progenitor Cells in Culture*. Retrieved from Pubmed: https://www.ncbi.nlm.nih.gov/pubmed/27821713

Devinsky O1, C. M.-R.-A.-O. (2014, 06). *Cannabidiol: pharmacology and potential therapeutic role in epilepsy and other neuropsychiatric disorders*. Retrieved from Pubmed: https://www.ncbi.nlm.nih.gov/pubmed/?term=Cannabidiol%3A+Pharmacology+and+potential+therapeutic+role+in+epilepsy+and+other+neuropsychiatric+disorders

Di Marzo V1, P. F. (2011). *Cannabinoids and endocannabinoids in metabolic disorders with focus on diabetes*. Retrieved from Pubmed: https://www.ncbi.nlm.nih.gov/pubmed/21484568

Di Marzo V1, P. F. (2011). *Cannabinoids and endocannabinoids in metabolic disorders with focus on diabetes*. Retrieved from Pubmed: https://www.ncbi.nlm.nih.gov/pubmed/21484568

Dionigi A1, G. P. (2017, 03). *A combined intervention of art therapy and clown visits to reduce preoperative anxiety in children*. Retrieved from Pubmed: https://www.ncbi.nlm.nih.gov/pubmed/27627730

Dirikoc S1, P. S. (2007). *Nonpsychoactive cannabidiol prevents prion accumulation and protects neurons against prion toxicity*. Retrieved from Pubmed: https://www.ncbi.nlm.nih.gov/pubmed/17804615

DP1., F. (2010, 08). *Endocannabinoid-mediated modulation of stress responses: physiological and pathophysiological significance.* Retrieved from https://www.ncbi.nlm.nih.gov/pubmed/19616342

Durst R1, D. H. (2007, 12). *Cannabidiol, a nonpsychoactive Cannabis constituent, protects against myocardial ischemic reperfusion injury.* Retrieved from Pubmed: https://www.ncbi.nlm.nih.gov/pubmed/17890433

Dutch Passion Seed Company. (2011, 09 22). *Cannabi Ruderalis.* Retrieved from Dutch Passion Seed Company: http://www.cannabisruderalis.com/

Duvall, C. (2014). *Cannabis.* Reakton Books.

Dvorak, J. (n.d.). *America's Harried Hemp History.* Retrieved from Hemphasis: http://www.hemphasis.net/History/harriedhemp.htm

E1., D. (2008). *Cannabidiol: a prion therapy for mice?* Retrieved from Pubmed: https://www.ncbi.nlm.nih.gov/pubmed/18338806

El-Remessy AB1, K. I.-M. (2003). *Neuroprotective effect of (-)Delta9-tetrahydrocannabinol and cannabidiol in N-methyl-D-aspartate-induced retinal neurotoxicity: involvement of peroxynitrite.* Retrieved from Pubmed: https://www.ncbi.nlm.nih.gov/pubmed/14578199

El-Remessy AB1, K. Y. (2010, 08). *Cannabidiol protects retinal neurons by preserving glutamine synthetase activity in diabetes.* Retrieved from Pubmed: https://www.ncbi.nlm.nih.gov/pubmed/20806080

Entheogenic use of cannabis. (n.d.). Retrieved from https://infogalactic.com/info/Entheogenic_use_of_cannabis

Escohotado, A. (2010). *The General History of Drugs.* Graffiti Milante Press.

Espejo-Porras F1, F.-R. J. (2013, 12). *Motor effects of the non-psychotropic phytocannabinoid cannabidiol that are mediated by 5-HT1A receptors.* Retrieved from Pubmed: https://www.ncbi.nlm.nih.gov/pubmed/23924692

Esposito G1, S. C. (2007, 08). *Cannabidiol in vivo blunts beta-amyloid induced neuroinflammation by suppressing IL-1beta and iNOS expression.* Retrieved from Pubmed: https://www.ncbi.nlm.nih.gov/pubmed/17592514

Farrimond JA1, W. B. (2012, 09). *Cannabinol and cannabidiol exert opposing effects on rat feeding patterns.* Retrieved from Pubmed: https://www.ncbi.nlm.nih.gov/pubmed/22543671

Farzaei MH, B. R. (2016). *A Systematic Review of Plant-Derived Natural Compounds for Anxiety Disorders*. Retrieved from Pubmed: https://www.ncbi.nlm.nih.gov/pubmed/26845556

Farzaei MH, B. R. (2016). *A Systematic Review of Plant-Derived Natural Compounds for Anxiety Disorders*. Retrieved from Pubmed: https://www.ncbi.nlm.nih.gov/pubmed/26845556

Fernández-Ruiz J1, M.-M. M.-C.-G.-C. (2011, 08). *Prospects for cannabinoid therapies in basal ganglia disorders*. Retrieved from Pubmed: https://www.ncbi.nlm.nih.gov/pubmed/21545415

Fernández-Ruiz J1, S. O.-O. (2013, 02). *Cannabidiol for neurodegenerative disorders: important new clinical applications for this phytocannabinoid?* Retrieved from Pubmed: https://www.ncbi.nlm.nih.gov/pubmed/22625422

Flowers of India. (Unlisted). *Marijuana*. Retrieved from http://www.flowersofindia.net/catalog/slides/Marijuana.html

Fundacion -canna.es. (n.d.). *The Endocannabinoid System*. Retrieved from Fundacion -canna.es: http://www.fundacion-canna.es/en/endocannabinoid-system

Ganon-Elazar E1, A. I. (2013, 09). *Cannabinoids and traumatic stress modulation of contextual fear extinction and GR expression in the amygdala-hippocampal-prefrontal circuit*. Retrieved from Pubmed: https://www.ncbi.nlm.nih.gov/pubmed/23433741

Garberg HT1, 2. H.-O. (2016, 11). *Short-term effects of cannabidiol after global hypoxia-ischemia in newborn piglets*. Retrieved from Pubmed: https://www.ncbi.nlm.nih.gov/pubmed/27441365

García-Arencibia M1, G. S.-R. (2007, 02). *Evaluation of the neuroprotective effect of cannabinoids in a rat model of Parkinson's disease: importance of antioxidant and cannabinoid receptor-independent properties*. Retrieved from Pubmed: https://www.ncbi.nlm.nih.gov/pubmed/17196181

Gaston TE1, F. D. (2017, 05). *Pharmacology of cannabinoids in the treatment of epilepsy*. Retrieved from Pubmed: https://www.ncbi.nlm.nih.gov/pubmed/28087250

George F. Koob, M. L. (2005). *Neurobiology of Addiction*. Academic Press.

Ghaly, S. J. (2015, 10 28). *Cannabis, Marijuana, Ganja, Weed – Where Did These Names Come From?* Retrieved from http://herb.co/2015/10/28/cannabis-marijuana-ganja-weed-where-did-these-names-come-from/

Giannini L1, N. S. (2008, 08). *Activation of cannabinoid receptors prevents antigen-induced asthma-like reaction in guinea pigs.* Retrieved from Pubmed: https://www.ncbi.nlm.nih.gov/pubmed/18266975

Glangetas C1, G. D. (2013). *Stress switches cannabinoid type-1 (CB1) receptor-dependent plasticity from LTD to LTP in the bed nucleus of the stria terminalis.* Retrieved from Pubmed: https://www.ncbi.nlm.nih.gov/pubmed/24336729

Gobira PH1, V. L. (2015, 09). *Cannabidiol, a Cannabis sativa constituent, inhibits cocaine-induced seizures in mice: Possible role of the mTOR pathway and reduction in glutamate release.* Retrieved from Pubmed: https://www.ncbi.nlm.nih.gov/pubmed/26283212

Godwin, H. (1967). *The Ancient Cultivation of Hemp.* https://www.cambridge.org/core/journals/antiquity/article/the-ancient-cultivation-of-hemp/F6CF0F71951AA094BF2A554524B1262F.

Goldman, R. F. (2013). *Race and Ethnicity in the Classical World: An Anthology of Primary Sources in Translation.* Hackett Publishing.

Gomes FV1, R. L. (2011, 02). *The anxiolytic-like effects of cannabidiol injected into the bed nucleus of the stria terminalis are mediated by 5-HT1A receptors.* Retrieved from Pubmed: https://www.ncbi.nlm.nih.gov/pubmed/20945065

Gomez O1, S.-R. A.-C.-H.-H. (2011, 08). *Cannabinoid receptor agonists modulate oligodendrocyte differentiation by activating PI3K/Akt and the mammalian target of rapamycin (mTOR) pathways.* Retrieved from Pubmed: https://www.ncbi.nlm.nih.gov/pubmed/21480865

Gonca E1, D. F. (2015, 01). *The effect of cannabidiol on ischemia/reperfusion-induced ventricular arrhythmias: the role of adenosine A1 receptors.* Retrieved from Pubmed: https://www.ncbi.nlm.nih.gov/pubmed/24853683

Gonçalves TC1, L. A. (2014, 12). *Cannabidiol and endogenous opioid peptide-mediated mechanisms modulate antinociception induced by transcutaneous electrostimulation of the peripheral nervous system.* Retrieved from Pubmed: https://www.ncbi.nlm.nih.gov/pubmed/25282545

Gorzalka BB1, H. M. (2008). *Regulation of endocannabinoid signaling by stress: implications for stress-related affective disorders.* Retrieved from Pubmed: https://www.ncbi.nlm.nih.gov/pubmed/18433869

Gorzalka BB1, H. M. (2011, 08). *Putative role of endocannabinoid signaling in the etiology of depression and actions of antidepressants.* Retrieved from Pubmed: https://www.ncbi.nlm.nih.gov/pubmed/21111017

Graham, K. (2015, 05 25). *Ancient Scythians Spread The Use of Cannabis Through Death Rituals.* Retrieved from Digital Journal: http://www.digitaljournal.com/science/gold-artifacts-of-ancient-scythians-reveals-bastard-war-and-drugs/article/434123

Greco R1, G. V. (2010, 07). *The endocannabinoid system and migraine.* Retrieved from https://www.ncbi.nlm.nih.gov/pubmed/20353780

Greco R1, M. A. (2011, 04). *Effects of anandamide in migraine: data from an animal model.* Retrieved from Pubmed: https://www.ncbi.nlm.nih.gov/pubmed/21331757

Green, J. (2002, 10 12). *Spoonfuls of paradise.* Retrieved from The Guardian: https://www.theguardian.com/books/2002/oct/12/featuresreviews.guardianreview34

GS1., W. (2017, 03). *Pediatric Concerns Due to Expanded Cannabis Use: Unintended Consequences of Legalization.* Retrieved from Pubmed: https://www.ncbi.nlm.nih.gov/pubmed/27139708

Gui H1, T. Q. (2015, 05). *The endocannabinoid system and its therapeutic implications in rheumatoid arthritis.* Retrieved from Pubmed: https://www.ncbi.nlm.nih.gov/pubmed/25791728

Gururajan A1, T. D. (2012, 08). *Cannabidiol and clozapine reverse MK-801-induced deficits in social interaction and hyperactivity in Sprague-Dawley rats.* Retrieved from Pubmed: https://www.ncbi.nlm.nih.gov/pubmed/22495620

GW1., B. (2011, 09). *Cannabidiol as an emergent therapeutic strategy for lessening the impact of inflammation on oxidative stress.* Retrieved from Pubmed: https://www.ncbi.nlm.nih.gov/pubmed/21238581

GW1., B. (2011). *Cannabidiol as an emergent therapeutic strategy for lessening the impact of inflammation on oxidative stress.* Retrieved from Pubmed: https://www.ncbi.nlm.nih.gov/pubmed/21238581

Haj-Dahmane S1, S. R. (2014, 10). *Chronic stress impairs α1-adrenoceptor-induced endocannabinoid-dependent synaptic plasticity in the dorsal raphe nucleus*. Retrieved from Pubmed: https://www.ncbi.nlm.nih.gov/pubmed/25355210

Hallak JE1, D. S.-d.-S. (2011). *The interplay of cannabinoid and NMDA glutamate receptor systems in humans: preliminary evidence of interactive effects of cannabidiol and ketamine in healthy human subjects.* Retrieved from Pubmed: https://www.ncbi.nlm.nih.gov/pubmed/21062637

Hamelink C1, H. A. (2005, 08). *Comparison of cannabidiol, antioxidants, and diuretics in reversing binge ethanol-induced neurotoxicity.* Retrieved from Pubmed: https://www.ncbi.nlm.nih.gov/pubmed/15878999

Hanus, L. O. (2008). *Pharmacological and Therapeutic Secrets of Plant and Brain (Endo)Cannabinoids).* Retrieved from Cannabis Plus: http://cannabisplus.net/cannabis-research-pdf/Cannabinoid%20Chemistry/Hanus%20Pharmacological%20and%20Therapeutic%20Secrets%20of%20Plant%20and%20Brain%20(Endo)Cannabinoids.pdf

Hao E1, 2. M. (2015, 01). *Cannabidiol Protects against Doxorubicin-Induced Cardiomyopathy by Modulating Mitochondrial Function and Biogenesis.* Retrieved from Pubmed: https://www.ncbi.nlm.nih.gov/pubmed/25569804

Harm van Bakel, J. M. (2011, 09 20). *The draft genome and transcriptome of Cannabis sativa.* Retrieved from Biomed Centra: https://genomebiology.biomedcentral.com/articles/10.1186/gb-2011-12-10-r102

Hartley JP, N. S. (1978). *Bronchodilator effect of delta1-tetrahydrocannabinol.* Retrieved from Pubmed: https://www.ncbi.nlm.nih.gov/pubmed/656294

Hayakawa K1, M. K. (2005, 10). *Cannabidiol prevents infarction via the non-CB1 cannabinoid receptor mechanism.* Retrieved from Pubmed: https://www.ncbi.nlm.nih.gov/pubmed/15640760

Hayakawa K1, M. K. (2007, 03). *Repeated treatment with cannabidiol but not Delta9-tetrahydrocannabinol has a neuroprotective effect without the development of tolerance.* Retrieved from Pubmed: https://www.ncbi.nlm.nih.gov/pubmed/17320118

Herb Museum. (2001). *In the Ancient World, Hemp was the Tree of Life.* Retrieved from http://www.herbmuseum.ca/content/ancient-world-hemp-was-tree-life

Herb Museum. (Unlisted). *Cannabis Origin and Evolution.* Retrieved from Herb Museum : http://www.herbmuseum.ca/content/cannabis-origin-and-evolution

Hernán Pérez de la Ossa D1, L. M.-A.-T.-S. (2013). *Local delivery of cannabinoid-loaded microparticles inhibits tumor growth in a murine xenograft model of glioblastoma multiforme.* Retrieved from Pubmed: https://www.ncbi.nlm.nih.gov/pubmed/23349970

Hernán Pérez de la Ossa D1, L. M.-A.-T.-S. (2013). *Local delivery of cannabinoid-loaded microparticles inhibits tumor growth in a murine xenograft model of glioblastoma multiforme.* Retrieved from Pubmed: https://www.ncbi.nlm.nih.gov/pubmed/23349970

Hicks, J. (2015). *The Medicinal Power of Cannabis: Using a Natural Herb to Heal Arthritis Nausea, Pain, and Other Ailments.* Skyhorse Publishing;.

Hiley CR1, H. P. (2007). *Oleamide: a fatty acid amide signaling molecule in the cardiovascular system?* Retrieved from Pubmed: https://www.ncbi.nlm.nih.gov/pubmed/17445087

Hill MN1, B. L. (2013, 10). *Reductions in circulating endocannabinoid levels in individuals with post-traumatic stress disorder following exposure to the World Trade Center attacks.* Retrieved from Pubmed: https://www.ncbi.nlm.nih.gov/pubmed/24035186

Hill MN1, G. B. (2009). *The endocannabinoid system and the treatment of mood and anxiety disorders.* Retrieved from Pubmed: https://www.ncbi.nlm.nih.gov/pubmed/19839936

Hill MN1, M. G. (2009, 09). *Circulating endocannabinoids and N-acyl ethanolamines are differentially regulated in major depression and following exposure to social stress.* Retrieved from Pubmed: https://www.ncbi.nlm.nih.gov/pubmed/19394765

Hill MN1, M. R. (2010). *Endogenous cannabinoid signaling is essential for stress adaptation.* Retrieved from Pubmed: https://www.ncbi.nlm.nih.gov/pubmed/20439721

Hill MN1, P. S. (2005, 03). *Downregulation of endocannabinoid signaling in the hippocampus following chronic unpredictable stress.* Retrieved from Pubmed: https://www.ncbi.nlm.nih.gov/pubmed/15525997

Hill MN1, P. S. (2010, 11). *Functional interactions between stress and the endocannabinoid system: from synaptic signaling to behavioral output.* Retrieved from Pubmed: https://www.ncbi.nlm.nih.gov/pubmed/21068301

Hillard CJ, L. Q. (2014). *Endocannabinoid signaling in the etiology and treatment of major depressive illness.* Retrieved from Pubmed: https://www.ncbi.nlm.nih.gov/pubmed/24180398

Hine B, T. M. (1975, 09). *Differential effect of cannabinol and cannabidiol on THC-induced responses during abstinence in morphine-dependent rats.* Retrieved from Pumbed: https://www.ncbi.nlm.nih.gov/pubmed/1237925

Hohmann T1, G. U. (2017, 01). *The influence of biomechanical properties and cannabinoids on tumor invasion.* Retrieved from Pubmed: https://www.ncbi.nlm.nih.gov/pubmed/27149140

Horatio C. Wood, J. (1896, Jan). *On the Medical ctivity of the Hemp Plant as Grown in North America.* Retrieved from Proceedings of the American Philosophical Society: http://www.jstor.org/stable/981465?Search=yes&resultItemClick=true&searchText=((CANNABIS)&searchUri=%2Faction%2FdoBasicSearch%3Ffc%3Doff%26acc%3Don%26prq%3D%2528%2528CANNABIS%2529%2BAND%2B%2528time%2529%2529%26amp%3D%26amp%3D%26amp%3D%26amp%3D%26amp%3D%26

How To Make Cannabis Balm. (2010, Feb 10). *How To Make Cannabis Balm.* Retrieved from Cannabis.info: https://www.cannabis.info/en/how-to-make-balm

Howard J1, A. K. (2005, 10). *Cannabis use in sickle cell disease: a questionnaire study.* Retrieved from Pubmed: https://www.ncbi.nlm.nih.gov/pubmed/16173972

https://en.wikipedia.org/wiki/Cannabis_in_India. (n.d.). Retrieved from Wikepedia.

https://www.ncbi.nlm.nih.gov/pubmed/22280340. (2012). *Cannabinoids: novel medicines for the treatment of Huntington's disease.* Retrieved from Pubmed: Sagredo O1, Pazos MR, Valdeolivas S, Fernandez-Ruiz J.

https://www.youtube.com/watch?v=RpEUqEIubkw, T. S. (Director). (2014). *Hemp's Beginnings - The Holy Annoining Oil - Hempology 101 - Video 7* [Motion Picture].

Hurd YL1, Y. M.-A. (2015, 10). *Early Phase in the Development of Cannabidiol as a Treatment for Addiction: Opioid Relapse Takes Initial Center Stage.* Retrieved from Pubmed: https://www.ncbi.nlm.nih.gov/pubmed/26269227

Hurd YL1, Y. M.-A. (2015, 10). *Early Phase in the Development of Cannabidiol as a Treatment for Addiction: Opioid Relapse Takes Initial Center Stage.*

Retrieved from Pubmed: https://www.ncbi.nlm.nih.gov/pubmed/26269227

Hwang YS1, K. Y. (2017, 06). *Cannabidiol upregulates melanogenesis through CB1 dependent pathway by activating p38 MAPK and p42/44 MAPK.* Retrieved from Pubmed: https://www.ncbi.nlm.nih.gov/pubmed/28601556

I1., K. (2015). *Cannabis and Endocannabinoid Signaling in Epilepsy.* Retrieved from Pubmed: https://www.ncbi.nlm.nih.gov/pubmed/26408165

Ibeas Bih C1, C. T. (2015, 10). *Molecular Targets of Cannabidiol in Neurological Disorders.* Retrieved from Pubmed: https://www.ncbi.nlm.nih.gov/pubmed/26264914

Infographic: What Are Cannabis Terpenes and How Do They Affect You? (n.d.). Retrieved from Leafly: https://www.leafly.com/news/cannabis-101/infographic-what-are-cannabis-terpenes-and-how-do-they-affect-you

Ingram, C. (2016, 09 23). *Crude Raw Supercritical Cannabis Extract – It's Power and Uses.* Retrieved from Cass Ingram: https://cassingram.com/crude-raw-supercritical-cannabis-extract-power-uses/

Ishiguro H1, H. Y. (2010, 05). *Brain cannabinoid CB2 receptor in schizophrenia.* Retrieved from Pubmed: https://www.ncbi.nlm.nih.gov/pubmed/19931854

ITN News Source. (2016, 03 29). *ISRAEL-CANNABIS U.S. firms eye Israeli cannabis R&D.* Retrieved from ITN: http://www.itnsource.com/en/shotlist/RTV/2016/03/29/RTV290316045/?s=cannabis

Iuvone T1, E. G. (2004, 04). *Neuroprotective effect of cannabidiol, a non-psychoactive component from Cannabis sativa, on beta-amyloid-induced toxicity in PC12 cells.* Retrieved from Pubmed: https://www.ncbi.nlm.nih.gov/pubmed/15030397

Iuvone T1, E. G. (2009). *Cannabidiol: a promising drug for neurodegenerative disorders?* Retrieved from Pubmed: https://www.ncbi.nlm.nih.gov/pubmed/19228180

Javed H1, A. S. (2016, 08). *Cannabinoid Type 2 (CB2) Receptors Activation Protects against Oxidative Stress and Neuroinflammation Associated Dopaminergic Neurodegeneration in Rotenone Model of Parkinson's Disease.* Retrieved from Pubmed: https://www.ncbi.nlm.nih.gov/pubmed/27531971

JL1., C. (2003). *Therapeutic potential of cannabinoids in CNS disease.* Retrieved from Pubmed: https://www.ncbi.nlm.nih.gov/pubmed/12617697

JM1., W. (2007). *Update on pharmacotherapy guidelines for treatment of neuropathic pain.* Retrieved from Pubmed: https://www.ncbi.nlm.nih.gov/pubmed/17504648

Jones NA1, G. S. (2012, 06). *Cannabidiol exerts anti-convulsant effects in animal models of temporal lobe and partial seizures.* Retrieved from Pubmed: https://www.ncbi.nlm.nih.gov/pubmed/22520455

Jones NA1, H. A. (2010, 02). *Cannabidiol displays antiepileptiform and antiseizure properties in vitro and in vivo.* Retrieved from Pubmed: https://www.ncbi.nlm.nih.gov/pubmed/19906779

Joyner, B. (2016, 4 14). *Could Cannabis Growing in the Garden of Eden Explain the Tree of Knowledge?* Retrieved from Pulse: https://www.marijuanapackaging.com/blog/cannabis-growing-in-garden-of-eden/

Juhasz G1, L. J. (2009, 09). *Variations in the cannabinoid receptor 1 gene predispose to migraine.* Retrieved from Pubmed: https://www.ncbi.nlm.nih.gov/pubmed/19539700

Juknat A1, P. M. (2012, 04). *Differential transcriptional profiles mediated by exposure to the cannabinoids cannabidiol and Δ9-tetrahydrocannabinol in BV-2 microglial cells.* Retrieved from Pubmed: https://www.ncbi.nlm.nih.gov/pubmed/21542829

Jürg Gertsch, 1. R. (2010, 06). *Phytocannabinoids beyond the Cannabis plant – do they exist?* Retrieved from Pubmed: https://www.ncbi.nlm.nih.gov/pmc/articles/PMC2931553/

Kaplan BL1, S. A. (2008, 15). *The profile of immune modulation by cannabidiol (CBD) involves deregulation of nuclear factor of activated T cells (NFAT).* Retrieved from Pubmed: https://www.ncbi.nlm.nih.gov/pubmed/18656454

Kaplan BL1, S. A. (2008). *The profile of immune modulation by cannabidiol (CBD) involves deregulation of nuclear factor of activated T cells (NFAT).* Retrieved from Pubmed: https://www.ncbi.nlm.nih.gov/pubmed/18656454

Karasu T1, M. T. (2011, 05). *The role of sex steroid hormones, cytokines and the endocannabinoid system in female fertility.* Retrieved from Pubmed: https://www.ncbi.nlm.nih.gov/pubmed/21227997

Karl T1, C. D. (2012, 04). *The therapeutic potential of the endocannabinoid system for Alzheimer's disease.* Retrieved from Pubmed: https://www.ncbi.nlm.nih.gov/pubmed/22448595

Karler R, T. S. (1981, 08). *The cannabinoids as potential antiepileptics.* Retrieved from Pubmed: https://www.ncbi.nlm.nih.gov/pubmed/6975285

Karlsborg M1, C. A. (2017, 02). *[Self-medication with cannabidiol oil in a patient with primary lateral sclerosis].* Retrieved from Pubmed: https://www.ncbi.nlm.nih.gov/pubmed/28397674

Karsak M1, G. E.-E. (2007, 06). *Attenuation of allergic contact dermatitis through the endocannabinoid system.* Retrieved from Pubmed: https://www.ncbi.nlm.nih.gov/pubmed/17556587

Katsidoni V1, A. I. (2013, 03). *Cannabidiol inhibits the reward-facilitating effect of morphine: involvement of 5-HT1A receptors in the dorsal raphe nucleus.* Retrieved from Pubmed: https://www.ncbi.nlm.nih.gov/pubmed/22862835

Kerbage H1, R. S. (2013, 02). *Non-Antidepressant Long-Term Treatment in Post-Traumatic Stress Disorder (PTSD).* Retrieved from Pubmed: https://www.ncbi.nlm.nih.gov/pubmed/?term=traumatic+and+Kerbage+H

Khare, C. (2004). *Indian Herbal Remedies: Rational Western Therapy, Ayurvedic and Other Traditional Usage, Botany.* Springer.

Kleiner D1, D. K. (2012, 04). *[The potential use of cannabidiol in the therapy of metabolic syndrome].* Retrieved from Pubmed: https://www.ncbi.nlm.nih.gov/pubmed/22430005

Kohli DR1, L. Y. (2010, 07). *Pain-related behaviors and neurochemical alterations in mice expressing sickle hemoglobin: modulation by cannabinoids.* Retrieved from Pubmed: https://www.ncbi.nlm.nih.gov/pubmed/20304807

Kwiatkoski M1, G. F.-B. (2012). *Cannabidiol-treated rats exhibited higher motor score after cryogenic spinal cord injury.* Retrieved from Pubmed: https://www.ncbi.nlm.nih.gov/pubmed/21915768

La Porta C1, B. S. (2014, 02). *Involvement of the endocannabinoid system in osteoarthritis pain.* Retrieved from Pubmed: https://www.ncbi.nlm.nih.gov/pubmed/24494687

Lafuente H1, P. M.-O. (2016, 07). *Effects of Cannabidiol and Hypothermia on Short-Term Brain Damage in New-Born Piglets after Acute Hypoxia-*

Ischemia. Retrieved from Pubmed: https://www.ncbi.nlm.nih.gov/pubmed/27462203

Lastres-Becker I1, M.-H. F.-R. (2005, 06). *Cannabinoids provide neuroprotection against 6-hydroxydopamine toxicity in vivo and in vitro: relevance to Parkinson's disease.* Retrieved from Pubmed: https://www.ncbi.nlm.nih.gov/pubmed/15837565

Le Foll B1, T. J. (2013, 05). *Cannabis and Δ9-tetrahydrocannabinol (THC) for weight loss?* Retrieved from Pubmed: https://www.ncbi.nlm.nih.gov/pubmed/23410498

Leaf Science. (2016, 12 14). *5 Essential Facts About Cannabis Oil.* Retrieved from http://www.leafscience.com/2016/12/14/5-essential-facts-cannabis-oil/

Leafly. (n.d.). *Myrcene, Linalool, and Bisabolol: What Are the Benefits of These Cannabis Terpenes?* Retrieved from https://www.leafly.com/news/cannabis-101/myrcene-linalool-and-bisabolol-what-are-the-benefits-of-these-can

Learn how terpenes work synergistically with cannabinoids. (Unlisted). Retrieved from Medical Jane: https://www.medicaljane.com/category/cannabis-classroom/terpenes/

Lee JL1, B. L. (2017, 03). *Cannabidiol regulation of emotion and emotional memory processing: relevance for treating anxiety-related and substance abuse disorders.* Retrieved from Pubmed: https://www.ncbi.nlm.nih.gov/pubmed/28268256

Leo A1, R. E. (2016, 05). *Cannabidiol and epilepsy: Rationale and therapeutic potential.* Retrieved from Pubmed: https://www.ncbi.nlm.nih.gov/pubmed/26976797

Levine, D. M. (2009, 04 24). *Human and Cannabis Coevolution.* Retrieved from Cannabis Culture: http://www.cannabisculture.com/content/2009/04/24/human-and-cannabis-coevolution

Leweke FM1, M. J. (2016, 04). *Therapeutic Potential of Cannabinoids in Psychosis.* Retrieved from Pubmed: https://www.ncbi.nlm.nih.gov/pubmed/26852073

Li C, J. P. (2011, 03). *Role of the endocannabinoid system in food intake, energy homeostasis and regulation of the endocrine pancreas.* Retrieved from Pubmed: https://www.ncbi.nlm.nih.gov/pubmed/21055418

Lin JG1, H. C. (2015, 06). *Analgesic Effect of Electroacupuncture in a Mouse Fibromyalgia Model: Roles of TRPV1, TRPV4, and pERK.* Retrieved from Pubmed: https://www.ncbi.nlm.nih.gov/pubmed/26043006

Lin JG1, H. C. (2015, 04). *Analgesic Effect of Electroacupuncture in a Mouse Fibromyalgia Model: Roles of TRPV1, TRPV4, and pERK.* Retrieved from Pubmed: https://www.ncbi.nlm.nih.gov/pubmed/26043006

Lin JG1, H. C. (2015, 06). *Analgesic Effect of Electroacupuncture in a Mouse Fibromyalgia Model: Roles of TRPV1, TRPV4, and pERK.* Retrieved from Pubmed: https://www.ncbi.nlm.nih.gov/pubmed/26043006

Linge R1, J.-S. L.-C. (2016, 04). *Cannabidiol induces rapid-acting antidepressant-like effects and enhances cortical 5-HT/glutamate neurotransmission: role of 5-HT1A receptors.* Retrieved from Pubmed: https://www.ncbi.nlm.nih.gov/pubmed/26711860

Liput DJ1, H. D. (2013, 11). *Transdermal delivery of cannabidiol attenuates binge alcohol-induced neurodegeneration in a rodent model of an alcohol use disorder.* Retrieved from Pubmed: https://www.ncbi.nlm.nih.gov/pubmed/24012796

Lisboa SF1, G. F. (2017). *The Endocannabinoid System and Anxiety.* Retrieved from Pubmed: https://www.ncbi.nlm.nih.gov/pubmed/28061971

Liu CS1, 2. C. (2015, 08). *Cannabinoids for the Treatment of Agitation and Aggression in Alzheimer's Disease.* Retrieved from Pubmed: https://www.ncbi.nlm.nih.gov/pubmed/26271310

Lizarraga KJ1, G. A. (2016, 03). *Molecular imaging of movement disorders.* Retrieved from Pubmed: https://www.ncbi.nlm.nih.gov/pubmed/27029029

Loflin M1, E. M. (2014, 03). *Subtypes of attention deficit-hyperactivity disorder (ADHD) and cannabis use.* Retrieved from Pubmed: https://www.ncbi.nlm.nih.gov/pubmed/24093525

Lupica CR1, H. Y. (2017, 04). *Cannabinoids as hippocampal network administrators.* Retrieved from Pubmed: https://www.ncbi.nlm.nih.gov/pubmed/28392266

M1., T. (2016). *THC:CBD Observational Study Data: Evolution of Resistant MS Spasticity and Associated Symptoms.* Retrieved from Pubmed: https://www.ncbi.nlm.nih.gov/pubmed/26901343

Maccarrone M1, D. E. (2010, 11). *Intracellular trafficking of anandamide: new concepts for signaling.* Retrieved from Pubmed: https://www.ncbi.nlm.nih.gov/pubmed/20570522

Mach F1, S. S. (2008, 05). *The role of the endocannabinoid system in atherosclerosis.* Retrieved from Pubmed: https://www.ncbi.nlm.nih.gov/pubmed/18426500

Maldonado R1, B. F. (2011, 05). *Neurochemical basis of cannabis addiction.* Retrieved from Pubmed: https://www.ncbi.nlm.nih.gov/pubmed/21334423

Malfait AM1, G. R. (2009, 08). *The nonpsychoactive cannabis constituent cannabidiol is an oral anti-arthritic therapeutic in murine collagen-induced arthritis.* Retrieved from Pubmed: https://www.ncbi.nlm.nih.gov/pubmed/10920191

Maor Y1, Y. J. (2012, 07). *Cannabidiol inhibits growth and induces programmed cell death in kaposi sarcoma-associated herpesvirus-infected endothelium.* Retrieved from Pubmed: https://www.ncbi.nlm.nih.gov/pubmed/?term=Cannabidiol+inhibits+growth+and+induces+programmed+cell+death+in+kaposi+sarcoma-associated+herpes+virus-infected+endothelium

Marco EM1, S. M. (2013, 10). *Emotional, endocrine and brain anandamide response to social challenge in infant male rats.* Retrieved from Pubmed: https://www.ncbi.nlm.nih.gov/pubmed/23660109?dopt=Abstract

Marcu JP1, C. R. (2010, 06). *Cannabidiol enhances the inhibitory effects of delta9-tetrahydrocannabinol on human glioblastoma cell proliferation and survival.* Retrieved from Pubmed: https://www.ncbi.nlm.nih.gov/pubmed/20053780

Marijuana - The First Twelve Thousand Years. (n.d.). Retrieved from http://druglibrary.org/Schaffer/hemp/history/first12000/1.htm

Mark Nesbitt, S. G. (2005). *The Cultural History of Plants.* Taylor and Francis.

Maroof N1, P. M. (2013, 12). *Endocannabinoid signalling in Alzheimer's disease.* Retrieved from Pubmed: https://www.ncbi.nlm.nih.gov/pubmed/24256258

Massi P1, S. M. (2015, 02). *Cannabidiol as potential anticancer drug.* Retrieved from Pubmed: https://www.ncbi.nlm.nih.gov/pubmed/22506672

Massi P1, V. A. (2004, 03). *Antitumor effects of cannabidiol, a nonpsychoactive cannabinoid, on human glioma cell lines.* Retrieved from Pubmed: https://www.ncbi.nlm.nih.gov/pubmed/14617682

Matt. (2016, 04 20). *Cannabis Ecology.* Retrieved from In Defence of Plants: http://www.indefenseofplants.com/blog/2016/4/20/cannabis-ecology

McPartland, J. M. (2001). *Cannabis and Eicosanoids: A Review of Molecular Pharmacology.* Retrieved from Journal of Cannabis Therapeutics: https://www.cannabis-med.org/data/pdf/2001-01-5.pdf

Medical Marijuana. (Copyrighted 2017). *Cannabinoids Treat Symptoms of Cystitis and Urethritis.* Retrieved from Medical Marijuana: https://www.medicalmarijuana.com/medical-marijuana-treatments-cannabis-uses/cannabinoids-treat-symptoms-of-cystitis-and-urethritis/

Merlin, R. C. (2013). *Cannabis: Evolution and Ethnobotany.* University of California Press.

Michele Ross, P. (2015, 10 15). *How Cannabis Helps Lupus.* Retrieved from Linked In: Michele Ross, PhD

Minns, E. H. (2011). *Scythians and Greeks: A Survey of Ancient History and Archaeology on the North Coast of the Euxine from the Danube to the Caucasus (Cambridge Library Collection - Archaeology).* Cambridge University Press.

Mishima K1, H. K. (2005, 05). *Cannabidiol prevents cerebral infarction via a serotonergic 5-hydroxytryptamine1A receptor-dependent mechanism.* Retrieved from Pubmed: https://www.ncbi.nlm.nih.gov/pubmed/15845890

Montgomery, N. M. (1995). *A Short History of Cannabis.* Retrieved from Channel 4: http://www.ukcia.org/research/potnight/pn4.htm

Morgan CJ1, D. R. (2013, 09). *Cannabidiol reduces cigarette consumption in tobacco smokers: preliminary findings.* Retrieved from Pubmed: https://www.ncbi.nlm.nih.gov/pubmed/23685330

Morrens M1, H. W. (2008). *[Psychomotor symptoms in schizophrenia: the importance of a forgotten syndrome].* Retrieved from Pubmed: https://www.ncbi.nlm.nih.gov/pubmed/18991232

Muldoon PP1, C. J.-S. (2015, 02). *Inhibition of monoacylglycerol lipase reduces nicotine withdrawal.* Retrieved from Pubmed: https://www.ncbi.nlm.nih.gov/pubmed/25258021

Murillo-Rodríguez E1, M.-A. D.-R.-C. (2006, 08). *Cannabidiol, a constituent of Cannabis sativa, modulates sleep in rats.* Retrieved from Pubmed: https://www.ncbi.nlm.nih.gov/pubmed/16844117

Murillo-Rodríguez E1, M.-A. D.-R.-C. (2008, 12). *The nonpsychoactive Cannabis constituent cannabidiol is a wake-inducing agent.* Retrieved from Pubmed: https://www.ncbi.nlm.nih.gov/pubmed/19045957

N1., S. (2010, 07). *Cannabinoid and cannabinoid-like receptors in microglia, astrocytes, and astrocytomas.* Retrieved from Pubmed: https://www.ncbi.nlm.nih.gov/pubmed/20468046

Nabissi M1, M. M. (2013). *Triggering of the TRPV2 channel by cannabidiol sensitizes glioblastoma cells to cytotoxic chemotherapeutic agents.* Retrieved from Pubmed: https://www.ncbi.nlm.nih.gov/pubmed/23079154

Nelson, R. A. (Unlisted). *A History of Hemp.* Retrieved from Rex Research: http://www.rexresearch.com/hhist/hhist1.htm

Nelson, R. (n.d.). *The eCS Therapy Companion Guide: A Reference Source for Your Endocannabinoid System.* 2012: Integral Education & Consulting, LLC.

NJ1., W. (2003). *The cellular energy crisis: mitochondria and cell death.* Retrieved from Pubmed: https://www.ncbi.nlm.nih.gov/pubmed/12544643

Norris C1, 2. L. (2016, 11). *Cannabidiol Modulates Fear Memory Formation Through Interactions with Serotonergic Transmission in the Mesolimbic System.* Retrieved from Pubmed: https://www.ncbi.nlm.nih.gov/pubmed/27296152

Nyishar: Health Products and Consulting. (2016, 10 28). *HOW CANNABIS WORKS – A Rudimentary Look At The Endocannabinoid System.* Retrieved from https://nyishar.com/2016/10/28/how-cannabis-works-a-rudimentary-look-at-the-endocannabinoid-system/

Oja SS1, J. R. (2000, 08). *Modulation of glutamate receptor functions by glutathione.* Retrieved from Pubmed: https://www.ncbi.nlm.nih.gov/pubmed/10812215

Oláh A, T. B. (2012, 09). *Cannabidiol exerts sebostatic and antiinflammatory effects on human sebocytes.* Retrieved from Pubmed: https://www.ncbi.nlm.nih.gov/pubmed/25061872

Onaivi ES1, C. O. (2008, 10). *Behavioral effects of CB2 cannabinoid receptor activation and its influence on food and alcohol consumption.* Retrieved from Pubmed: https://www.ncbi.nlm.nih.gov/pubmed/18991890

Osbourne, H. (2015, 05 21). *Scythian Bongs Discovered in Russia.* Retrieved from International Business Times: http://www.ibtimes.co.uk/solid-gold-scythian-bongs-cannabis-opium-discovered-russia-1503725

O'Shaughnessy, W. B. (1843). *On the Preparations of the Indian Hemp, or Gunjah**. Retrieved from Pubmed: https://www.ncbi.nlm.nih.gov/pmc/articles/PMC2490264/

P., K. (2003, 08). *Th1/Th2 balance: the hypothesis, its limitations, and implications for health and disease.* Retrieved from Pubmed: https://www.ncbi.nlm.nih.gov/pubmed/12946237

P., K. (2003, 08). *Th1/Th2 balance: the hypothesis, its limitations, and implications for health and disease.* Retrieved from Pubmed: https://www.ncbi.nlm.nih.gov/pubmed/12946237

Pagano E1, C. R. (2016, 10). *An Orally Active Cannabis Extract with High Content in Cannabidiol attenuates Chemically-induced Intestinal Inflammation and Hypermotility in the Mouse.* Retrieved from Pubmed: https://www.ncbi.nlm.nih.gov/pubmed/27757083

Pagotto U1, M. G. (2006, 02). *The emerging role of the endocannabinoid system in endocrine regulation and energy balance.* Retrieved from Pubmed: https://www.ncbi.nlm.nih.gov/pubmed/16306385

Pan H1, M. P. (2009, 03). *Cannabidiol attenuates cisplatin-induced nephrotoxicity by decreasing oxidative/nitrosative stress, inflammation, and cell death.* Retrieved from Pubmed: https://www.ncbi.nlm.nih.gov/pubmed/19074681

Pandolfo P1, S. V.-R. (2011). *Cannabinoids inhibit the synaptic uptake of adenosine and dopamine in the rat and mouse striatum.* Retrieved from Pubmed: https://www.ncbi.nlm.nih.gov/pubmed/21266173

Parolaro D1, R. N. (2010, 07). *The endocannabinoid system and psychiatric disorders.* Retrieved from Pubmed: https://www.ncbi.nlm.nih.gov/pubmed/20353783

Parray HA1, Y. J. (2016, 05). *Cannabidiol promotes browning in 3T3-L1 adipocytes.* Retrieved from Pubmed: https://www.ncbi.nlm.nih.gov/pubmed/27067870

Passie T1, E. H. (2012, 07). *Mitigation of post-traumatic stress symptoms by Cannabis resin: a review of the clinical and neurobiological evidence.* Retrieved from Pubmed: https://www.ncbi.nlm.nih.gov/pubmed/22736575

Patel S1, H. M. (2017, 04). *The endocannabinoid system as a target for novel anxiolytic drugs.* Retrieved from Pubmed: https://www.ncbi.nlm.nih.gov/pubmed/28434588

Patel S1, H. M. (2017, 05). *The endocannabinoid system as a target for novel anxiolytic drugs.* Retrieved from Pubmed: https://www.ncbi.nlm.nih.gov/pubmed/28434588

Paudel KS1, H. D. (2010, 09). *Cannabidiol bioavailability after nasal and transdermal application: effect of permeation enhancers.* Retrieved from Pubmed: https://www.ncbi.nlm.nih.gov/pubmed/20545522

Pava MJ1, d. H.-C. (2014, 02). *Endocannabinoid modulation of cortical up-states and NREM sleep.* Retrieved from Pubmed: https://www.ncbi.nlm.nih.gov/pubmed/24520411

Pava MJ1, M. A. (2016, 03). *Endocannabinoid Signaling Regulates Sleep Stability.* Retrieved from Pubmed: https://www.ncbi.nlm.nih.gov/pubmed/27031992

Pazos MR1, C. V.-R.-O. (2012, 10). *Cannabidiol administration after hypoxia-ischemia to newborn rats reduces long-term brain injury and restores neurobehavioral function.* Retrieved from Pubmed: https://www.ncbi.nlm.nih.gov/pubmed/22659086

Pertwee, R. (August 21, 2014). *Handbook of Cannabis.* OAP Oxford.

Ph.D., J. G. (2011, 06 16). *History of Cannabis in India.* Retrieved from Psychology Today: https://www.psychologytoday.com/blog/the-teenage-mind/201106/history-cannabis-in-india

Pini A1, M. G.-G. (2012, 06). *The role of cannabinoids in inflammatory modulation of allergic respiratory disorders, inflammatory pain and ischemic stroke.* Retrieved from Pubmed: https://www.ncbi.nlm.nih.gov/pubmed/22420307

Plattner F1, H. K. (2015). *The role of ventral striatal cAMP signaling in stress-induced behaviors.* Retrieved from Pubmed: https://www.ncbi.nlm.nih.gov/pubmed/26192746

Plattner F1, H. K. (2015, 08). *The role of ventral striatal cAMP signaling in stress-induced behaviors.* Retrieved from Pubmed: https://www.ncbi.nlm.nih.gov/pubmed/26192746

Pokrywka M1, G. J. (2016, 08). *Cannabinoids - a new weapon against cancer?* Retrieved from Pubmed: https://www.ncbi.nlm.nih.gov/pubmed/28100841

Porter BE1, J. C. (2013, 12). *Report of a parent survey of cannabidiol-enriched cannabis use in pediatric treatment-resistant epilepsy.* Retrieved from Pubmed: https://www.ncbi.nlm.nih.gov/pubmed/24237632

Pr Ntr Kmt - (Holy Place of The Divine Ancient Egypt. (Unlisted). *Cannabis*. Retrieved from Pr Ntr Kmt: http://www.prntrkmt.org/herbs/cannabis.html

Preston, A. (2016, 06 28). *Terpenoids in Hemp: Alpha-Pinen.* Retrieved from Elexinol: https://elixinol.com/blog/terpenoids-hemp-alpha-pinene/

Price, M. (Unlisted). *What Is Hemp? Understanding The Differences Between Hemp and Cannabis.* Retrieved from Medical Jane: https://www.medicaljane.com/2015/01/14/the-differences-between-hemp-and-cannabis/

Pucci M1, R. C. (2013, 08). *Epigenetic control of skin differentiation genes by phytocannabinoids.* Retrieved from Pubmed : https://www.ncbi.nlm.nih.gov/pubmed/23869687

Putnam SE1, S. A. (2007, 02). *Natural products as alternative treatments for metabolic bone disorders and for maintenance of bone health.* Retrieved from Pubmed: https://www.ncbi.nlm.nih.gov/pubmed/17106868

Rabinak CA, P. K. (2014). *Cannabinoid modulation of fear extinction brain circuits: a novel target to advance anxiety treatment.* Retrieved from Pubmed: https://www.ncbi.nlm.nih.gov/pubmed/23829364

Rabinski, G. (2015, 08 17). *WHAT ARE CANNABIS TRICHOMES AND WHY ARE THEY SO IMPORTANT?* Retrieved from whaxy.com: https://www.whaxy.com/learn/what-are-trichomes

Racz I1, N. X.-A. (2008, 11). *Interferon-gamma is a critical modulator of CB(2) cannabinoid receptor signaling during neuropathic pain.* Retrieved from Pubmed: https://www.ncbi.nlm.nih.gov/pubmed/19005078

Racz I1, N. X.-A. (2011, 08). *Interferon-gamma is a critical modulator of CB(2) cannabinoid receptor signaling during neuropathic pain.* Retrieved from Pubmed: https://www.ncbi.nlm.nih.gov/pubmed/19005078

Rahn, B. (2014). *Cannabinoids 101: What Makes Cannabis Medicine?* Retrieved from Leafly: https://www.leafly.com/news/cannabis-101/cannabinoids-101-what-makes-cannabis-medicine

Rajesh M1, M. P. (2010, 10). *Cannabidiol attenuates cardiac dysfunction, oxidative stress, fibrosis, and inflammatory and cell death signaling pathways in diabetic cardiomyopathy.* Retrieved from Pubmed: https://www.ncbi.nlm.nih.gov/pubmed/21144973

Ramer R1, H. B. (2016, 10). *Antitumorigenic targets of cannabinoids - current status and implications.* Retrieved from Pubmed: https://www.ncbi.nlm.nih.gov/pubmed/27070944

Ramer R1, H. K. (2013, 01). *COX-2 and PPAR-γ confer cannabidiol-induced apoptosis of human lung cancer cells.* Retrieved from Pubmed: https://www.ncbi.nlm.nih.gov/pubmed/23220503

Ramot Y1, S. K. (2013, 02). *A novel control of human keratin expression: cannabinoid receptor 1-mediated signaling down-regulates the expression of keratins K6 and K16 in human keratinocytes in vitro and in situ.* Retrieved from Pubmed: https://www.ncbi.nlm.nih.gov/pubmed/23638377

Rautsh, C. (2001). *Marijuana Medicine: A World Tour of the Healing and Visionary Powers of Cannabis.* Bear and Company.

Regina Nelson: https://www.youtube.com/watch?v=QgAfqy2ycVM (Director). (2015). *The Science of Cannabis (AHA Conference 2015)* [Motion Picture].

Ren Y1, W. J.-M. (2009, 11). *Cannabidiol, a nonpsychotropic component of cannabis, inhibits cue-induced heroin seeking and normalizes discrete mesolimbic neuronal disturbances.* Retrieved from https://www.ncbi.nlm.nih.gov/pubmed/19940171

Renard J1, N. C. (2017, 04). *Neuronal and molecular effects of cannabidiol on the mesolimbic dopamine system: Implications for novel schizophrenia treatments.* Retrieved from Pubmed: https://www.ncbi.nlm.nih.gov/pubmed/28185872

Revolutionary Health Committee of Hunan Province . (n.d.). *A Barefoot Doctor's Manual.*

Rezapour-Firouzi S1, A. S.-M. (2012, 10). *Alteration of delta-6-desaturase (FADS2), secretory phospholipase-A2 (sPLA2) enzymes by Hot-nature diet with co-supplemented hemp seed, evening primrose oils intervention in multiple sclerosis patients.* Retrieved from Pubmed: https://www.ncbi.nlm.nih.gov/pubmed/26365444

Riebe CJ1, W. C. (2011). *Endocannabinoids and stress.* Retrieved from Pubmed: https://www.ncbi.nlm.nih.gov/pubmed/21663537

Rocha FC1, D. S. (2014, 06). *Systematic review of the literature on clinical and experimental trials on the antitumor effects of cannabinoids in gliomas.* Retrieved from Pubmed: https://www.ncbi.nlm.nih.gov/pubmed/24142199

Ron Marczyk, R. W. (2011, 07 19). *Humans Discover Hemp 10,000 years ago.* Retrieved from Toke of The Town: http://www.tokeofthetown.com/2011/07/worth_repeating_humans_discover_hemp_10000_bc.php/

Rosenthal, M. F. (1978). *Marijuana Grower's Guide*. Retrieved from Walnet: http://www.walnet.org/rosebud/ancienthistory.html

Rossi F1, B. G., & Endocannabinoid Research Group (ERG), I. (2011, 05). *The endovanilloid/endocannabinoid system: a new potential target for osteoporosis therapy.* Retrieved from Pubmed: https://www.ncbi.nlm.nih.gov/pubmed/21237298

Rossignoli MT1, L.-A. C.-J.-S.-F.-P. (2017, 05). *Selective post-training time window for memory consolidation interference of cannabidiol into the prefrontal cortex: Reduced dopaminergic modulation and immediate gene expression in limbic circuits.* Retrieved from Pubmed: https://www.ncbi.nlm.nih.gov/pubmed/28344069

RS1., R. (2009). *Role of the endocannabinoid system in abdominal obesity and the implications for cardiovascular risk.* Retrieved from Pubmed: https://www.ncbi.nlm.nih.gov/pubmed/19641317

Rubin, V. D. (1975). *Cannabis and Culture*. Mouton.

Russo EB1, G. G. (2007, 08). *Cannabis, pain, and sleep: lessons from therapeutic clinical trials of Sativex, a cannabis-based medicine.* Retrieved from Pubmed: https://www.ncbi.nlm.nih.gov/pubmed/?term=Cannabis%2C+pain%2C+and+sleep%3A+lessons+from+therapeutic+clinical+trials+of+Sativex%2C+a+cannabis-based+medicine

Russo, E. (2001). Cognoscenti of Cannabis I: Jacques-Joseph Moreau (1804-1884). *Journal of Cannabis Therapeutics, Vol. 1(1) 2001*. Retrieved from Cannabis Med: https://www.cannabis-med.org/data/pdf/2001-01-6.pdf

Russo, E. (2007, 08 21). *History of Cannabis and Its Preparations in Saga, Science, and Sobriquet.* Retrieved from Wiley Online: http://onlinelibrary.wiley.com/doi/10.1002/cbdv.200790144/full

Russo, E. (2008, 04 28). *Clinical endocannabinoid deficiency (CECD): can this concept explain therapeutic benefits of cannabis in migraine, fibromyalgia, irritable bowel syndrome and other treatment-resistant conditions?* Retrieved from Pub Med: https://www.ncbi.nlm.nih.gov/pubmed/18404144

RW1., G. (1999). *Cancer cachexia and cannabinoids.* Retrieved from Pubmed: https://www.ncbi.nlm.nih.gov/pubmed/10575285

Ryan D1, D. A. (2007). *Interactions of cannabidiol with endocannabinoid signalling in hippocampal tissue.* Retrieved from Pubmed: https://www.ncbi.nlm.nih.gov/pubmed/17419758

Sl., D. (2013). *Medical use of cannabis. Cannabidiol: a new light for schizophrenia?* Retrieved from Pubmed: https://www.ncbi.nlm.nih.gov/pubmed/23109356

Sl., R. (1996). *Th1 and Th2 in human diseases.* Retrieved from https://www.ncbi.nlm.nih.gov/pubmed/8811042

Sl., R. (1996, 09). *Th1 and Th2 in human diseases.* Retrieved from Pubmed: https://www.ncbi.nlm.nih.gov/pubmed/8811042

Sagredo O1, P. M.-R. (2011, 09). *Neuroprotective effects of phytocannabinoid-based medicines in experimental models of Huntington's disease.* Retrieved from Pubmed: https://www.ncbi.nlm.nih.gov/pubmed/21674569

Sagredo O1, R. J.-R. (2007, 08). *Cannabidiol reduced the striatal atrophy caused 3-nitropropionic acid in vivo by mechanisms independent of the activation of cannabinoid, vanilloid TRPV1 and adenosine A2A receptors.* Retrieved from Pubmed: https://www.ncbi.nlm.nih.gov/pubmed/17672854

Sarijuana. (2016, 05 30). *Cannabis Medicine – It isn't only about the Endocannabinoid System.* Retrieved from Cannagramma: http://cannagramma.com/2016/05/30/cannabis-medicine-it-isnt-only-about-the-endocannabinoid-system/

Sarris J1, M. E. (2013, 04). *Plant-based medicines for anxiety disorders, part 2: a review of clinical studies with supporting preclinical evidence.* Retrieved from Pubmed: https://www.ncbi.nlm.nih.gov/pubmed/23653088

Scavone JL1, S. R. (2013, 08). *Impact of cannabis use during stabilization on methadone maintenance treatment.* Retrieved from Pumbed: https://www.ncbi.nlm.nih.gov/pubmed/23795873

Scherma M, F. L. (2014). *The role of the endocannabinoid system in eating disorders: neurochemical and behavioural preclinical evidence.* Retrieved from Pubmed: https://www.ncbi.nlm.nih.gov/pubmed/23829365

Schiavon AP1, S. L. (2014, 11). *Protective effects of cannabidiol against hippocampal cell death and cognitive impairment induced by bilateral common carotid artery occlusion in mice.* Retrieved from Pubmed: https://www.ncbi.nlm.nih.gov/pubmed/24532152

Schier AR1, R. N. (2012, 06). *Cannabidiol, a Cannabis sativa constituent, as an anxiolytic drug.* Retrieved from Pubmed: https://www.ncbi.nlm.nih.gov/pubmed/22729452

Schmall, J. (2010, 10 7). *The Health Benefits of Hemp Butter.* Retrieved from Cannabis Culture: http://www.cannabisculture.com/content/2010/10/07/health-benefits-hemp-butter

Schubart CD1, S. I.-P. (2014). *Cannabidiol as a potential treatment for psychosis.* Retrieved from Pubmed: https://www.ncbi.nlm.nih.gov/pubmed/24309088

Schuelert N1, M. J. (2011, 08). *The abnormal cannabidiol analogue O-1602 reduces nociception in a rat model of acute arthritis via the putative cannabinoid receptor GPR55.* Retrieved from Pubmed: https://www.ncbi.nlm.nih.gov/pubmed/21683763

Science Explains How Cannabis Kills Cancer Cells | CBD-Healthcare News (2015). [Motion Picture]. Retrieved from https://www.youtube.com/watch?v=5RtRil2ND-E

Scripture, E. W. (1893, 10 27). *Consciousness Uner The Influnce of Cannabis Indica.* Retrieved from https://archive.org/details/jstor-1766346

Scuderi C1, S. L. (2014, 03). *Cannabidiol promotes amyloid precursor protein ubiquitination and reduction of beta amyloid expression in SHSY5YAPP+ cells through PPARγ involvement.* Retrieved from Pubmed: https://www.ncbi.nlm.nih.gov/pubmed/24288245

Segev A1, R. A.-L. (2014, 03). *Cannabinoid receptor activation prevents the effects of chronic mild stress on emotional learning and LTP in a rat model of depression.* Retrieved from Pubmed: https://www.ncbi.nlm.nih.gov/pubmed/24141570

Senst L1, B. J. (2014, 01). *Neuromodulators, stress and plasticity: a role for endocannabinoid signalling.* Retrieved from Pubmed: https://www.ncbi.nlm.nih.gov/pubmed/24353209

Seshata. (2014, 12 02). *Cannabis in Archaeology & Palaeobotany.* Retrieved from Sensi Seeds: https://sensiseeds.com/en/blog/cannabis-archaeology-palaeobotany/

Shivapk1. (Unlisted). *Cannabis and Religion - Hindus and Rastas.* Retrieved from http://www.thehempire.com/index.php/cannabis/cannabis_hemp/cannabis_and_religion_hindus_and_rastas

Shoval G1, S. L. (2016). *Prohedonic Effect of Cannabidiol in a Rat Model of Depression.* Retrieved from Pubmed: https://www.ncbi.nlm.nih.gov/pubmed/27010632

Shuso Takeda, K. M. (2008, Sept). *Cannabidiolic Acid as a Selective Cyclooxygenase-2 Inhibitory Component in Cannabis.* Retrieved from Drug Metabolism and Disposition: http://dmd.aspetjournals.org/content/36/9/1917

Silva N Jr1, S. C. (2014, 02). *Searching for a neurobiological basis for self-medication theory in ADHD comorbid with substance use disorders: an in vivo study of dopamine transporters using (99m)Tc-TRODAT-1 SPECT.* Retrieved from Pubmed: https://www.ncbi.nlm.nih.gov/pubmed/23856832

Simpson CR1, A. W. (2002). *Coincidence of immune-mediated diseases driven by Th1 and Th2 subsets suggests a common aetiology. A population-based study using computerized general practice data.* Retrieved from Pubmed: https://www.ncbi.nlm.nih.gov/pubmed/12002734

Sircus, M. (2011, 10 21). *Transdermal and Oral Cannabis.* Retrieved from Dr. Sircus: http://drsircus.com/medical-marijuana/transdermal-oral-cannabis/

Smith SC, W. M. (2014). *Clinical endocannabinoid deficiency (CECD) revisited: can this concept explain the therapeutic benefits of cannabis in migraine, fibromyalgia, irritable bowel syndrome and other treatment-resistant conditions?* Retrieved from Pubmed: https://www.ncbi.nlm.nih.gov/pubmed/24977967

Smith, O. (n.d.). *Using Cannabis OIl on Your Skin.* Retrieved from https://cannabisdigest.ca/topical-cannabis-oil/

Solinas M1, M. P. (2012, 11). *Cannabidiol inhibits angiogenesis by multiple mechanisms.* Retrieved from Pubmed: https://www.ncbi.nlm.nih.gov/pubmed/22624859

Solinas M1, M. P. (2013). *Cannabidiol, a non-psychoactive cannabinoid compound, inhibits proliferation and invasion in U87-MG and T98G glioma cells through a multitarget effect.* Retrieved from Pubmed: https://www.ncbi.nlm.nih.gov/pubmed/24204703

Solinas M1, M. P. (2013, 10). *Cannabidiol, a non-psychoactive cannabinoid compound, inhibits proliferation and invasion in U87-MG and T98G glioma cells through a multitarget effect.* Retrieved from Pubmed: https://www.ncbi.nlm.nih.gov/pubmed/24204703

Soroceanu L1, M. R. (2013, 03). *Id-1 is a key transcriptional regulator of glioblastoma aggressiveness and a novel therapeutic target.* Retrieved from Pubmed: https://www.ncbi.nlm.nih.gov/pubmed/23243024

Stanley CP1, H. W. (2013, 02). *Is the cardiovascular system a therapeutic target for cannabidiol?* Retrieved from Pubmed: https://www.ncbi.nlm.nih.gov/pubmed/22670794

Steffens S1, M. F. (2006, 10). *Cannabinoid receptors in atherosclerosis.* Retrieved from Pubmed: https://www.ncbi.nlm.nih.gov/pubmed/16960500

Støving RK1, A. A. (2009, 02). *Leptin, ghrelin, and endocannabinoids: potential therapeutic targets in anorexia nervosa.* Retrieved from Pubmed: https://www.ncbi.nlm.nih.gov/pubmed/18926548

Stumm C1, H. C. (2013, 11). *Cannabinoid receptor 1 deficiency in a mouse model of Alzheimer's disease leads to enhanced cognitive impairment despite of a reduction in amyloid deposition.* Retrieved from Pubmed: https://www.ncbi.nlm.nih.gov/pubmed/?term=Cannabinoid+receptor+1+deficiency+in+a+mouse+model+of+Alzheimer%E2%80%99s+disease+leads+to+enhanced+cognitive+impairment+despite+of+a+reduction+in+amyloid+deposition

Sulak, H. -C. (Director). (2015). *https://www.youtube.com/watch?v=xVdyFM_CR54* [Motion Picture].

Syed YY1, M. K. (2014, 04). *Delta-9-tetrahydrocannabinol/cannabidiol (Sativex®): a review of its use in patients with moderate to severe spasticity due to multiple sclerosis.* Retrieved from Pubmed: https://www.ncbi.nlm.nih.gov/pubmed/24671907

Sylantyev S1, J. T. (2013, 03). *Cannabinoid- and lysophosphatidylinositol-sensitive receptor GPR55 boosts neurotransmitter release at central synapses.* Retrieved from Pubmed: https://www.ncbi.nlm.nih.gov/pubmed/23472002

Szaflarski JP1, B. E. (2014, 12). *Cannabis, cannabidiol, and epilepsy--from receptors to clinical response.* Retrieved from Pubmed: https://www.ncbi.nlm.nih.gov/pubmed/25282526

TAO CHEN2, 3. S. (2014, 02 25). *Identification of Cannabis Fiber from the Astana Cemeteries,Xinjiang, China, with Reference to Its Unique Decorative Utilization.* Retrieved from www.botany.hawaii.edu: http://www.botany.hawaii.edu/plant/wp-content/uploads/2014/04/Ancient-Cannabis-Fiber-as-an-artificial-Horsetail.pdf

The Chemistry of Cannabis & Synthetic Cannabinoids. (2015, 05 26). Retrieved 03 01, 2017, from Compound Interest: http://www.compoundchem.com/2015/05/26/cannabinoids/

The Seven Booksof Paulus Aegineta: In 3 Vol, Volume 3. (Translated 1847).

Tomida I1, A.-B. A. (2006, 10). *Effect of sublingual application of cannabinoids on intraocular pressure: a pilot study.* Retrieved from Pubmed: https://www.ncbi.nlm.nih.gov/pubmed/16988594

Tosch, E. (2016, 04 27). *Ayurvedic Cannabis.* Retrieved from everydayayurveda.org: http://everydayayurveda.org/ayurvedic-cannabis/

Tóth BI1, D. N. (2011, 05). *Endocannabinoids modulate human epidermal keratinocyte proliferation and survival via the sequential engagement of cannabinoid receptor-1 and transient receptor potential vanilloid-1.* Retrieved from Pubmed: https://www.ncbi.nlm.nih.gov/pubmed/21248768

TV, P. (Director). (2014). *Kaneh Bosm: The Hidden Story of Cannabis in the Old Testament* [Motion Picture].

Tzadok M1, U.-S. S.-S.-Z. (2016, 02). *CBD-enriched medical cannabis for intractable pediatric epilepsy: The current Israeli experience.* Retrieved from Pubmed: https://www.ncbi.nlm.nih.gov/pubmed/26800377

Tzadok M1, U.-S. S.-S.-Z. (2016, 02). *CBD-enriched medical cannabis for intractable pediatric epilepsy: The current Israeli experience.* Retrieved from Pubmed: https://www.ncbi.nlm.nih.gov/pubmed/26800377

V1., D. M. (2008, 08). *The endocannabinoid system in obesity and type 2 diabetes.* Retrieved from Pubmed: https://www.ncbi.nlm.nih.gov/pubmed/18563385

Vaccani A1, M. P. (2005, 04). *Cannabidiol inhibits human glioma cell migration through a cannabinoid receptor-independent mechanism.* Retrieved from Pubmed: https://www.ncbi.nlm.nih.gov/pubmed/15700028

Valadez, L. (2014, 11 02). *Asterion The God of Cannabis.* Retrieved from The Cave of Oracle - Musings of A Mad Prophet: https://caveoforacle.wordpress.com/2014/02/11/asterion-the-god-of-cannabis/

Valdeolivas S1, 2. S.-R. (2017). *Effects of a Sativex-Like Combination of Phytocannabinoids on Disease Progression in R6/2 Mice, an Experimental Model of Huntington's Disease.* Retrieved from Pubmed: https://www.ncbi.nlm.nih.gov/pubmed/28333097

Valdeolivas S1, N. C. (2015, 01). *Neuroprotective properties of cannabigerol in Huntington's disease: studies in R6/2 mice and 3-nitropropionate-lesioned mice.* Retrieved from Pubmed: https://www.ncbi.nlm.nih.gov/pubmed/25252936

Valdeolivas S1, S. V.-R. (2012, 05). *Sativex-like combination of phytocannabinoids is neuroprotective in malonate-lesioned rats, an inflammatory model of Huntington's disease: role of CB1 and CB2 receptors.* Retrieved from Pubmed: https://www.ncbi.nlm.nih.gov/pubmed/22860209

Van Klingeren B, T. H. (1976). *Antibacterial activity of delta9-tetrahydrocannabinol and cannabidiol.* Retrieved from Pubmed: https://www.ncbi.nlm.nih.gov/pubmed/1085130

van Rijn CM1, P. M. (2011). *Endocannabinoid system protects against cryptogenic seizures.* Retrieved from Pubmed: https://www.ncbi.nlm.nih.gov/pubmed/21441624

Vicente-Valor MI1, G.-L. P. (2013, 02). *Cannabis derivatives therapy for a seronegative stiff-person syndrome: a case report.* Retrieved from Pubmed: https://www.ncbi.nlm.nih.gov/pubmed/22726074

Walsh SK1, H. C. (2010, 07). *Acute administration of cannabidiol in vivo suppresses ischaemia-induced cardiac arrhythmias and reduces infarct size when given at reperfusion.* Retrieved from Pubmed: https://www.ncbi.nlm.nih.gov/pubmed/20590615

Watzl B1, S. P. (1991). *Marijuana components stimulate human peripheral blood mononuclear cell secretion of interferon-gamma and suppress interleukin-1 alpha in vitro.* Retrieved from Pubmed: https://www.ncbi.nlm.nih.gov/pubmed/1667651

Watzl B1, S. P. (1991). *Marijuana components stimulate human peripheral blood mononuclear cell secretion of interferon-gamma and suppress interleukin-1 alpha in vitro.* Retrieved from Pubmed: https://www.ncbi.nlm.nih.gov/pubmed/1667651

Way of Infinite Harmony. (2017, 03 09). *Her Infinite Holiness - Magu.* Retrieved from Way of Infinite Harmony: http://www.wayofinfiniteharmony.org/

Weston-Green K1, H. X. (2012). *Alterations to melanocortinergic, GABAergic and cannabinoid neurotransmission associated with olanzapine-induced weight gain.* Retrieved from Pubmed: https://www.ncbi.nlm.nih.gov/pubmed/22438946

What is CBD Cannabidiol Hemp OIl. (2016, 10 3). Retrieved from Medical Marijuana: http://www.medicalmarijuanainc.com/what-is-cbd-hemp-oil/

Wilcox, A. (Unlisted). *The Origin of the Word "Marijuana".* Retrieved from Leafly: https://www.leafly.com/news/cannabis-101/where-did-the-word-marijuana-come-from-anyway-01fb

Wilkinson JD1, W. E. (2007, 02). *Cannabinoids inhibit human keratinocyte proliferation through a non-CB1/CB2 mechanism and have a potential therapeutic value in the treatment of psoriasis.* Retrieved from Pubmed: https://www.ncbi.nlm.nih.gov/pubmed/17157480

Wu LT1, B. K., & Workgroup., N. A. (03, 2014). *Cannabis use disorders are comparatively prevalent among nonwhite racial/ethnic groups and adolescents: a national study.* Retrieved from Pubmed: https://www.ncbi.nlm.nih.gov/pubmed/24342767

www.zambeza.com. (2016, 01 13). *The Difference Between Cannabis Sativa Indica-and Ruderalis.* Retrieved from www.zambeza.com: https://www.zambeza.com/blog-difference-between-cannabis-sativa-indica-and-ruderalis-n13

Xie S1, D. L. (2012, 06). *Implications of Th1 and Th17 cells in pathogenesis of oral lichen planus.* Retrieved from Pubmed: https://www.ncbi.nlm.nih.gov/pubmed/22684574

Yamada D1, T. J. (2014, 07). *Modulation of fear memory by dietary polyunsaturated fatty acids via cannabinoid receptors.* Retrieved from Pubmed: https://www.ncbi.nlm.nih.gov/pubmed/24518289

Yamada T1, U. T. (2010, 08). *TRPV2 activation induces apoptotic cell death in human T24 bladder cancer cells: a potential therapeutic target for bladder cancer.* Retrieved from Pubmed: https://www.ncbi.nlm.nih.gov/pubmed/20546877

Yoshihara S1, M. H. (2005, 09). *Endogenous cannabinoid receptor agonists inhibit neurogenic inflammations in guinea pig airways.* Retrieved from Pubmed: https://www.ncbi.nlm.nih.gov/pubmed/16103691

Young, R. T. (2013). *Essential Oil Safety: A Guide for Health Care Professionals.* Elsever Helath Sciences.

Zheng WH1, Q. R. (2004, 05). *Comparative signaling pathways of insulin-like growth factor-1 and brain-derived neurotrophic factor in hippocampal neurons and the role of the PI3 kinase pathway in cell survival.* Retrieved from Pubmed: https://www.ncbi.nlm.nih.gov/pubmed/15140184

Zlebnik NE1, C. J. (2016, 07). *Beyond the CB1 Receptor: Is Cannabidiol the Answer for Disorders of Motivation?* Retrieved from Pubmed: https://www.ncbi.nlm.nih.gov/pubmed/27023732

Zoerner AA1, S. D. (2011, 09). *Allergen challenge increases anandamide in bronchoalveolar fluid of patients with allergic asthma.* Retrieved from Pubmed: https://www.ncbi.nlm.nih.gov/pubmed/21716266

Zuardi A1, C. J. (2010). *Cannabidiol was ineffective for manic episode of bipolar affective disorder.* Retrieved from Pubmed: https://www.ncbi.nlm.nih.gov/pubmed/18801823

Zuardi AW1, C. J. (2006, 04). *Cannabidiol, a Cannabis sativa constituent, as an antipsychotic drug.* Retrieved from Pubmed: https://www.ncbi.nlm.nih.gov/pubmed/16612464

Zuardi AW1, C. J. (2009, 12). *Cannabidiol for the treatment of psychosis in Parkinson's disease.* Retrieved from Pubmed: https://www.ncbi.nlm.nih.gov/pubmed/18801821

Zuardi AW1, C. J.-S. (2012). *A critical review of the antipsychotic effects of cannabidiol: 30 years of a translational investigation.* Retrieved from Pubmed: https://www.ncbi.nlm.nih.gov/pubmed/22716160

Zweig RM1, D. E. (2016, 02). *Cognitive and Psychiatric Disturbances in Parkinsonian Syndromes.* Retrieved from Pubmed: https://www.ncbi.nlm.nih.gov/pubmed/26614001

Zweig RM1, D. E. (2016). *Cognitive and Psychiatric Disturbances in Parkinsonian Syndromes.* Retrieved from 02: https://www.ncbi.nlm.nih.gov/pubmed/26614001

Руденко, С. И. (n.d.). *Frozen Tombs of Siberia: The Pazyryk Burials of Iron Age Horsemen.* University of California Press.

www.ingramcontent.com/pod-product-compliance
Lightning Source LLC
Chambersburg PA
CBHW082201220526
45470CB00010B/3008